INVOKING YOUR INNER THERAPIST IN HEART FAILURE

UNTOLD PATIENT EXPERIENCES FROM PREVENTION TO END STAGE

KRIS VIJAY

FOREWORD BY DR. MARC SILVER

Spotlight PUBLISHING

Goodyear, AZ

INVOKING YOUR INNER THERAPIST IN HEART FAILURE: Untold Patient Experiences From Prevention to End Stage

Paperback ISBN: 978-1-7354690-8-9
Hardcover ISBN: 978-1-953806-01-7
eBook ISBN: 978-1-953806-00-0
Library of Congress Control Number: 2020918212

First Published in the USA in 2020
Publisher: Spotlight Publishing™ https://spotlightpublishing.pro
Book Cover: Kennedy Evans
Editor: Nina Durfee http://NinaDurfee.com
Formatting: Soumi Goswami

For information contact:
Kris Vijay
https://elevatebi.com/KrisVijay

INVOKING YOUR INNER THERAPIST IN HEART FAILURE

UNTOLD PATIENT EXPERIENCES FROM PREVENTION TO END STAGE

KRIS VIJAY

FOREWORD BY DR. MARC SILVER

CONTENTS

Acknowledgments

I am indeed honored to have been able to get this book together. I am indebted to the publisher, their team and, especially to Becky Norwood of Spotlight Publishing whose talent and support made this book a reality. I am extremely grateful to Angie for designing the cover of the book which required special skills. I am very thankful to the publishing team and editors for making a user-friendly text that will allow for easier navigation through the entire book to gain powerful motivational messages from many patients I have encountered over the years.

I am beholden to all patients who have allowed me to help in their healing and to have given me enough armaments to gain knowledge to write and bring this book to fruition.

A great deal of thanks goes to Dr. Marc Silver for accepting to write the Foreword for this book. Marc is one of the pioneers in the field of Heart Failure. He was one of the founding members of the Heart Failure Society of America, author of HFSA and ACC/AHA heart failure guidelines for over a decade and served as Editor-in-Chief of Congestive Heart Failure Journal for 15 years. He has authored *Success with Heart Failure*, now in the 4th edition. Marc has been a great mentor for me and an amazing friend. He has taught me so many aspects in Heart Failure and beyond. He epitomizes the paradigm of heart-rending *Humanism* in most poignant ways.

So many deserve thanks and kudos. Without your help, this book would not have made it to print. To Cesar Delgado for being the scribe for me over the last year and typing up every word, as I dictated to him. This was challenging due to my accent, medical jargon, and complicated words in the motivational domain.

To Desiree Little for her help as both a nurse and nurse practitioner for so many patients, she has helped heal along the way. Desiree also wrote and the chapter on Nursing Perspectives.

To Kennedy Evans for her creative and imaginative artwork for the cover page as well as many medical illustrations that are interspersed throughout this book.

To Teresa Mercer for being part of the team of our Cardiorenal Center and helping out as a nurse over the last year.

To Tammy Querrey for her continued support as Service Line Director at Abrazo health network.

To Dr. Aye Win for covering me during my absence helping many heart failure patients at the clinic.

To Sarah Wilmowski, our Nurse Navigator for being there always at times of need.

To Dr Tim Byrne for his unrelenting support of our Heart Failure Program at Abrazo/Tenet in Phoenix, Arizona

To Dr. Rick Kirchner, Heart Surgeon, for helping so many of my patients achieve a great outcome after bypass or valve surgery over the years.

Dr. Ayman Jamal for helping with invasive procedures on so many of my patients.

Romelia Laborin, my Medical Assistant, whose energy, kindness, and competence, allows me to perform my work most efficiently.

To all the healthcare team at Scottsdale Cardiovascular Center for their invaluable contributions in patient care and helping many of my patients reach their therapeutic goals. To name a few, Nancy Avila, my Medical Assistant, Norma Jean my Administrative Assistant, Margo our Nuclear Tech, Reese Draemel and Debbie Batchelder (our ECHO techs), Jan Skinner, Office manager, and Doctors Scott Robertson, Philip Gideon, Alan Tenaglia, Brad Oswood for their hard work, inspiration and motivation for more than 15 years tolerating my idiosyncrasies loaded with philosophical deliberations!!

To Drs. Mattioni, David Riggio and Renzo Cataldo. Marwan Bahu and Akash Makkar for their strong support from electrophysiology point of view over the years.

I am extremely grateful to Charles Paltzer for helping with so many aspects to bring this book to fruition. He is instrumental in getting the videos recorded and edited (the ones you see in the QR codes throughout this book), and helping with social media and beyond.

I have to thank many of my mentors without whose help and support, I would not have become a cardiologist, or have had the benedictions to be of help to the needy and susceptible. To the late Dr. Ken Desser who was the director of the fellowship program at Good Samaritan Medical Center in Phoenix. Dr. Stan Pearson, Medical Director at Cigna, who gave me the approval to pursue my Master's in Research at the School of Public Health at the University of Michigan. And to the late Dr. Sridhar who was the first person we met when we came to Arizona. Dr. Sridhar has been an amazing influence in my life!!

And finally, to many in my family whose tolerance, acceptance, patience, understanding, and dealing with days and weeks of my absences from their lives, enabling me to reach out to my patients at times of need and at their times of vulnerable situations. A heartfelt appreciation to my wife Jayanthi for her unconditional love, generosity, mercy, and compassion, and courage to deal with grueling situations with grace, to our two sons who have continuously brought us happiness through their passion, touch and embrace, humor and constructive criticisms.

As someone in my 60s, I have felt a little unsteady dealing with technology. Many times, I have been asked by my family if I grew up in deep remote village, as they raised questions about my brain function! And last but certainly not least, to my father-in-law and mother-in-law whose respect, admiration, and boundless blessings have allowed for a magical and wondrous journey of life.

WATCH NOW

Every Life is divine. With all the stressors of life, with accumulation of all the negative layers of anxiety, fear, humiliation, isolation, sadness, conflicts, greed, jealousy, anger and hatred, this divinity is masked. My meaning and purpose of life is to attain peace, to peel these layers one by one, so I can see my own divinity.

I will have to peel these layers through work or worship, through psychic control and mindfulness or through philosophy and unconditional love for all. I should be able to see the holiness in every person, benevolence in every animal and sacrosanctity in everything that is "nature" around me.

I should be able to put my hands together at every encounter in "Namaste" fashion to say, "I salute the Godliness in You". As I peel the layers every day by doing a good deed, getting to the core of my consciousness, only then shall I experience my own spirituality, and invoke my own divinity that I envision to be so dazzling to the sight, bright with splendor of the fiery sun blazing from all sides.

WATCH NOW

You will notice that each chapter has "Watch Now" QR Codes.

With your smartphone, click on your camera. A link will appear, click on it and up on your screen will come a video with Dr. Kris Vijay speaking. His short videos will capture the essence of the incredible man who wrote this book. What he shares in these short videos will be inspiring and informative.

Foreword

By

Dr. Marc Silver

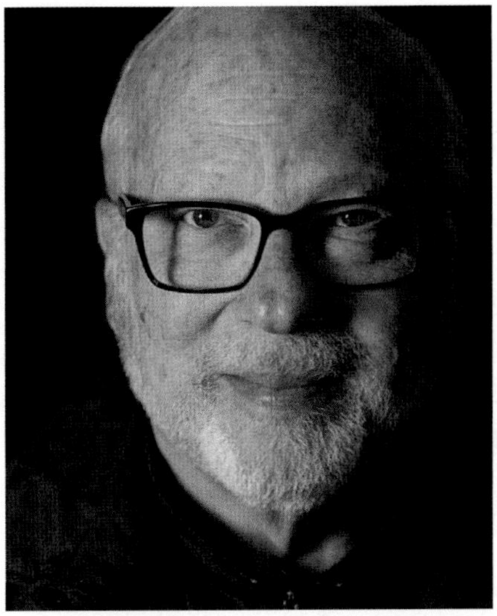

It is both simple and difficult to describe for you the roots of the book you are now reading, and the spirit and dedication of my dear friend Kris Vijay.

The difficult part would be to distill a lifetime of exceptional and selfless work, both in youth and through maturity, to become more learned and wiser, all the while keeping his eye on the goal of helping and serving patients and families with medical and social ills. He had an entire career in the UK before coming to the US and proceeding through and overcoming the hurdles and barriers that faced him. Because of who he is, he emerged successful, grateful, and rose to leadership in every position he has been in. His resume is exhaustive and filled with scientific endeavor, leadership, growth in many areas and extreme volunteerism.

The simple part is to describe Kris as an Old Soul. One who is filled with wisdom, fairness, justness, kindness, and altruism. Reading his story at the start of the book is advised to place a frame around what you are about to read from this remarkable force in our time.

Somehow, we met. I actually don't recall the first introduction, but I soon came to call him my friend, colleague, and collaborator. We shared patients from each of our distant practices, ideas, work in healthcare and beyond. One belief that resonates within both of us equally, is that patients themselves must have knowledge and ownership of their healthcare. I will tell you that if you have the fortune to interact with Dr. Vijay you will emerge a more joyful and better person.

Which brings me to his book, Invoking Your Inner Therapist in Heart Failure: Untold Patient Experiences From Prevention to End Stage. Like all things Kris, it is comprehensive and overflowing with detail and compassion. I would dare to say that you will feel his love for all of you emerge from the pages.

And it is his style, his relentless focus on the patient and all that encompasses anyone who suffers, that makes this book unique and a treasure.

Heart failure is an unrelenting US and Worldwide epidemic. One of my bonds with Kris has been our great disappointment that we and our colleagues have not attenuated or halted this disease. We both have learned that there are missing pieces in the process and care of heart failure patients and their families that go beyond the office, emergency room or hospital bed. It takes a keen observer to discern these nuances that compose the secret sauce of caring.

I am envious of the experience you are about to immerse yourselves in. There is much to absorb and learn and reflect upon in its pages. Enjoy, and as always, wishing you success!

Marc A. Silver, MD, FACP, FACC, FAHA, FHSA
Clinical Professor of Medicine, University of Illinois
Founding member, "Heart Failure Society of America"
Author, *Success with Heart Failure* and *Strategic Heart Failure*.

WATCH NOW

Endorsements

One of the essential qualities of the clinician is interest in humanity,
for the secret of the care of the patient is in caring
for the patient.

~ Francis W. Peabody, 1927

Dr. Kris Vijay has always been known by colleagues worldwide as one of the most heralded and heavily credentialed leaders and teachers in a huge spectrum of cardiology-related areas. He travels worldwide to share his perspectives on a wide variety of topics and often takes leadership positions for underserved populations and important areas of medicine where few have wandered (e.g. cardiorenal). In Heart Failure Management: From Prevention to End Stage, he has just created a contemporary and practical patient-centered personal guide to heart failure prevention, diagnosis and treatment that could only be written by him.

The book could have many titles including a "Humanistic (or spiritual or holistic) approach to Heart Failure" and yet it contains a wide spectrum of useful technical information accessible to the intelligent layperson. As a physician, I am impressed by how carefully he selects examples of heart failure conditions and illuminates key lessons. The classifications of heart failure conditions and causes are well-organized and will be easily recognized by patients as to relevance. I am more astounded by how Dr. Vijay respects the non-medical aspects and relates them to the overall health and future of his patients. Completely non-judgmental, Dr. Vijay is an astute observer and carefully listens to the patient's full life story. In fact, he is the best example I know of a "medical detective" incorporating all facets of relevant patient history and conditions.

Each section contains a superb example of how a spiritually-based, compassionate, careful, clinician/detective approaches an individual with a medical problem. Dr. Vijay spends the time to understand the relationships and medical relevance of family life, psychological and spiritual outlook, social circumstances, lifestyle considerations, financial stresses, and worldview. With his natural respect for the human condition, he examines each life journey finding illness an opportunity to understand, teach and to serve—intervening with great technical knowledge and experience suffused with abundant compassion, respect, and humanity.

Despite his considerable training and authority developed after a very humble upbringing in India, his care and his attitude towards serving others is absolutely inspiring. He understands the limitations of science and can be counted on to reveal the very latest drugs, tests, and devices for each aspect of cardiovascular disease.

Each section has inspiring quotes and superbly selected true cases. The subsequent well-organized discussions each reveal an important category or cause of heart failure from a most respectful physician/scientist/teacher.

Most physicians asked to review a book choose to skim, get an idea of the flow and quality and present their review and perspectives. Each section of this tome inspired me—I found myself reading the book and every example twice. Frankly, regardless of future aspirations in medicine, I believe it should be required reading for all medical and nursing students. Beyond the technical aspects, we all need to be reminded of the special privilege of serving others—and the value of understanding the patient far beyond the obvious medical problems. Dr. Vijay reveals the enormous value of each person, but sadly, in today's world, few feel special to a busy physician. The extra time to listen and observe and to care about the life story often makes the difference between a healthy future and a bleak outlook. We often talk about the "art and science of medicine", "holistic care" and "integrative medicine". How fortunate for Dr. Vijay's patients that these concepts and his ability to integrate "east-west medicine" have been embedded in his DNA decades before they became part of our vocabulary. Cardiology fellows will find his selection of cases to be wonderful teaching tools on rounds and for patients. And it will remind them of the importance of being a careful observer who knows and respects his patients.

This book is an absolute gem—I love how Dr. Vijay gives the reader up-to-date information (including Covid), explanations of the relationships between organ systems and the introduction to all the modern tools and therapies related to heart failure. But it is the balance he achieves by being an international observer of the human condition—someone who always values and respects the human condition, one's spiritual life, and our uniqueness in his quest to promote the health and well-being of everyone he encounters.

James Ehrlich, MD
Clinical Asst Professor, Division of Endocrinology, University of Colorado (Anschutz campus)
Board Certified, Anesthesiology
Board Certified, Obesity Medicine
Co-founder of 3 Cardiovascular Societies
Former Medical Director, Colorado Heart Imaging, HeartScan Houston, Washington DC, Indianapolis
Medical Director, Monitored Telemedicine
Medical Director, Prosperity Health

Winston Churchill once said, "Likes and dislikes are of little consequence, just do what needs to be done, it may not be happiness, but it is greatness." I shared this quote within a note of appreciation that I presented to Dr. Vijay in 2001 after completing my third-year medical school cardiology rotation with him. The quote by Mr. Churchill was most appropriate for Dr. Vijay as he has spent his life's work doing clinically what needed to be done for those most vulnerable. His clinical and academic prowess rendered him a leading expert in the governance of the heart and more specifically in the management of heart failure. His passion to help this particular sector of humanity has allowed longevity in his chosen field and thus, wisdom associated with time.

I had placed my previously mentioned thank you note in a book titled, The Power of One. This is a text written by Bryce Courtenay that speaks of the life and struggles of an amateur boxer in South Africa. It talks of the balance between the head and the heart while navigating life. Dr. Vijay, through his intellect and caring has served tens of thousands of patients. His journey of health advocacy alongside his patients and their families has taught him both clinical and life lessons and this book is the product of these lessons. His aim is to educate those both internal and external to medicine on methods to avoid heart failure and/or to prevent the advancing of it. He graciously shares personal anecdotes along the way which makes the book an easy read and also allows those infirmed to know that they are not alone. Through his words, Dr. Vijay demonstrates the influence that the power of one can have by doing what needs to get done, with love and compassion.

Dr. Alan Schalscha
Associate Professor
University of Texas Dell Medical School
Chief Medical Officer
Community Care Health Clinics
Acting Chief Medical Officer
Travis County Hospital District

There are multiple books for patients with cancer or diabetes but very few for those suffering from congestive heart failure which affects over 6 million in the United States alone. Yet more than ever patients want information and to understand their disease so they can make important choices and be partners in their health care. Dr. Vijay has produced such a work that will be a tremendous resource for patients and their families. It comes from his decades long experience with this serious ailment and is rich with information, compassion, and wisdom. I will certainly recommend it to my patients and their loved ones.

J. Thomas Heywood MD
Director, Advanced Heart Failure and Mechanical Circulatory Support
Scripps Clinic
La Jolla, Ca

I met Dr. Vijay in May 2010 and I didn't know it would change my life.

My Father was on vacation in Scottsdale, Arizona and suffered a sudden, serious stroke. In addition to neurological consultation and the involvement of many other specialists, Dr. Vijay became involved in directing my Father's care due to his complex cardiac history, and its overriding impact on his overall health and prognosis. I can only say this was divine intervention.

Having a serious health emergency is never a good thing, and that is amplified and made even more difficult when it is thousands of miles from home. The shock, distress, unease, and fear that families go through is well known, and easily understood by common experience.

What was completely uncommon was when I met Dr. Vijay in the ICU of the region's Level 1 Trauma Centre. It was one of the most important things that has ever happened to my family. It was instantly evident that Dr. Vijay was clearly expert in complex cardiology. However, his approach to his patients, and their loved ones, was anything but solely clinical. His presence was instantly calming yet brimming with knowledge and a quiet, powerful, and ethereal confidence. He was able to share his technical expertise in a manner which was respectful and empathetic, all the while demonstrating his mastery of his field. I have had the opportunity and fortune to meet some amazing medical practitioners in Canada and the US, in private and public settings, and I can say unequivocally that Dr. Vijay has the perfect, and unique, blend of bedside manner and medical and technical excellence, and is one of the finest doctors I know.

Dr. Vijay has a singularly remarkable ability to deliver his diagnosis, evaluation and options for treatment in a way that I can only describe as if he were your own family. He speaks to you with benevolence, grace and kindness. This mix of compassion and knowledge coupled with caring and endless patience possessed by Dr. Vijay reflects an embodiment of who he is and his journey in life. All too often those blessed with his intellect and knowledge are unable to bestow their gifts or share them with others – whether they may be colleagues, patients, students, or peers. Dr. Vijay transcends all the cardiological medical fraternity stereotypes and is the genuine article.

Dr. Vijay saved my father's life with his unique intellect and capacity for creativity, rigour, and discipline to principle—which may seem counterintuitive however which is frankly ingenious. This special characteristic of Dr. Vijay's practise approach is recounted in his ego-less book, time and again and all and only for his patient's welfare, and of course their concerned families. He earned our trust seemingly effortlessly, and extended the life of my beloved Father for nearly a decade with his dedication to patient outcomes, and his innate ability to ensure his patients truly believe that they can and will, influence their own outcomes. Dr. Vijay and his lovely wife have become lifelong friends of our family, and along with my *both* my parents, were honoured guests at my wedding.

Dr. Vijay now codifies and shares his vision of medicine and care in this magnificent book, which encapsulates all of which I have experienced in person: his special blend of humanity, knowledge, compassion and amazing medical experience and intellect. As he does in life with his patients, he does in this book – seamlessly blend medicine and non-medicine for his readers, regardless of whether you are a doctor or a patient, and all those fortunate enough to read this outstanding and unique treatise. I would urge anyone interested in health outcomes, regardless of affliction, patient, and practitioner alike, to read and *absorb* the lessons Dr. Vijay shares within. Dr. Vijay not only wants to make a difference, he does so every day. Society needs many, many more doctors like him.

Rob Doman
Founder and President of Waterstone Partners Inc.,
Former member of the Board of Governors of the British Columbia Institute of Technology
Former Chair of Governance Committee of BCIT
B. Comm (Bachelor of Commerce, University of British Columbia (UBC)
MBA (Master of Business Administration, UBC); LL. B/JD (Bachelor of Laws/Juris Doctor, University of Victoria)

INTRODUCTION

PERSONAL STORY

WATCH NOW

I grew up in Bombay and remember waking up at 5 am to stand in line to get a gallon of milk for my family, or rice and sugar during the rationing days. The line would be hours long simply to get cooking supplies.

The struggles of getting from point A to point B were real as well. I would commute to the college by train and, often the rain, mud, heat, and floods that would prevent me from even getting to the train station. There were times when the water would be up to my chest, and there was no way to reach the train station. Frequently, the train would be canceled, and I would end up missing the chemistry lab and have to make up the class on another day. Many students came from far away while others would walk long distances to get to class. The stress of both high school and college was real because so many who were competing to get into medical school. It was a struggle to get good scores to qualify to get into medical school.

Sometimes, lower socio-economic strata students would not have the resources to be competitive and would not get in. There were so many who could not get into medical school because they did not make it by one point, which resulted in them having to change their career. The stories in terms of the struggle, and having to endure the physical and mental trauma of not making it by the skin of your teeth were nothing compared to the endless hours of sleep deprivation that one would experience during residency after the medical school was over and done.

When the total recovery of someone expected to die is juxtaposed with the unexpected death of another happening during the same day multiple times over the years, one starts to wonder about the inevitability of it all.

In January 1977, my father had just come home from Harkisandas Hospital after being discharged from congestive heart failure. He was treated by one of the finest cardiologists of that time, Dr. J. K Mehta. I left without concern to return to medical school which was 1,000 miles away. My final exam was coming up in May, and a week before my exam I had a hunch that my father was not well and had fallen through the cracks. He had passed away a week before my final exam.

To be a doctor was one thing, but the trials and tribulations of internship and residency were a totally different animal. The angst that is etched in their mitochondria is very palpable. Perhaps, it is this very ordeal that gives the wherewithal and the chutzpah to make it through and perform at times of crisis or an emergency.

Perhaps it is the richness of existence and the bountiful experience that is gained over the years with mental and physical trauma and sleep deprivation being part and parcel of this journey that makes one stronger.

As I walked into our home, my brothers were looking at me with grief and I broke down in tears. My father had been ill so many times over the last four years of his life that every time he would be hospitalized, there was a fear that he may not come back alive. While it was not a major surprise when he died, it was tough to handle his absence. I knew that my father was there for me and he was a great mentor. He embodied the Gandhian philosophy of nonviolence, equality, freedom, truth, and religious tolerance and acceptance.

After coming back to Bombay, I completed my internship and residency but always had cardiology in the back of my mind as a specialty of interest. The internship itself was strenuous and the catecholamine surge of being in the emergency room the first week of internship carried me through to treating patients with end-stage malignancy to cirrhosis, lung disease, end-stage kidney disease, and cancer. It felt as if the curriculum in the real-world scenario involved endless learning with overwhelming uncertainty of it all which was exhausting. There were days where I wanted to quit and believe that it was not worth it at all. So many questions were flocking through the chambers of my hippocampus.

Time and again, some of the darkest moments would spring along the course and one had to be resilient. I had to suddenly shake off everything I was going through and empathize with what my patients were going through. I had to believe that my life was a picnic as opposed to my patient's lives. From their perspective, I had to be there for reassurance and be there for them regardless of my struggles. I had to say to myself constantly "I will bring all of my knowledge and expertise to the extent that I can and take the message from everything I have learned to take the patient's fears away and make them comfortable." And I would say to myself "Just for today, I shall be cheerful" on a daily basis even when all about me would be going wrong!!

The inexorable nature of suffering and tales of images of unexpected beauty bring contrast and congruence, and visibility and indistinctness about our own existence. It begs the question about the meaning and purpose of our daily lives with warts and all, fractured, unscathed, or both. After 40 years since medical school, one thing that is very appealing to me is the stories of the person behind the disease and the struggles they have gone through and the inconceivable things they have accomplished.

> We know that when a single child in Kenya goes to sleep hungry, the entire planet is malnourished. We know that when the ocean of homeless people roams through the streets of Damascus or Dhaka, then our conscience is indelibly disturbed. We know that when the heart stops beating in Ukraine or in Uruguay, silence engulfs the whole world.

I believe that invoking conversations about these achievements in and of itself is partly a panacea for healing their physical and mental maladies. Certainly, there remains a big gap in the human touch and the treasured values of kindness and caring we must uphold at all times. The touchy-feely aspect of healing and reconciliation with the suffering and sunlight that is often found around it has to be highlighted. No doubt there are many unsettling questions of right vs wrong vs shades of gray. One has to expand its vision to include all the different values that are sustained, reflected, and continues to resonate over time in the foundation of humankind.

I have been told by my inner therapist to visit a world, entirely other than myself on a diligent basis and have an unquenchable human urge to strive for a better life for the patients that I encounter daily. I have learned that I must be global, national, diverse, technologically advanced, compassionate, and must bring to all a sense of healing.

I believe that I am fortunate to be alive and blessed to be given an incredible opportunity to serve the underserved and have been given a road map of thinking about our changing world.

I must marry the knowledge and experience that I have gained through my patients with precise realism that will resonate with intricate and disturbing echoes because this world is textured and complex while the stories are intimate and universal.

To believe that science is perfect is foolhardy, as there are many uncertainties in medicine, and to believe that we can cure every heart disease or cancer would befall on the ludicrous. While we aspire to help patients reach their highest level of quality and functionality, and if they happen to live longer than expected, then we will be humble to accept the outcome, will praise the Lord, have faith and worship the higher power that has bestowed the elixir of life upon us.

In the next few pages of this book, I share stories with tremendous tenderness, respecting the dignity of my patients who are struggling or have struggled with heart disease, yet always had a sense of hope and dream to live, love, and be loved for one more day. Allow me to unlock your hidden potential and empower your neurocognitive signs, expand your knowledge, and shape your future in ways unimaginable.

SECTION I

Introduction

CHAPTER 1

The Electrical, The Circulatory, and The Pump

WATCH NOW

Do you remember your mother telling you when you were older, when she was pregnant with you at 16 weeks since inception, the doctor told your mother that he/she heard a heartbeat? Have you ever thought about where this heartbeat was the day before? A week before? Was it even there? What makes it start the beating process at that time?

At 16 weeks, that tissue at the top of your right atrium called the sinus node, started off with one cell at the time of inception, then 2, then 4 then 16 then 256 and beyond. And suddenly at 16 weeks, it has grown to millions of cells and reaches a critical mass. This critical mass is reached not only at the sinus node but also at the junction of the right top chamber, atrium, and bottom chamber, ventricle, called the AV node. There is another tissue called the right bundle and it goes towards the bottom of the right ventricle. Another tissue, called the left bundle divides into the anterior and posterior fascicles and goes to the left side of the heart.

> Did you ever know that once your heart kicks off at 16 weeks, it never stops until you die? Did you know that your heart beats about 100,000 times a day? So, the question that keeps coming up for me on a regular basis is,
>
> *"If my heart is the powerhouse that sustains me and keeps me going with awareness the minute I wake up with a certain level of consciousness about my existence, then do I not have an obligation to cherish it, nurture it, preserve it and prevent it from getting hurt: Physically? Emotionally? Spiritually?"*

Now, at 16 weeks, when these nodes and bundles reach critical mass simultaneously, something happens, like lightning, like electricity, like rubbing two stones against each other. What happens when you rub two stones against each other? We know that suddenly we get fire, we get electricity. And that exactly is energy, it is electricity. That is precisely what happens in your heart. These electrical issues are your superpowers. You may want to believe that these are simply basic biochemical, biomechanical, and anatomical phenomenon that gives you the opportunity of life. But the bottom line is this: the minute they reach that critical mass and evoke electricity, the current descends like lightning, and the force of electricity that goes downstream from the top chamber to the bottom chamber, from the sinus node to the AV node initiates the opening and closing of the mitral and tricuspid valves as well as the aortic and pulmonic valves and the first heartbeat has just begun!!.

And swiftly, the blood is now flowing from the Left Ventricle, which is the pump, through the aorta and to the rest of the body along every blood vessel supplied by this force that gushes out of the heart to sustain all tissues with adequate blood flow and oxygen to perform their functions.

So, it is indeed like electricity first, followed by mechanical functioning; it is like lightning followed by thunder. It is like your spirit has allowed your physical construct, and your physical abilities decode your intellectual prowess which then sends a cosmic vibratory impulse though your body that now allows you to perform in some compelling fashion.

You have just been gifted with a sense of power to create, a sense of empowerment and a sense that emboldens you towards an impeccable code of conduct. You have just received glory from above that is casting light at the end of your complex maze. It has given you that healing power from your own inner therapist to follow a path strewn with a positive outlook which should make you perform and accomplish great things as you understand the meaning and purpose of life.

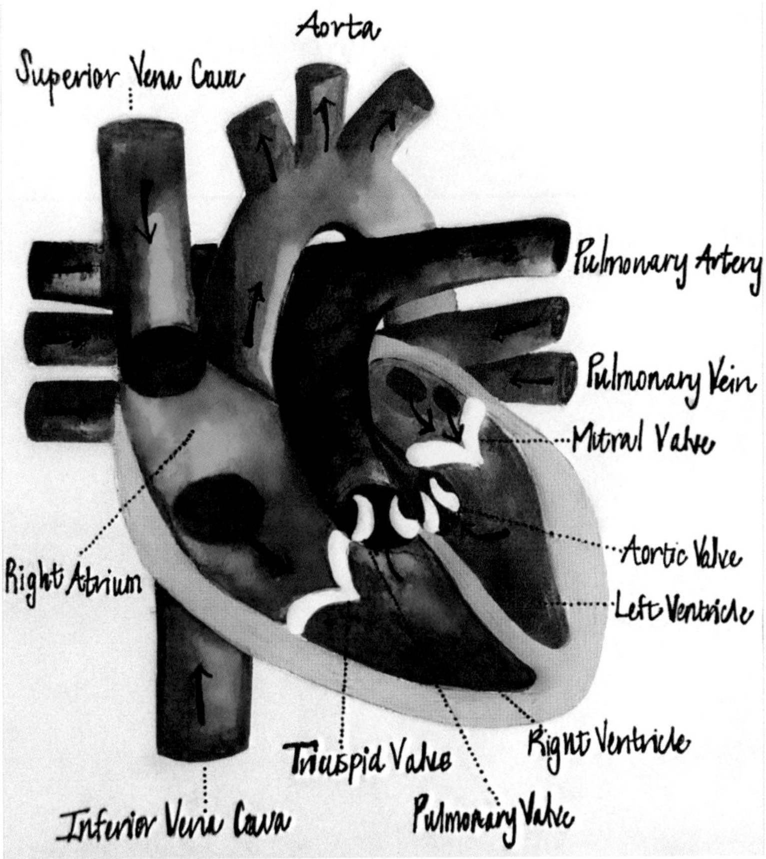

Normal Heart Fig. 1

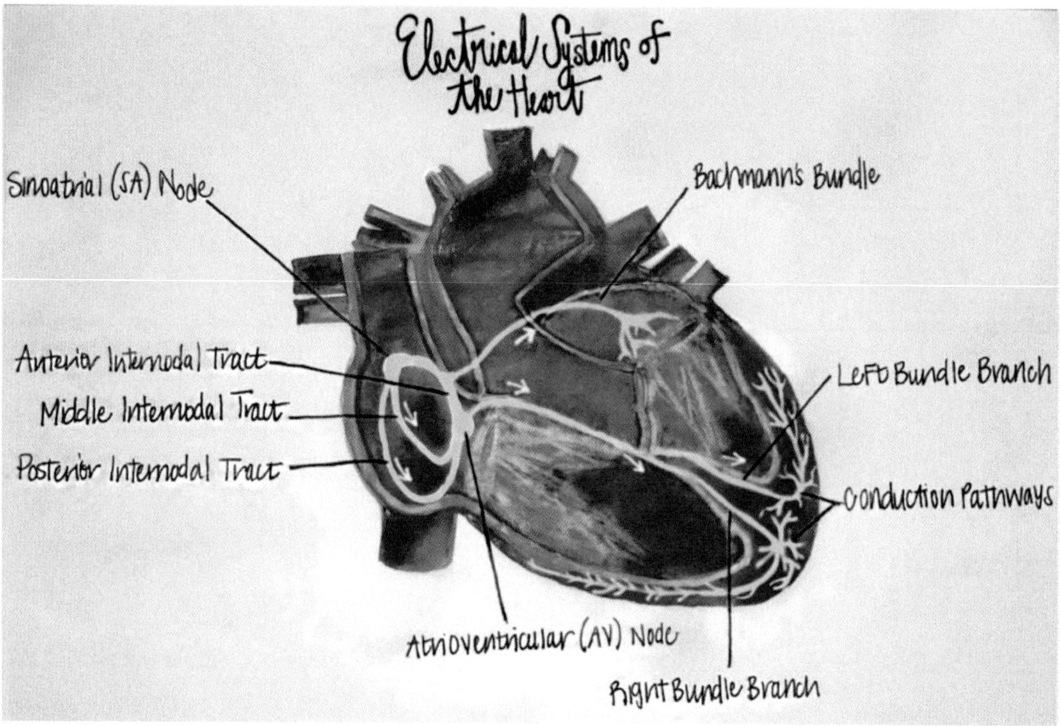

Electrical Systems of the Heart Fig. 2

CHAPTER 2

Heart Failure Around the World: Global Burden of Heart Failure

When thou examinest the obstruction in his abdomen and thou findest that he is not in a condition to leap the Nile, his stomach is swollen and his chest asthmatic, then say thou to him: "It is blood that has got itself fixed and does not circulate."

Do thou cause and emptying by means of a medicinal remedy?

Make him, therefore:
Wormwood 1/8, Elderberries 1/16, Sebesten 1/8, Sasa-chips 1/8, Cook in Beer-that-has-been-brewed-from many-ingredients, strain into one, thoroughly, and let the patient drink.

— Egyptian Papyrus...around 1400 B.C.

One of the cardiologists was very emotional in his experiences when he said that many patients who have multivessel coronary artery disease were presenting to the hospital with heart failure as the initial manifestation.

It was in the early 2000s when I was invited to attend the first Society of Heart Failure in India's meeting where we had many cardiologists from India and the US where we discussed the prevalence of heart failure around the world. At the time, we realized that while the heart failure prevalence and epidemiology is well recognized in the United States and over 6 million people in the US with heart failure, the prevalence in India was undetermined. The data was not there yet but there were multiple registries. At the same time, capturing much of this data was flawed and it was almost impossible at the time to determine what the true prevalence of this issue was.

It has been interesting over the years to see what the underlying reasoning has been beyond the increased prevalence of heart failure. It has been a challenge to truly determine how many people suffer from heart failure around the world, but it appears that about 26 million people have heart failure as of 2019 but there is a projection of 77 million by 2040 around the world. It has been mentioned even in the *Egyptian Papyrus in the 1400s B.C.*, many centuries ago.

WATCH NOW

So, what is **Heart Failure** then? Heart failure is a condition in which the heart is not able to pump enough blood to meet the body's requirements to function properly.

This may be due to a weakness of the pump or low Left ventricular Ejection Fraction (normal is more than 50%). This is called systolic heart failure or HFrEF. In some cases, the heart is not able to fill with enough blood despite a normal forward pump or left ventricular ejection fraction. This is called diastolic heart failure or HFpEF. Many patients have both problems. Left-sided heart failure with preserved or reduced ejection fraction gives rise to symptoms of shortness of breath due to fluid accumulation in the lungs. In other cases, the right side of the heart fails and does not pump enough blood into the pulmonary arteries to get to the lungs to pick up oxygen.

This is called Right Heart Failure. Right-side heart failure may cause fluid to build up in the feet, ankles, legs, liver, abdomen, and the veins in the neck. Right-side and left-side heart failure also may cause shortness of breath and fatigue.

The term "heart failure" does not mean that your heart has stopped or is about to stop working. However, heart failure is a serious condition that requires medical care. Heart failure is a quite common condition affecting more than 6 million people in the United States. Both children and adults can have the condition, although the symptoms and treatments differ. Currently, heart failure has no cure. However, treatments—such as medicines, device therapy, and lifestyle changes—can help people who have the condition live longer and function better being more active. Researchers continue to study new ways to treat heart failure and its complications.

The WHO has been trying to assess the epidemiological concepts of heart failure around the world but has difficulty in teasing it out.

> The more important goal that we need to have is to prevent the onset of heart failure itself.

When you look at the prevalence of risk factors that leads to this issue, then we have to think about coronary artery disease as the number one reason. CAD is significantly high in western countries such as the United States or Europe but is trickling down to other developing countries including Asia, Australia, and Africa.

Clearly, the risk factors of heart failure need to be addressed around the world. Hypertension seems to be highly prevalent in China. I remember being in a meeting regarding the global burden of cardiovascular disease and a professor from China was presenting on the prevalence of hypertension. It looks like in 2010, the prevalence of hypertension was present in almost ⅓ of the population over the age of 18 in China. But in recent years, it is now well known that hypertension has been recognized as an issue attributed to high salt intake. The prevalence was then reduced to 23% in 2018, however, the prevalence of prehypertension is close to 41% and is present in almost 500 million people.

The risk factors of hypertension as a progressive disease towards heart failure is accepted all over the world. There does not appear to be a significant difference in Urban and Rural population in these countries. The prevalence of diabetes is another issue that leads to heart failure. In India, diabetes prevalence seems to be increasing significantly along with metabolic syndrome and cardiovascular disease. The prevalence of diabetes seems to be about 24% in some Indian studies.

The prevalence of prediabetic state is 33% to 40% among the South Asian population over the age of 18; so, clearly the globalization concepts, increased restaurant openings, lack of exercise may be contributors to metabolic syndrome. Lack of exercise is an example of globalization and mechanization concepts with more people owning cars and taking public transportation and not walking enough. Along with this, comes an increase in pollution and is intertwined in the pursuit of financial stability in developing countries. This is also true in the US. Diabetes and hypertension have increased while smoking prevalence has decreased in the US. However, smoking prevalence has increased in Europe and other developing countries. Coronary artery disease is obviously a reflection of the above-mentioned risk factors. There is also nonischemic cardiomyopathy with a nonatherosclerotic disease which can be secondary to infectious etiology. There are many lessons that I have been learning about the global increase in heart failure. The aging population around the world is on the rise and it appears that the incidence of heart failure will slowly increase, and hospitalizations or healthcare costs will follow.

Many of the developing countries outside of Western civilization are beginning to adopt Western culture. While there are some amazing positives about westernization and adopting many of these nuances, many countries and population are resorting to the negative aspects of Western culture. This includes dietary indiscretions with high saturated fat and high carbs consumption and lack of exercise, thus increasing their body mass index, some disproportionately in different parts of the body leading to the Metabolic Syndrome of Globalization. This may contribute to a pandemic of heart failure moving forward. Also, the concept of heart failure with preserved ejection fraction is poorly understood and investigated with no effective therapies yet. Hence, the global burden of heart failure is going to be a significant public health problem that we will need to face and mitigate with the prevention of risk factors at primary, secondary, and primordial levels.

Heart Failure is a condition where the heart does not pump adequately, or it does not relax properly which will then turn into a state where there is fluid retention. The fluid can accumulate in the lower extremities or the abdomen, or the lungs, or outside the lungs in pleural space. Patients can become short of breath very easily, they can become fatigued, or weak and inability to function seeps in.

There are more than 6 million people in the US with heart failure, more than a million get admitted to the hospital due to heart failure. Out of which about 40-50% of them have normal pump function or what is called "ejection fraction". They might have what is called HFpEF which is heart failure which preserved ejections, which means that the pump is squeezing adequately but not relaxing properly. The other half of the population will have what is called "reduced ejection" or HFrEF; this means the pump function is inadequate and ejection fraction may be reduced. So, what is normal ejection fraction? Well, any number that is more than 50% is normal, perhaps up to 80% I would say.

Again, when we say 50-80%, it means that this amount of blood is being pumped out of the heart and there is a need for blood to be left behind when the heart is relaxing so that there is an adequate filling of the coronary arteries that supply the heart muscle during relaxation of the heart. The arteries that supply the heart muscle are called "coronary arteries" and they fill and perfuse the heart when the heart is relaxing during diastole through what is called a "recoil mechanism" which usually follows a heart squeeze or what is called "systole".

Out of the 6-7 million people with heart failure, the lifetime risk of getting heart failure is about 20-45% at age 75 years. The incidence is higher with African Americans compared to Caucasians. Although we have made some inroads in improving survival, it is important to know that this disease has an extremely high mortality. So far as we know, about 50-75% of the patients die within 5 years of being diagnosed. But this statistic is also changing and in addition, the functional capacity or what is known as "quality of life" is a lot more important than death itself.

Hence, improving the quality of life through medical management and keeping them on the dryer side without fluid retention is critical in managing heart failure.

Over the past few years, the cost of heart failure management has skyrocketed. We are spending close to $77 billion on just managing heart failure. Of this about $ 35M is being spent in inpatient care.

Much of the cost is reflected by hospitalization within 30 days of the previous admission. Medicare has come with a penalty to the hospital if the patient is readmitted within 30 days. Unfortunately, the hospital may not be the culprit but may still get penalized. The doctor does not get penalized. But at the same, in many systems, the doctors do have an incentive not to readmit the patient within 30 days and keep patients out of the hospital in addition to making them feeling better and living longer.

The worldwide prevalence of heart failure is not clearly known. Many countries do not have enough data but what is known is that the prevalence is increasing significantly as we improve our statistics in preventing heart attacks. Around the world, when patients come in through the hospital ER for chest pain and they are diagnosed with a heart attack or blocked artery that supplies the heart muscle called "coronaries" then there is a lot more opportunity for doctors to make sure that the patient is quickly stabilized by opening a blood vessel or two.

Additionally, many of these systems around the world have bypass surgery available as an option in some facilities, and resources in operating rooms have become available more recently. Clearly, as we improve heart attacks and open blood vessels, perform bypass surgeries, longevity seems to have improved but most of these patients will end up in heart failure. Hence, the prevalence of heart failure has increased significantly. While we have helped one condition and made them feel better and hopefully live longer, we have now transferred the epidemiological burden of coronary disease to a higher burden of heart failure and mortality thereof.

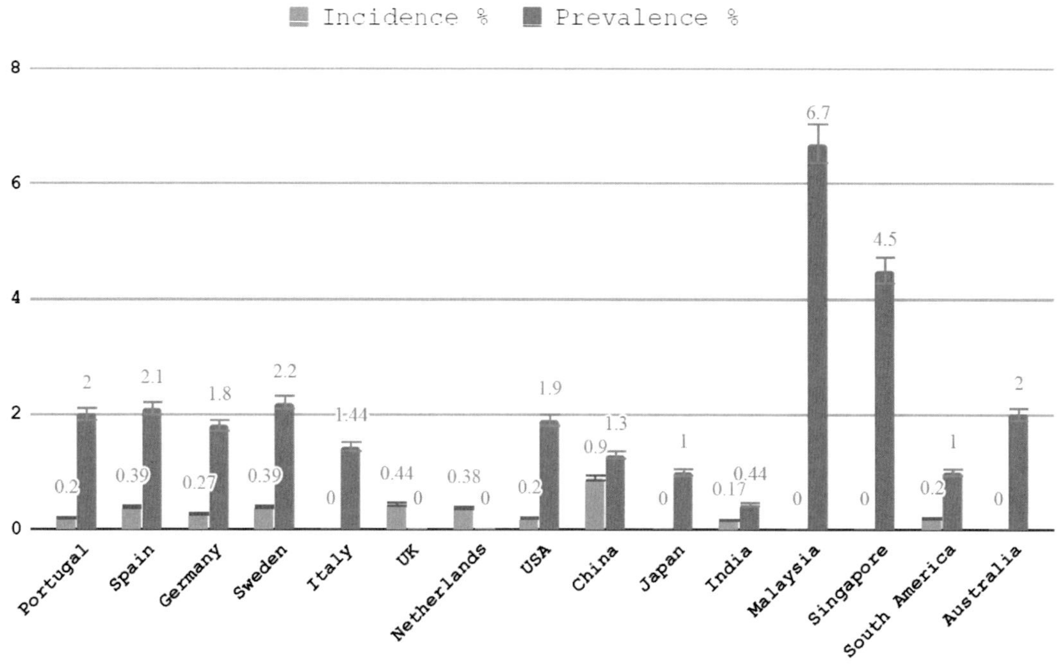

Fig. 3

I've known Doctor Kris Vijay for almost 20 years now and I must say that he is not only a very well trained, top of the line cardiologist but he exemplifies the concept of the word "doctor". Kris is truly a hardworking man of science with many accolades to his name from colleagues, patients, and society at large. Always able and available to take care of the sickest of the sick from a scientific point of view, he has consistently gone beyond the expectations of a person of medical knowledge to be that person that all patients always want in a doctor. He exudes the *humanity* that we should all strive for in our profession. He is an analyst and a synthesist, the kind of listener that brings any one patient's experience home as well as someone with a bird's eye view of patients at large. I was honored to have been chosen to be part of his medical missions and his non-profit organization, but mostly to be considered part of his inner circle of colleagues and friends.

Renzo Cataldo, MD FHRS FACC
Director, Electrophysiologist, Mountain Heart, Flagstaff, Arizona
Professional Photographer
Multilinguist

CHAPTER 3

Causes of Heart Failure

WATCH NOW

Patient Story: Takotsubo Syndrome

Ms. SR is a 38-year-old female who had come to see me for a panic disorder. She told me the story of her husband being in a UHAUL while they were moving into Arizona from Oregon. She and her 2 daughters were in the car. Her husband had a head-on collision with a semi-truck and died while they were on the way. There were so many trials and tribulations that she had to face with the support of multiple family members and friends.

They arrived in Arizona and after the cremation of her husband, she has been having to deal with multiple other issues that one deals with after spousal demise. This is so sad and unfortunate with her feeling confused, irritated, and angry with herself. She was having panic attacks on a daily basis with her HR in the 120s and she just could not bring it down.

She assumed all of this was anxiety related. Her blood pressure has been on the lower side with dizziness which she attributes all of this to her husband's death.

> She turned into a happier person than she had ever imagined. She clearly is sad about the loss of her husband but now has a meaning and purpose in her life to fill a gap that her husband left behind and is working towards fulfilling those needs. It is almost as if she has plugged into a cosmic energy source in pursuit of a mission. She is thankful to us for detecting her condition and treating it, but truly she has taught us how to take control of one's own physical, intellectual, and mental health. You can harness your own brain's power to change your life for the better.

After evaluating her with an echocardiogram, it was clear that she had a "broken heart syndrome" or Takotsubo Syndrome. She was monitored in the hospital, underwent an angiogram and luckily, she had no blockages in her arteries. The apex of her left ventricle was not moving and had ballooned out. This is typical of Takotsubo or apical ballooning syndrome with no heart attacks. She had presented with chest tightness which she attributed to emotional stress. Clearly, the emotional stress had taken a toll on the heart and the movement abnormality of the left ventricle with ballooning of the apex was a typical symptom or sign of this condition. The stress hormones probably stunned the heart and triggered all the changes in the heart muscle, leading to the apical portion of the heart being akinetic or dyskinetic, hence, her symptoms were probably secondary to the broken heart syndrome.

She was placed on beta-blockers, a small dose of ACE inhibitors with a touch of diuretic and potassium supplement. With time, her panic disorder was slowly dissipating, and her heart rate was now in the '70s or '80s. She did not require any anti-anxiety medications. Slowly she took charge of her life and became more revitalized in activating her other desires to feel alive. She took control of her life and took care of her 2 daughters and developed a sense of connection with newer friends or family. She compelled herself to believe that she had the emotional intelligence and a strive to accomplish by getting a new job and staying mentally occupied. With exercise and cardiac rehab, her heart returned to normal anatomy and function.

Causes of Heart Failure

We know that the risk factors that cause heart failure such as blocked arteries may not be the only reason many patients go into heart failure. It could be due to uncontrolled high blood pressure and the incidence and prevalence of high blood pressure are increasing around the world both in rural and urban areas. Increased salt consumption, decreased exercise, and the availability of different kinds of processed food, as well as stress levels that go with mechanization and globalization, is contributing to a significantly higher prevalence of heart failure. The other risk factors that are also contributing to heart failure include diabetes.

Viral cardiomyopathy can lead to heart failure as well. But what does this mean? This truly means that a viral infection such as pneumonia or the flu or some other kind of virus affecting the body, including SARS-COV-2 can also directly affect the heart muscle.

> Diabetes doubles the risk of heart failure and frequently exists in conjunction with other risk factors such as blood pressure or blocked arteries called "coronary disease" as well as obesity. Smoking is obviously a major risk factor for coronary artery disease which can consequently lead to heart failure.

This toxicity of the heart muscle can lead to poor functioning of the muscles at a cellular level. This translates to a reduction in ejection fraction and can lead to congestive heart failure. Anther reasons why some patients can go into heart failure include alcoholism; alcohol is a direct toxin to the heart muscle and may be a primary cause of heart failure. Abstinence from alcohol can reverse this cardiomyopathy. High thyroid function can also lead to heart failure. High thyroid function can also lead to atrial fibrillation, which is a rapid heartbeat originating from the top chamber of the heart called "the left atrium."

The origin of atrial fibrillation is usually at the mouth of the pulmonic vein which drains into the left atrium. This can worsen heart failure. The heart rate becomes very rapid because of atrial fibrillation. This can lead to what is called "tachycardia-induced cardiomyopathy" or persistent high heart rate can put the heart at distress and fatigue will ensue very soon. Inflammation of the heart muscle can be from an autoimmune disease or fungal, or parasitic infections; they can all lead to heart failure.

There is a condition called peripartum cardiomyopathy which is secondary to childbirth or around childbirth. The underlying reasoning is not quite clear, but there could be some underlying genetic basis in patients who have developed peripartum cardiomyopathy. Other systemic disorders that can cause heart failure include amyloidosis. This is a condition where deposits of insoluble proteins in different parts of the body can happen. If it affects the heart, then it is called amyloid cardiomyopathy. The reason why we need to be focusing on the detection of amyloid cardiomyopathy more so now than ever is that a couple of treatment strategies are available in this condition at the present time. In addition, there are other conditions that can cause infiltration of the heart muscle with different kinds of proteins. One of them is called sarcoidosis. This autoimmune disease is due to a fungus-like ball causing inflammation that can get deposited in the heart muscle called granulomas. There is another condition called hemochromatosis which is secondary to iron overload, and that can either cause HFpEF or HFrEF due to deposition of iron in the heart muscle or myocardium. This can also occur because of repeated blood transfusions.

There are certain kinds of hereditary anemias which can also lead to cardiomyopathy. There is a very distinct genetic condition called hypertrophic cardiomyopathy which is caused by gene mutations and it can run in families. In this condition, the septal portion of the heart muscle, mainly the left ventricle becomes very thick in a very asymmetric fashion and due to this, the mitral valve leaflet can get suctioned into the outflow tract of the left ventricle. When the left ventricle is trying to squeeze across the aortic valve into the aorta, one of the leaflets of the mitral valve can get suctioned into this outflow tract and close that door. The left ventricle is suddenly stunned because the door is closed and is not able to push the blood into the aorta. This can lead to sudden cardiac arrest because of no blood flow going to the brain.

Another condition called Arrhythmogenic Right Ventricular Dysplasia which is characterized by fibrofatty deposition of myocardium mainly in the right ventricle which is also genetically mediated can lead to heart failure. Another condition called ventricular noncompaction results during the development of the embryo. In this condition, there is a sudden arrest in the heart muscle development into a contractile muscular structure. Instead, it produces spongy architecture without the trabeculation of the heart muscle. Other conditions such as Duchenne muscular dystrophy or Becker muscular dystrophy or genetic disorders are characterized by progressive weakness in the heart muscle, as well as in a skeletal muscle.

Other causes of heart failure include inflammation of the heart muscle itself called "myocarditis. Inflammation of the envelope that surrounds the heart muscle called pericardium can also lead to pericarditis, a pericardial inflammation, which leads to restriction of the heart muscle and lead to heart failure. Valvular heart disease such as the mitral valve, aortic valve, tricuspid valve, or pulmonic valve which are the valves inside the heart, can have dysfunction. It can be narrowed which is called stenosis or leaky which is called regurgitation. Valvular heart disease, if it becomes moderate or severe, can lead to congestive heart failure. Other causes include congenital heart disease.

Some people are born with an abnormal heart muscle or due to abnormal great vessels such as the aorta, pulmonary artery becoming transposed or there could be a hole in the heart leading to enlargement of the heart and heart failure. All these will be discussed in greater detail in the congenital heart disease section. Irregular heartbeat such as atrial fibrillation can also lead to worsening heart failure. The disease of the aorta, as well as the pulmonary artery, can also lead to congestive heart failure. We talked about pregnancy itself taking a toll on the heart and if there are other issues inside the heart that may be mild in severity, to begin with, then pregnancy can actually worsen that specific condition such as valvular heart disease and place the patient at higher risk during pregnancy and delivery.

Of course, there are other genetic variations, that may also lead to congestive heart failure. There are toxic substances such as heroin, methylamphetamine, cocaine, alcohol, and chemotherapeutic agents such as Adriamycin, cyclophosphamide can lead to congestive heart failure. Other toxic agents include sulfonamides, lead, arsenic, cobalt, phosphorus. In terms of nutritional deficiency, there is thiamine protein deficiency which is also called vitamin B1 that can lead to a condition called "Beriberi" which can subsequently lead to heart failure. Protein malnutrition, selenium deficiency, other nutritional deficiencies can contribute as well. Some of the electrolyte disorders include low calcium levels called "hypocalcemia", low phosphate levels called "hypophosphatemia", low sodium and potassium can all be contributors to heart failure as well.

There are other systemic diseases such as collagen vascular disease, lupus, rheumatoid arthritis, systemic sclerosis which can also lead to heart failure. There are other rare conditions called polyarteritis nodosa, Takayasu arteritis, polymyositis which are all conditions that affect connective tissues in the body such as bones, joints, and muscles. Many of them can be related to the heart indirectly through elevation of the pressure in the artery that supplies the lung called "pulmonary artery" and leads to pulmonary hypertension. This can lead to congestive heart failure.

Many of these are indirectly related. We talked about some endocrine diseases called diabetes mellitus, thyroid disorders with low functioning thyroid disease called hypothyroidism or high functioning thyroid disease called hyperthyroidism which can also lead to heart failure. Hypoparathyroidism which is a low functioning of a gland around the thyroid gland in the neck called parathyroid can also lead to heart failure with low calcium levels. There is a condition called pheochromocytoma which is a tumor in the core of the adrenal glands in the medulla which releases catecholamines, also called "adrenaline" and "noradrenaline" and lead to higher sympathetic activity contributing to heart failure. There is a condition called acromegaly secondary to an increase in growth hormone levels which can enlarge the heart and lead to heart failure.

But let us assume that the grass is not green but there is enough water and the irrigation tubes are open and there is adequate flow and yet the grass is yellow.

This will then start to make you think whether the grass is receiving enough nourishment, enough sunshine, if there is toxicity of the grass because the cat next door has cancer and is excreting all over your patch of grass or is because there is toxicity underneath with different kinds of worms attacking the grass or is it because there is some type of genetic variation in the type of grass you placed that causes it to not grow properly. So, the same thing can be applied to the heart muscle where you start thinking if it is not getting enough blood flow because of a blocked artery then the ideal thing to do is getting the artery opened up. If indeed, the arteries are open, then we start wondering what the underlying reason is or "etiology" is. What could be the etiology when the arteries are open? Well, we talked about multiple underlying reasoning as mentioned above, and start addressing the culprit. The treatment strategy now has not changed regardless of what the underlying reasoning is for the most part. In the next chapter, we will discuss the neurohormonal basis for why the heart muscle may not be functioning adequately regardless of the underlying coronary anatomy.

Table 1. – Causes for Heart Failure

Common:

Coronary Artery Disease	**Hypertension**	**Valvular Heart Disease**
Idiopathic Cardiomyopathy Viral/Bacterial/Fungal/Parasitic		

Less Common:

Arrhythmias: Tachycardia, Bradycardia, Sick Sinus Syndrome, Heart Block.	**Toxic Cardiomyopathy:** Alcohol, Cocaine, Radiation, Methamphetamine, Chemotherapy	**Kidney Disease:** Glomerulonephritis, Nephrotic Syndrome, Chronic Kidney Disease, End-Stage Kidney Disease Anemia
Hypertrophic Cardiomyopathy	**Postpartum Cardiomyopathy**	**Congenital Heart Disease**
Takotsubo Cardiomyopathy	Myocarditis	Pericarditis
Endocrine Disorders: Diabetes, Thyroid, and Adrenal	**Genetic Cardiomyopathy** Non-Compaction, Fabry's Disease	**Collagen Vascular Disease** Lupus Scleroderma
Lung Disease: Pneumonia, COPD, Pulmonary Embolism, Sleep Apnea	**Arrhythmogenic Right Ventricular Dysplasia**	**Vitamin/Mineral Deficiency** such as Thiamine, Selenium, Etc.
Medication-induced such as Non-Steroidal overuse of Ibuprofen Antidiabetic Medications such as Pioglitazone, saxagliptin, Excess Licorice, Steroids, Androgen		

SECTION II

Epidemiology, Pathophysiology, and Categories in Heart Failure

CHAPTER 4

Role of Neurohormones

WATCH NOW

Patient story

Mr. JB is a 40-year-old male who came into the hospital with chest pain and was noted to have multiple blocked vessels and had a heart attack. 3 major blood vessels supply the heart muscle LAD, circumflex, and RCA which seemed to have 90-95% narrowing and the heart muscle itself had been damaged probably acutely and one of the vessels may have been opened up spontaneously. But the damage may have been sustained and he was struggling with fluid overload. His heart pump was about 10%. Hence the surgeon felt he was too high of a risk for open-heart surgery to get a 3-vessel bypass. JB was totally distraught that he would be unable to get bypass surgery.

He suddenly realized that there is a battle in his own body and that winning or losing this war was up to him. After explaining the underlying reasons for his atherosclerotic disease and how neurohormones are like hamburgers to quench your hunger; but after you eat more than a couple of double cheese whoppers, it starts to affect your body negatively.

Some neurohormones are good in the short run while they are not upregulated too much, but once they start increasing above the threshold level, they attack the heart negatively. After explaining to him that the medications we use in heart failure are either blockers or inhibitors such as beta-blockers, angiotensin receptor blockers or aldosterone receptor blockers, and ACE inhibitors, it suddenly made sense to JB that these medications are blocking the neurohormones that are damaging his heart.

He had no insurance and was struggling in the hospital with fluid overload in spite of all the medications. He did get discharged finally after 2 weeks with medications but could not afford all his medications and was not taking them as he was advised. He did not follow up in the outpatient setting and his family was struggling to get him back and get some kind of insurance to at least get medications while he qualified for a heart transplant. Finally, JB showed up in the office a few months later with fluid retention and shortness of breath. He still did not have insurance and it was a struggle to explain to him why he needed medications to keep him from dying or getting hospitalized multiple times.

We spent a long time talking about the disease state and explained to him the reason why he had arterial occlusions due to his diabetes and obesity; as well as non-compliance with medications or diets suggested by physicians. The educational component was difficult as he had recently lost his job and we embraced him in our heart failure center and slowly increased his medications and placed him in cardiac rehab. His family was able to pay a little to sustain again and have him continue medications and pay out of pocket for cardiac rehab. We have a program where they can contribute $15 a week and continue cardiac rehab for a longer time.

When we discussed the concept of neurohormones and the fight between neurohormones that are slowly damaging his heart and the medications are to prevent this from happening.

Slowly, his heart started to improve with the cardiac rehab program and his ejection fraction increased from 10% to 20% in 4 to 6 weeks, and within 3 months, it was up to 30%. He was advised a Lifevest but was not wearing it. He could not get a pacemaker or ICD due to lack of insurance. However, he eventually got Medicaid and had an angiogram which showed the left main was close to 60% occluded and he did qualify to get bypass surgery. He underwent this surgery without complications and his ejection fraction went up to 45% and he did not require ICD or pacemaker. He has become positive on his outlook on life and working towards developing new skills and looking for a job opportunity.

> This is a success story for the patient and from my point of view as to how the patient's life was dramatically changed. He had the power to embolden himself and transcend further in life. He has been a tough titan in spite of all the risk factors and illnesses that he has had embraced, and yet had the courage to believe in his own healing process.

He was seeking a loan through one of the nonprofit organizations that I recommended and is totally ecstatic about suddenly changing his life for the better with a healthy lifestyle.

Cellular and Molecular Basis and Role of Neurohormones

> *Now, I am no scientist, but I know what endorphins are. They are tiny little magical elves that swim through your bloodstream and tell funny jokes to each other. When they reach your brain, you hear what they're saying and that boosts your health and happiness. "Knock Knock... Who's There? Little endorphin. Little endorphin who? Little Endorphin Annie." And then the endorphins laugh and then you laugh. See? Its Science.*
>
> *– Ellen De Generes*

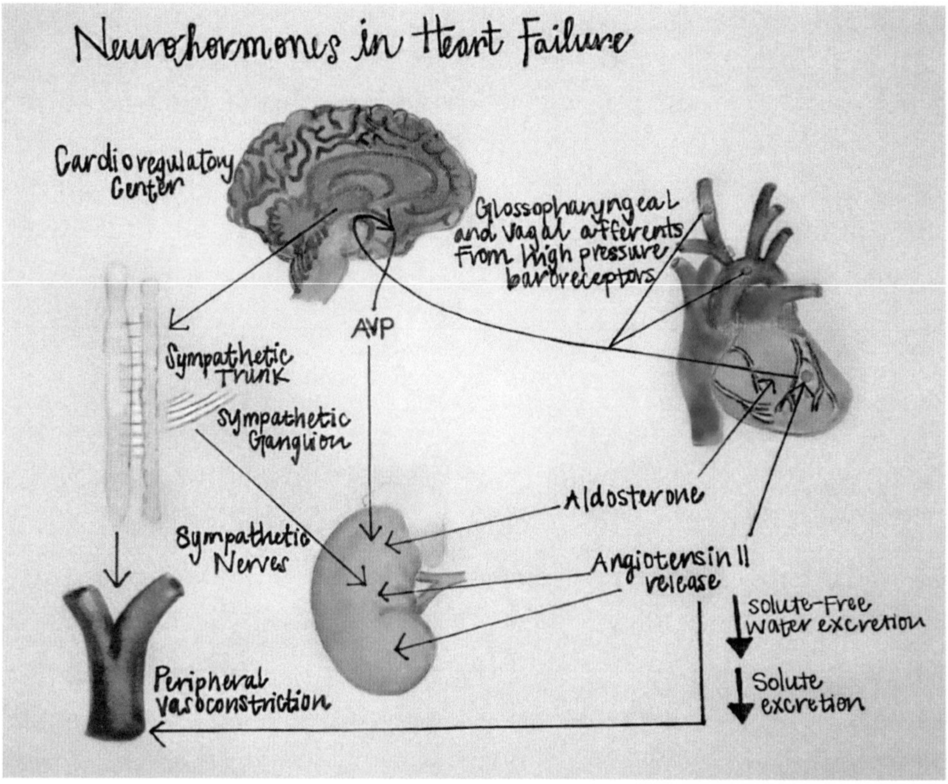

Fig. 4

The heart is an overly complex anatomical organ. Optimum regulation of the circulation of the heart and the blood going from the head to the toe is dependent on two major reflexes: One is called the arterial baroreflex, and the other is cardiopulmonary baroreceptors. These two reflexes are beautifully balanced in a physiological state. The arterial baroreflexes are in the neck in an area called the carotid sinus. The aorta arches around the pulmonary artery and goes behind the heart. At this level of the arch, there are tissues that are called baroreceptors. These two locations trigger the arterial baroreflexes and respond to an initial discharge caused by an increase in arterial blood pressure.

These reflexes react to maintain the blood pressure in its normal range. The cardiopulmonary baroreceptors are located inside the atrium, around the area where the superior and inferior vena cava pour into the right atrium and around the pulmonary veins which pour into the left atrium. These reflexes are discharged during contraction of the heart and the rate of their discharge is causally related to the force of the squeeze or contraction of the heart muscle. They are also related to the filling of the heart itself. The principal functions of these two receptors are to balance the sympathetic neural outflow and parasympathetic outflow.

The signals from both these receptors reach nucleus solitarius in the brain stem. This is where the sympathetic and parasympathetic nervous system originates. The action of the sympathetic nervous system is to increase blood pressure and heart rate. The action of the parasympathetic nervous system is to decrease blood pressure and heart rate. The actions of the sympathetic nervous system and parasympathetic nervous system result in a beautifully balanced function of the sinus node which controls the heart rate, and the resistance inside the vascular system which controls the blood pressure. Hence, these two receptors control the vital signs: the heart rate and blood pressure specifically. This happens with a normally functioning heart muscle.

Let us now imagine that there is congestive heart failure due to one of the reasons discussed. Now, because of this, there is an alteration in the baroreceptors and since the heart is very resilient, it tries to balance the sympathetic and parasympathetic nervous system by the mediation of the receptor activity to defend the heart and protect it in the most amazing ways. If there is an imbalance because of congestive heart failure that reaches a point beyond a certain limit, these sympathetic activations may start to dominate and can lead to the release of multiple neurohormones. These neurohormones also try to defend the heart to some extent, however, after a while, these neurohormones start overflowing beyond a certain threshold which will consequently affect the heart negatively and cause symptomatic heart failure. These symptoms include shortness of breath, fatigue, and retention of fluid in the legs, abdomen, or lungs.

Neurohormonal Mechanisms in Heart Failure

As we discussed above, because of alteration in the cardiovascular reflexes, neurohormonal stimulation plays a major role in doing the balancing act of heart failure. The neurohormones that are detrimental to the heart muscle include the release of the molecules by the renin-angiotensin-aldosterone system (RAAS) and the sympathetic nervous system. Activation of these systems release angiotensin, aldosterone, and catecholamines or adrenaline/noradrenaline. Additionally, other neurohormones may also be released such as vasopressin, thromboxane, endothelin, bad cytokines or tumor necrosis factor-alpha, and many others. These are essentially balanced by the good neurohormones for the most part. There is an ongoing balancing act.

These good neurohormones include natriuretic peptides, kallikreins, prostaglandins (prostacyclin), dopamine, and nitric oxide. The negative neurohormones cause constriction of the blood vessels, increase in HR, increase in sympathetic outflow, increase thickening of the heart muscle initially followed by thinning of the heart muscle which causes dilation of the heart over time. Active fibroblasts and collagen take over the role of the heart muscle and the contractile function of the heart muscle deteriorates due to a reduction in myocyte number, density, and function. This can contribute to ventricular remodeling of the heart muscle or alteration in the geometric shape, size, and function. Many of these neurohormones also affect other parts of the body such as the kidneys, adrenal glands, brain, sympathetic nervous system, and vascular smooth muscle. In a sense, when the imbalance occurs with the bad neurohormones dominating the good neurohormones, problems arise. Hence, many of the treatment strategies include inhibitors or blockers of these neurohormones such as beta-blockers or ACE inhibitors, ARBs, aldosterone blockers. So, if you ask yourself what these medications are doing, they are all blocking or inhibiting a certain biochemical process.

In a sense, the main root function of these medications is to block these negative neurohormones to protect the heart and let it heal over time. In addition, there are agents such as neprilysin inhibitor which inhibits a certain enzyme which leads to the production of good neurohormones and thus protecting the heart. There are other agents used in heart failures, such as hydralazine which is a vasodilator and controls blood pressure while protecting the heart and kidneys. In combination with hydralazine, there is a medication called isosorbide or nitroglycerin or nitrates which also have an interesting vasodilatory effect that dilates both the veins and arteries to improve the symptoms of heart failure. There are agents like diuretics which removes excess water from the system caused by water retention secondary to heart failure.

Congestive heart failure is essentially a chronic condition leading to a reduction in the filling of the heart that increases the signaling of these reflexes causing constriction of blood vessels and increasing vascular resistance. This increase in vascular resistance along with suppression of the inhibitory action of the beta receptor leads to an enhanced sympathetic or adrenal activity. This leads to stimulation of sodium retention and reabsorption increases in the kidneys which leads to water retention. If you leave salt in the open air it will attract water and become crystal. So, salt attracts water. This is one of the reasons that a treatment strategy of congestive heart failure with fluid retention is to reduce salt intake to avoid water retention. We also mentioned tumor necrosis factor-alpha as a bad actor, but studies with agents that suppress this neurohormone have not really panned out in making a favorable health outcome.

In addition, research performed with agents that suppress "endothelin" which is a negative neurohormone, called endothelium receptor antagonist, did not prove itself in heart failure but showed promise in the treatment of pulmonary hypertension. This will be discussed in a later chapter.

CHAPTER 5

Systolic, Diastolic, and Right Heart Failure

*"If the clinician, as an observer, wishes to see things as they really are, he must make a **tabula rasa** of his mind and proceed without any preconceived notions whatever."*

– Jean-Martin Charcot

WATCH NOW

Patient Story

MG is a 32-year-old male who came to my office crying for being rejected by his surgeon who felt he was at high risk for mitral valve surgery. He was referred by a cardiologist to the surgeon to replace his mitral valve due to severe mitral regurgitation. He was rejected because of his weak pump and having an ejection fraction of 10% (normal is more than 50%). The surgeon said if he operated on him, he would die on the operating table and he did not want to risk it. He had an angiogram to assess if his arteries were open and to his relief, they were open, but his heart pump was weak which ruled him out as a candidate for the surgery.

When I asked more about the details of his substance abuse, he had indulged in cocaine habit and started talking about his life as an air condition technician and was making a good living. He then met a group of friends who told him to get into this route; he was lost.

I explained to him that it was not his fault and it was a situation where he had entered into a jungle for a hike with the hope that he would have fun but got lost in the maze of the jungle and it had engulfed him and pulled him in like a whirlpool in the middle of an ocean with nothing to hold on to come up to the surface. When I explained to him that we will not judge him for his missteps or his actions, but we will address the "what" and "how" we can do to make a difference and change his life.

He also was not a candidate for left ventricular assist device or heart transplant due to substance abuse disorder and was disappointed, continued to feel fatigued and shortness of breath, but did not have significant fluid retention. He felt lonely and shaken; he realized that it was his cocaine habit that was killing him. We had a long discussion about management from medical therapy and to seek therapy from cardiac rehab, pain management, and primary care doctor. He had his mother with him and had 2 small kids, but his wife was not with him and he was taking care of his children. He was humiliated about his actions and deeds and was frustrated. We had an interesting conversation about why he resorted to this habit and how his heart got affected by it. He realized that his actions had totally taken a toll on his physical abilities and mental state.

After an hour-long discussion, he was ready to be initiated on a long-standing follow up weekly with medical optimization and slowly increase beta-blocker, with up-titration over time, and getting him on a good exercise program. He was optimized on RAAS blockers, beta-blockers, MRA. He was given a life vest and wore it frequently. Within 3 months, his ejection fraction had gone up from 10 to 22% and he was very encouraged by this. He accepted his flaws and found his calling because he saw that there was an improvement in his condition subjectively and objectively. He realized that he had to be turbocharged and have a longing to heal. I sensed his vibrant exuberance for medical optimization and although he qualified for a defibrillator and a pacemaker, he wanted to wear the Lifevest a little longer. He had given up his drug habits and removed himself from bad company of friends who were enabling him on his cocaine habit.

He clearly began with a blank slate, the "tabula rasa" in what he expressed. The idea of the tabula rasa is that humans have an uninformed mind at birth and acquired beliefs through experienced sensation and reflection. While the mind is capable of maintaining or developing its own notions in creating more complex thoughts from simpler ones, no thought is written in stone. Hence, the fact that he had no inflexible perceptions allowed him to open his mind from a blank sheet of paper waiting to be filled with powerful ideas and fill it with a rekindled passion for life.

He was open to the vibrant exuberance of the beauty of life and to experience every minute of the day, the magical aspects of it all.

Another 3 months later, his EF had gone up to 36% and he did not require the Lifevest or a defibrillator. He was so thrilled. With significant improvement in his heart pump, he returned back to work as a technician. I suggested a chamber of commerce as another avenue to get a loan so he can pursue his dream and start a company. After another year, his ejection fraction had gone up to 60%. He received a loan and started his own air conditioning company with 5 employees. He reminded me of someone who did not have any idea which direction his life would have gone had he continued his cocaine habit or not sought help.

His mother was there for him and every time they would come to see me, I would explain how he has come a long way in transcending his own weaknesses and emboldening himself to achieve a normalized ejection fraction of his heart with medical therapy, exercise, and a psychosocial will. It gave him much satisfaction and belief in the healing process. Now he is a spokesperson for multiple organizations in the community talking about his personal experience and he has overcome his weaknesses to encourage other people to seek a better life with a sense of hope and dream.

Systolic, Diastolic, and Right Heart Failure

Heart failure is a common endpoint of a wide variety of cardiovascular diseases as previously discussed. One of the largest epidemiological studies, called the Framingham Heart Study, revealed that high BP was the leading factor in the development of heart failure.

Seventy-five percent of patients with heart failure had an element of hypertension. In addition, blocked arteries have become the main cause of heart failure In the US and other parts of the world. A blocked artery can be secondary to high cholesterol, high BP, obesity, diabetes mellitus, genetic factors, and smoking. This can affect the heart muscle directly which leads to a reduction in EF or amount of blood squeezed out of the left ventricle.

There is another entity called dilated cardiomyopathy which causes systolic heart failure. Many of the causes for this form of cardiomyopathy can be attributed to infections, genetic predisposition, rheumatic fever, infiltrative disease, toxic conditions, nutritional deficiencies, electrolyte disorders, collagen vascular disease, endocrine factors, metabolic factors, arrhythmias such as atrial fibrillation, valvular heart disease, pregnancy, myocarditis, pericarditis, and aortic diseases.

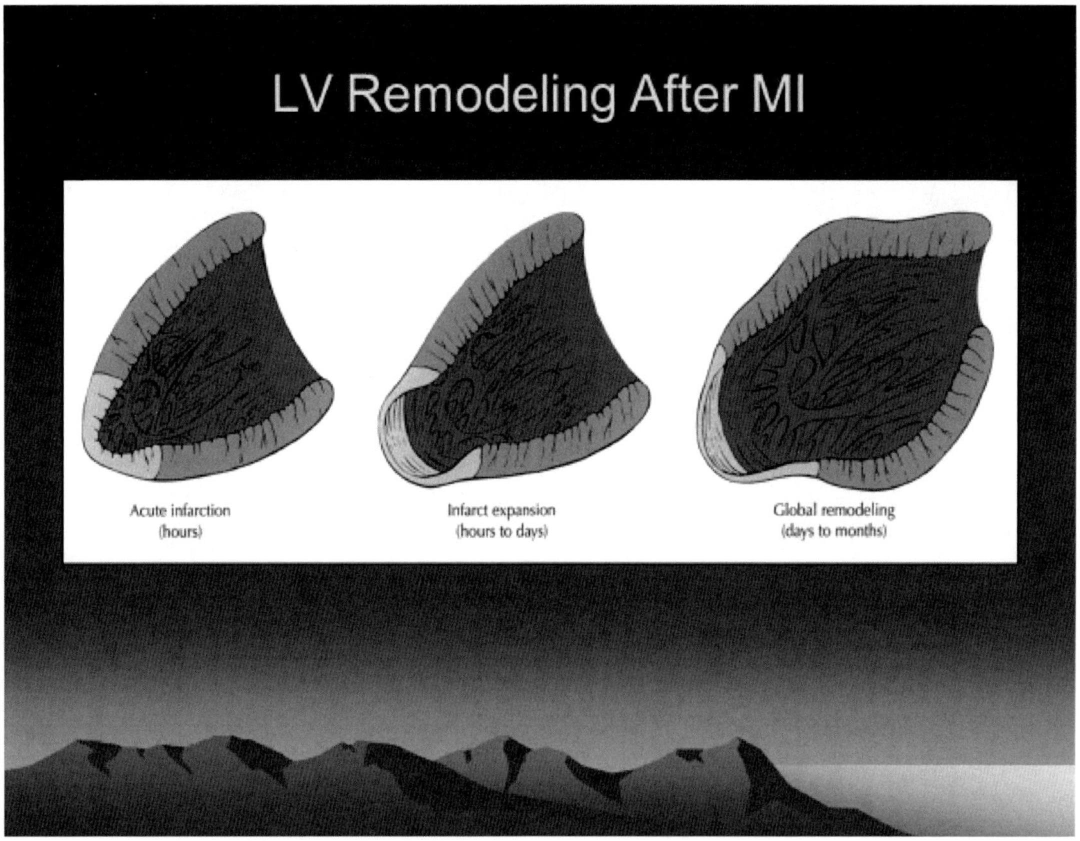

Fig. 5

Poor Prognostic Factors

The causes for worsening heart failure and poor prognosis include ischemia as the underlying substrate, because, once there is a blocked artery, the risk of recurrence after treatment is dramatically high if all the risk factors are not adequately managed; specifically the environmental factors that caused this occlusion in the first place. Many of the patients require bypass surgery as a life-saving measure; and yet, this intervention itself can lead to damage to the heart muscle if the risk factors are not controlled adequately after the bypass surgery and possibly lead the patient down a slippery slope with worsening heart failure over time. The other poor prognostic factors include advanced age, duration of symptoms, low ejection fraction below 25%, and poor functional capacity as detected by NYHA class.

(NYHA) has shown to be quite effective in gauging the metrics of the patient's functionality. Class I is someone who is not symptomatic, class II is someone who is mildly symptomatic with moderate exertional activity, class III is someone who is moderately symptomatic with mild functional activity, and class IV is someone who is severely symptomatic with no activity.

New York Heart Association (NYHA) Classification of Heart Failure

Class	Patient Symptoms
Class I (Mild)	No limitation of physical activity. Ordinary physical activity does not cause undue fatigue, rapid/irregular heartbeat (palpitation) or shortness of breath (dyspnea).
Class II (Mild)	Slight limitation of physical activity. Comfortable at rest, but ordinary physical activity results in fatigue, rapid/irregular heartbeat (palpitation) or shortness of breath (dyspnea).
Class III (Moderate)	Marked limitation of physical activity. Comfortable at rest, but less than ordinary activity causes fatigue, rapid/irregular heartbeat (palpitation) or shortness of breath (dyspnea).
Class IV (Severe)	Unable to carry out any physical activity without discomfort. Symptoms of fatigue, rapid/irregular heartbeat (palpitation) or shortness of breath (dyspnea) are present at rest. If any physical activity is undertaken, discomfort increases.

Fig. 6

Many times, class IV patients land up in a hospital setting which then becomes a critical situation with poor prognosis. Once a heart failure patient is hospitalized, the chances of subsequent admissions are 4-fold higher and cumulative risk of death becomes higher as well. Aggressive management strategy is needed, and this can be done with medical optimization, device strategies, intervention with a possible invasive approach such as opening up arteries or bypass surgery, pacemaker/defibrillator implantation and some needing advanced circulatory device therapy or heart transplant. Clearly, advances over the past 20 years have been significant from pharmacological and device therapy. Hence, patients are now living longer, but at the same time, the prevalence of risk factors such as high cholesterol, obesity, diabetes mellitus lack of exercise has been proven to increase the risk of the overall population. Metabolic syndrome is the nemesis of the baby boomer generation.

The other poor prognostic factors include reduced exercise duration and reduced oxygen consumption. A pO2 value less than 14 ml/kg per minute can make one eligible for a ventricular assist device and a possible heart transplant. There is another metric we evaluate in Heart Failure centers. It is a 6-minute walking distance. Less than 350 meters walking distance in 6 minutes is a red flag for poor prognosis. Of course, we talked about neurohormonal factors earlier in chapter 4. Increased levels of bad neurohormones such as norepinephrine, renin aldosterone angiotensin, brain natriuretic peptide, vasopressin, endothelin, tumor necrosis factor-alpha can also be a poor prognostic factor. Other poor prognostic factors are sudden cardiac arrest with arrhythmias called ventricular tachycardia secondary to poor contractile disorder.

Patient story – Diastolic Heart Failure

Ms. VC is a 58-year-old female who has been admitted to the hospital multiple times with fluid retention. She would take medications to remove the water and indulge in salt and sugar consumption and land up in the hospital with a significant amount of fluid retention in the lungs, abdomen, and lower extremities. She also had morbid obesity with weighing 480 pounds and was extremely difficult for her to lose weight. Interestingly, she was a diabetic, but, not on any medications!

She had tried metformin in the past but stopped due to gastrointestinal issues. She was taking a lot of diuretics and her kidney function began to deteriorate and was getting dehydrated and she would not take medications that would keep her water from accumulating. Being a complex issue for her, we started following her at the congestive failure clinic and was told that she had to visit us weekly to improve her medications and keep the water out of the system. We also recommended a dietician and bariatric assessment that she sought attention for but was feeling depressed and thought there was no recourse. We initiated a GLP1 agonist that has been approved for obesity. She was advised cardiac rehab, but insurance does not cover for patients with HFpEF, so she had to pay out of pocket.

The patient was not being hospitalized anymore for heart failure as she was compliant with her medications and lost over 60 pounds but hit a plateau state. The bariatric center was overly impressed with her motivation and suggested bariatric surgery. She now felt that there was some hope and her weight reduction may improve her health comorbidities. After the surgery, her success was significant with a weight loss of over 160 pounds, and her only complaint was that she had to change her entire wardrobe!

> The lesson she has given us and the learning point for me has been that heart failure with preserved ejection fraction might be different for everyone, but the weight loss program seems to have a major impact on stabilizing her heart failure and improving it.

What was interesting is that her weight reduction also helped her heart failure with no fluid retention and as she continued to take her medications to control her blood pressure, she had not been hospitalized.

Diastolic Heart Failure

Diastolic heart failure is when the forward pump function itself is normal, but the relaxation of the heart becomes abnormal and the left atrium becomes enlarged and abnormally functioning. The left atrium is the one that is actively pushing the blood into the left ventricle. There are 2 components to the filling from the left atrium to the left ventricle: early filling, and late filling. The left ventricle fills passively in the early phase and atrium is contracting actively in the late phase in normal conditions.

However, in heart failure, secondary to preserved left ventricular ejection fraction, there may be a problem with early and/or ate filling. If the left atrium is enlarged or pressure is high, or the left ventricle itself may be abnormal, not relaxing properly, then the pressure in the left ventricle at the end of relaxation becomes significantly high. When the mitral valve is open the pressure in the left ventricle which is now high, transmits to the left atrium, and the left atrium now becomes enlarged. The left atrium is connected to the 4 pulmonary veins that pour blood forward into the left atrium in normal conditions. However, in subjects with diastolic heart failure or HFpEF, there is a backward flow into the pulmonic veins. This can lead to fluid pouring into the interstitial spaces in the lungs which may cause pulmonary edema and lead to significant shortness of breath either suddenly or slowly.

If this is a slow process, then the pressure increases in the pulmonary capillary system that is connected to the pulmonary arterial system, and the pulmonary artery pressure increases which are connected to the right ventricle. The right ventricle pressure increases which are connected to the right atrium. Increased right atrial pressure, which is connected to the inferior vena cava, transmits a higher venous pressure in the abdomen and lower extremities leading to abdominal distension and leg swelling due to fluid oozing out into the tissues.

Causes for HFpEF include valvular heart diseases such as the mitral valve narrowing, tricuspid valve narrowing, aortic valve narrowing/stenosis, pulmonic valve stenosis, mitral valve regurgitation, and aortic valve regurgitation. One of the common causes of HFpEF is atrial fibrillation when the left atrium loses its ability to squeeze adequately leading to increased pulmonic venous pressures and HFpEF. Other causes of heart failure with normal ejection fraction or "diastolic heart failure" include restrictive cardiomyopathies such as infiltration with amyloidosis, sarcoidosis, Fabry's disease, hemochromatosis, eosinophilic infiltration, radiation exposure, and tumor infiltration. Other reasons include lack of blood flow to the right side of the heart secondary to a blocked artery, conduction system abnormality to the right side of the heart and, hypertrophic cardiomyopathy which will be discussed in detail in one of the chapters.

Both diastolic and systolic heart failure can be symptomatic with shortness of breath with or without exertional activity, and reduced exercise tolerance. One would have been able to exercise for a couple of miles on a daily basis and slowly, one may realize that their exercise tolerance is decreasing and they may not be able to walk for more than half a mile now and are getting short-winded. One also must consider what is called a deconditioned state when a patient may be increasing their weight for different reasons altogether. In the nighttime, when the person is lying down there is return of blood flow from the legs to the right side of the heart and this increased blood flow can be a strain on the heart muscle which can affect the heart negatively because of increased filling pressures and this can lead to shortness of breath while lying down at night. The patient may require a few pillows and may cause a person to sit upright.

This is called paroxysmal nocturnal dyspnea; other symptoms include fatigue, fluid retention in the legs, abdomen, abdominal distention, and at times failure, palpitations, lightheadedness, syncope secondary to low blood pressure. This low pressure may be a result of low ejection fraction or squeezing of the blood to the brain which can lead to the symptoms mentioned above. Sometimes when the heart muscle is not functioning properly and the flow is not adequate, it can accumulate clots inside the heart muscle. If they have atrial fibrillation, it can accumulate clots in the left atrial appendage and if this gets dislodged into the left ventricle, it can pump it to the brain leading to a stroke.

In addition, if the pump is weak and ejection fraction is low, this itself can lead to clot accumulation in the apex of the left ventricle. If this gets dislodged, it can also travel to the brain and cause a stroke. If it skips the carotid artery, the other arteries that come out the aorta consist of arteries traveling to the arm, kidneys, liver, and legs. Many times, these clots can propagate to the mentioned anatomical organs/appendages in the body causing blocked arteries.

Patient Story – Right Heart Failure

Ms. DH is a 49-year-old female who had presented with shortness of breath a few months ago and an echocardiogram revealed a large fluid collection around the heart which had to be removed in the hospital. While trying to determine the cause of this fluid retention, we discovered that she was positive for lupus and the right side of her heart was enlarged while the left side was normal. She had extremely high pulmonary hypertension with pulmonary pressure of 90'mmHg, (normal is less than 25mmHg.) All of these may have been contributing to her shortness of breath.

The treatment of right heart failure is different than left heart failure and we had to explain to her in great detail the need for heart biopsy, heart catheterization, or heart transplant. It appeared that she had secondary pulmonary hypertension from lupus but also had another antibody-positive which essentially added to her immunocompromised state. Currently, she is awaiting heart and lung transplant but the lesson we learned from her is that when one encounters right-sided heart failure, one might have to probe into the trenches more to determine the root cause of the problem because some of these issues are treatable.

The right-sided heart failure leads to liver enlargement, pericardial effusion, pleural effusion, ascites, lower extremity fluid retention. Therefore, we have to be cognizant of the symptoms and the underlying reason why someone may present with right-sided heart failure but a normal left side of the heart and still be very symptomatic. By excavating deeper, one may unravel treatable conditions and give new life and new hope to someone who may have lost the battle to live.

CHAPTER 6

Pulmonary Hypertension

Humanitas:

Ability to see the humanness in each individual, to personally connect one to the other, to chip in and participate, to be content to be themselves, and to uniquely tip the balance of life towards the warmth of togetherness.
"When a people person enters the room, it feels better, happier, safer."

—Bhagavat Gita

WATCH NOW

Patient Story – Pulmonary Hypertension

Mr. DD was another patient I met a few years ago who was from Canada and had a house in Paradise Valley. Mr. DD had a stroke, coronary artery disease, ischemic cardiomyopathy, and pulmonary hypertension. We were watching him closely with echocardiograms and improving his pulmonary hypertension with medications. He was also requiting O2 at home and had a caretaker who was taking care of him along with his family. He was a wonderful human being who had the opportunity to make a significant impact on people's lives through achievements in real estate. He and his family brought congruence and visibility to many fractured lives in Canada.

Mr. DD had helped numerous people along his journey of life between Canada and Arizona He was one of those men that was so value-driven and always was kind, caring, and compassionate. He was very realistic and knew the limitations of his lifespan and yet he was seeking lasting rewards through caring for his family by his balanced approach to life and being an incredible human being. He taught me to revisit what William Osler once said: *"It is more important to know what kind of a patient has a disease than what kind of disease a patient has*".

The humanism, personal stories, and the element of success about every patient is emphasized in this statement. I had the pleasure of meeting his family as well who have amazing principles and values. Mr. DD passed away last year and there was a wonderful celebration of his life by his family that truly was very touching and inspirational.

Pulmonary Hypertension

This is an especially important topic that is becoming more commonly detected primarily because of the diagnostic capacity that is available today. In addition. There are new treatments on the market today for pulmonary hypertension. Hence, the awareness is increasing in detecting this disease earlier to avail of the treatments to change the outcome favorably. What is pulmonary hypertension? This is a condition where the pressure in the pulmonary artery is significantly elevated. To understand the anatomy of the pulmonary artery we will first need to understand the anatomy of the heart. The superior and inferior vena cava are filling into the right atrium, which is one of the four chambers of the heart.

From here, through the tricuspid valve, the blood goes into the right ventricle, from the right ventricle, the pulmonary artery emerges, and through the pulmonic valve, the pulmonary artery gets filled. The blood is pushed into the lungs to get oxygenated. With every breath that one takes the oxygen is now combined with the blood flow in the lungs. This is now sent back through all the small pulmonary venous vessels and capillaries and alveoli where oxygenated blood goes to the left side of the heart.

There are four pulmonary veins that drain into the left atrium, from where the blood crosses through the mitral valve into the left ventricle. From the left ventricle, the blood goes through the aortic valve to reach the large blood vessel in the body called the aorta. The aorta supplies oxygenated blood to the entire body, first to the brain through the carotid arteries, then behind the heart to supply blood to the upper limbs all the way to the liver, kidneys, and all the special organs in the body. In addition, oxygenated blood flows all the way to the lower extremities including the toes.

This occurs so that every tissue can get oxygenated blood on a continuum and perform its functions. Having said this from an anatomical perspective, pulmonary hypertension is when the pressure in the pulmonary artery is elevated. Normal pressures range from 8-25 mmHg with no exertional activity, however, when it exceeds 25 mmHg then it can be identified as systolic pulmonary hypertension. When the diastolic pressure in the pulmonary artery is more than 8 mmHg, then it is considered elevated. There are categories from mild to moderate to severe. Severe pulmonary hypertension can range from 70-150 mmHg from a systolic pulmonary artery pressure perspective.

When the pressure is elevated then symptoms of shortness of breath or pulmonary edema can occur. This can lead to fatigue, coughing, significant liver enlargement, and swelling of the legs. There are five subsets of pulmonary hypertension which include: pulmonary venous HTN, hypoxic pulmonary hypertension, arterial obstruction of pulmonary bed, left or right shunt with a hole in the heart, and primary pulmonary hypertension. Hypoxic pulmonary hypertension is usually secondary to low oxygenation in the lungs which can occur among individuals with lung diseases such as chronic obstructive pulmonary disease (COPD).and in some subjects with morbid obesity. Hypoxia can be caused by COPD and a high level of red blood cells secondary to long term smoking and obstructive sleep apnea (OSA).

Recurrent pulmonary thromboembolic embolism can happen from clots that keep forming secondary to genetically mediated abnormal clotting factor or activation of some vasoconstricting components such as serotonin, or thromboxane. Sometimes cystic fibrosis, bronchiectasis, and granuloma from valley fever can affect the lung tissue that can all lead to this condition including interstitial fibrosis. The underlying sickle cell disease or connective diseases like lupus can also lead to arterial occlusion which results in pulmonary hypertension. There is a condition called schistosomiasis which is an infectious parasitic disease mainly seen in the middle eastern region of the world. Left to right or right to left shunts occur if there is a hole in the heart.

This can lead to alteration in chamber dimensions and pressure inside the chambers. A shunt that occurs between the aorta and pulmonary artery is known as patent ductus arteriosus. It usually closes in a few days after birth, but when it remains persistent then this can lead to low oxygenation, blue baby syndrome and may require surgical intervention. There is also a condition where the aortic sinus ruptures that can form a fistula in the pulmonary artery which can result in shunts. Two other conditions such as a ventricular septal defect or a hole within the bottom portion of the heart or atrial septal defect which is a hole in the top portion of the heart can lead to shunting which allows blood flow from the left side of the heart to the right contributing to a significant amount of pulmonary hypertension.

Primary pulmonary hypertension was once a rare condition but is now becoming more prevalent as technology is improving and is becoming easier to diagnose with imaging techniques. It is more common in women with the women to men ratio known to be 1.7:1 and more common among African Americans with a mean age of 35 years and ranging from infancy to 80 years of age. Familial clusters have been reported in 5-10% of cases. The artery totally becomes altered in its pliability, flexibility, shape, size, and dimension called plexiform vasculopathy. This condition is rare and yet it may represent multiple underlying, unsuspecting substrate. The etiology, for the most part, remains unknown, however, one may be able to figure out if there is a correctable reason.

Some of the possible causes of primary pulmonary hypertension include recurrent clotting secondary to genetic abnormalities, such as factor 5 Leiden, connective tissue disorders, toxins such as grapeseed oil, l-tryptophan, inadequate detoxification of proteins, enzymes, hormones in association with cirrhosis of the liver that leads to pulmonary hypertension and portal hypertension. There are hormonal factors predominantly in females, hence, one raises the suspicion that female hormones may be a contributor to this condition. There is also suspicion of contribution from oral contraceptive medications as well. There is evidence that the primary pulmonary hypertension can be from a congenital defect of the valves on the right ventricle.

Diagnostic procedures to identify pulmonary hypertension include chest X-rays, electrocardiograms, echocardiograms which all have a role in detecting this condition. Catheters that can be inserted into the right side of the heart which can be pushed into the pulmonary artery and detect abnormal pressures from both the left and right side of the heart. Some patients with primary pulmonary hypertension may benefit from medications that are called vasodilators such as calcium channel blockers such as nifedipine, diltiazem, which may be helpful to improve symptoms and hemodynamics. Sildenafil used in small doses seem to help.

Hence, the underlying reasoning behind increasing high pulmonary pressures needs to be deciphered, and once decoded, then the treatment strategy can be given towards the underlying condition which may improve overall longevity, survival, symptoms, functional capacity, and quality of life.

There are agents such as prostacyclin that are also used as subcutaneous injectables and seem to be significantly helpful in improving functional capacity and quality of life. Nitroglycerin which is also helpful as well as endothelin receptor antagonists that have been found to be an agent of choice and seem to improve survival/longevity with improvement in quality and function as measured by 6-minute walk test. If the underlying cause is known, then it needs to be fixed based on the duration and severity. The correction will change the course of the disease and make it reversible. If there is a clot, then a patient will need to be on long term anticoagulation such as warfarin or newer anticoagulant medications. If they have connective tissue disease, then there are other therapies such as immunosuppressants and oral steroids that may be helpful.

Causes of Pulmonary Hypertension

Group 1:

Idiopathic- (unknown) or primary	Hereditary	Congenital heart disease
Drug-induced: meth, cocaine, desatinib, phen/fen	HIV associated	Systemic sclerosis/connective tissue disease
Schistosomiasis	Newborn persistent PH	

Group 2:

Systolic Heart Failure	Diastolic Heart Failure	Valvular Heart Failure

Group 3:

COPD	Sleep Apnea	Pulmonary Fibrosis

Group 4:

Chronic thromboembolic: e.g. Recurrent DVT or pulmonary embolism

Group 5:

Thyroid Disease	Sarcoidosis	Blood Disorder e.g. sickle cell anemia

Dr. Vijay's holistic and motivational book provides an understandable and comprehensive coverage of heart failure that is an invaluable resource for individuals who have, or seek to prevent, heart failure. It is based on countless experiences with patients over a lifetime combined with research and clinical trials. Actual patient stories are used to encourage lifestyle changes that address the root causes of heart disease. His humanistic approach to patient care continues to inspire both medical professionals and patients.

Thomas E. McWilliams, D.O., FACOFP
Advisor to the President – A.T. Still University
Founding Associate Dean – Midwestern University – Arizona College of Osteopathic Medicine & A.T. Still University – School of Osteopathic Medicine in Arizona
Former Interim Dean – ATSU/SOMA

CHAPTER 7

Acute Decompensated Heart Failure

WATCH NOW

Patient Story

Ms. J.H. is a 77-year-old female who was initially referred for severe fluid retention in her legs, abdomen, and inability to respond the oral diuretics. She had had Aortic and mitral valve replacements just more than a year ago and has been dwindling with severe right-sided heart failure since. It was felt that she would need what is called Aquapheresis or ultrafiltration (UF) after placing a tunneled catheter into the heart through a vein in her neck. After evaluation, it was felt that she was decompensated and needed hospitalization for intravenous therapy to get the fluid out of her body.

She did better after 4 days on hospitalization, got a lot of fluid out of her body with mild worsening of her kidney function, but not requiring Aquapheresis/UF or dialysis. After discharge, she followed up with us twice a week initially and then once a week while needing intravenous therapies as an outpatient. She was noted to have severe anemia with a hemoglobin of 6 grams (normal is 13-16 gms) and needed either blood transfusion or iron infusions. She was referred to a hematologist, her blood thinners were stopped (no obvious bleeding from the GI tract was noted) and specialized blood tests were performed. It turns out that she was not eating properly and lacked iron in the most severe way.

She was given anti-ulcer meds, iron infusions regularly and her heart failure improved remarkably. She had come to us a few months ago in a wheelchair with leg ulcers from fluid retention, blocked arteries and poor circulation in her legs, and profound weakness and loss of any mental stamina to live. In less than 4 months, to see that she started walking with a cane without a wheelchair was so heartwarming. The lessons we learned in the process is that while a patient may have been getting mentally ready for an invasive procedure such as UF/dialysis if we dug a little deeper to assess the multi-modality of causes for decompensation, we might come up with a different answer; such as severe anemia and need for iron infusion, intravenous therapy to get the water out and yet salvage the kidneys. Clearly, Ms. JH is incredibly pleased with her progress and outcome so far.

Acute Decompensated Heart Failure

Heart failure is becoming a common condition with more than a half-million new cases diagnosed in the United States every year. It is estimated that more than 6 million Americans have congestive heart failure and mortality is close to 300,000 which is common in the older population aged 65 years or older. The annual health care cost is more than $77 billion, of which more than half is spent at the hospital setting. HFrEF and HFpEF seem to have similar prevalence with HFpEF somewhere around 40-45% and HFrEF being somewhere around 55-60%. There is a new category called heart failure with mid-range ejection fraction with EF of 40-50% which is mildly reduced but not severely reduced. Many subjects may not have any signs or symptoms of the disease. Hence, this mid-range is important to detect because as there are newer therapies such as neprilysin inhibitor with valsartan combination that seems to show some benefit in this midrange reduction of ejection fraction and further discussion will be held in the treatment section.

So, what is acute decompensated heart failure? When somebody crashes with sudden onset of shortness of breath and lands up with significant fluid retention in the lungs due to pulmonary edema, this is defined as acute decompensation with low oxygenation of the blood and many times with low blood pressure from cardiogenic shock. Some patients may manifest with low blood pressure and one can pass out or have low volume intravascularly but fluid retention in the extravascular space. These subjects may reveal swelling of the abdomen and lower extremities, dizziness, syncope, fatigue, and lightheadedness. Some of these are signs and symptoms of acute decompensation of heart failure.

Why would someone end up in trouble so acutely? Most common reasons are acute heart attack or lack of blood flow to the heart muscle due to partially or completely blocked coronary arteries with or without a plaque rupture inside the blood vessel, noncompliance with diet therapy (an increased salt loaded diet), atrial fibrillation with heart rate running over 130 beats per minute, systemic infections from urinary tract infections reaching the blood causing sepsis, pneumonia contributing to worsening breathing, a clot in the lung called pulmonary embolism, high cardiac output states such as anemia, pregnancy, or hyperthyroidism.

In addition, if kidney function may be failing in some patients, so they land up in an acute decompensated state with high potassium levels, high BUN, high creatinine which can result in reduced urinary output which will cause increased fluid retention in the lungs. Blood pressure of more than 220 systolic can lead to this condition as well with what is called "flash pulmonary edema". Toxins such as significant alcohol consumption, methamphetamine, cocaine abuse, inappropriate drug therapy with sodium/water retention, acute rupture of the ventricular septum secondary to a heart attack, acute mitral valve leak, large pericardial fluid with restriction of blood filling to the right side of the heart called " tamponade" can all be contributory to the acute decompensation.

What can we do if there is acute decompensation? Obviously, one needs to be admitted to the hospital directly, call 911, and reach an emergency room as soon as possible. ER doctors can quickly assess history, physical examination, electrocardiogram, chest X-ray, emergent echo-cardiography, and if needed activate emergently the cath lab for cardiac catheterization to open up any acute blockage that may have happened giving rise to a heart attack or what is called" myocardial infarction". This condition is also called cardiogenic shock when they are completely decompensated suddenly and some of them need to in intensive care unit, some may need a tube inserted into the lungs through the mouth and trachea where they can be connected to a breathing machine and supported in intensive care while trying to decipher underlying reasoning for the decompensated state.

Treatment strategy includes clearing water from the lungs with diuretics intravenously or if a patient has severe kidney failure, then, they will need acute dialysis. Many will respond quickly after they get supported in the intensive care unit while they are trying to figure out the etiology of why the crash happened. All further discussion regarding treatment plans will be discussed in the treatment section.

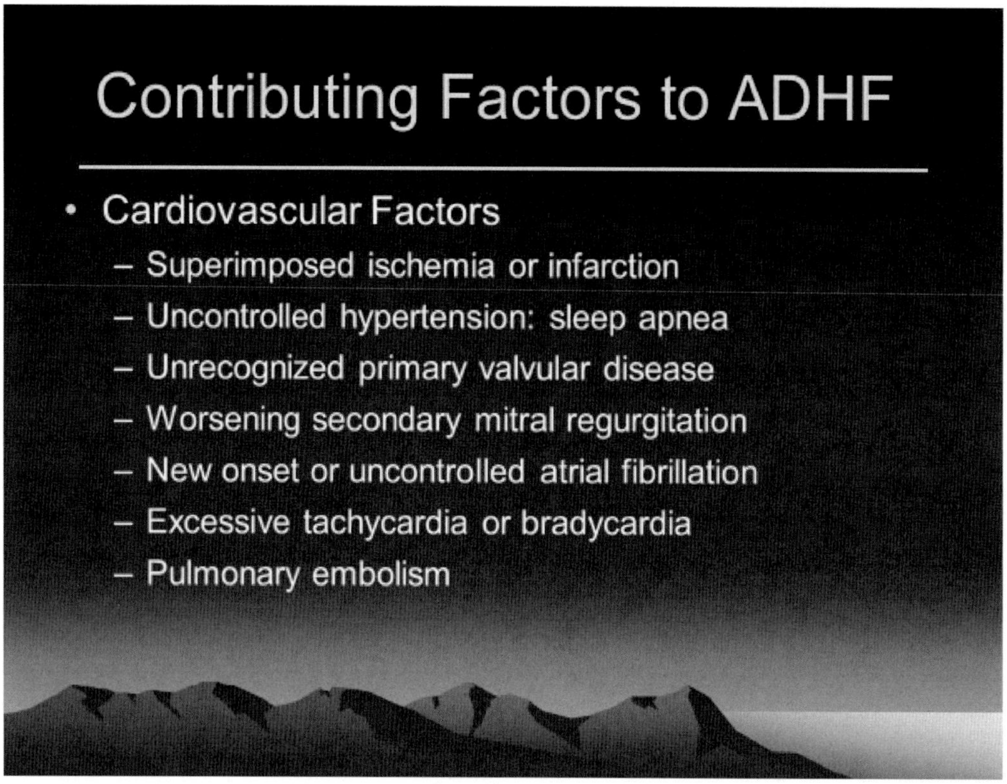
Contributing Factors to ADHF
• Cardiovascular Factors
– Superimposed ischemia or infarction
– Uncontrolled hypertension: sleep apnea
– Unrecognized primary valvular disease
– Worsening secondary mitral regurgitation
– New onset or uncontrolled atrial fibrillation
– Excessive tachycardia or bradycardia
– Pulmonary embolism

Fig. 7

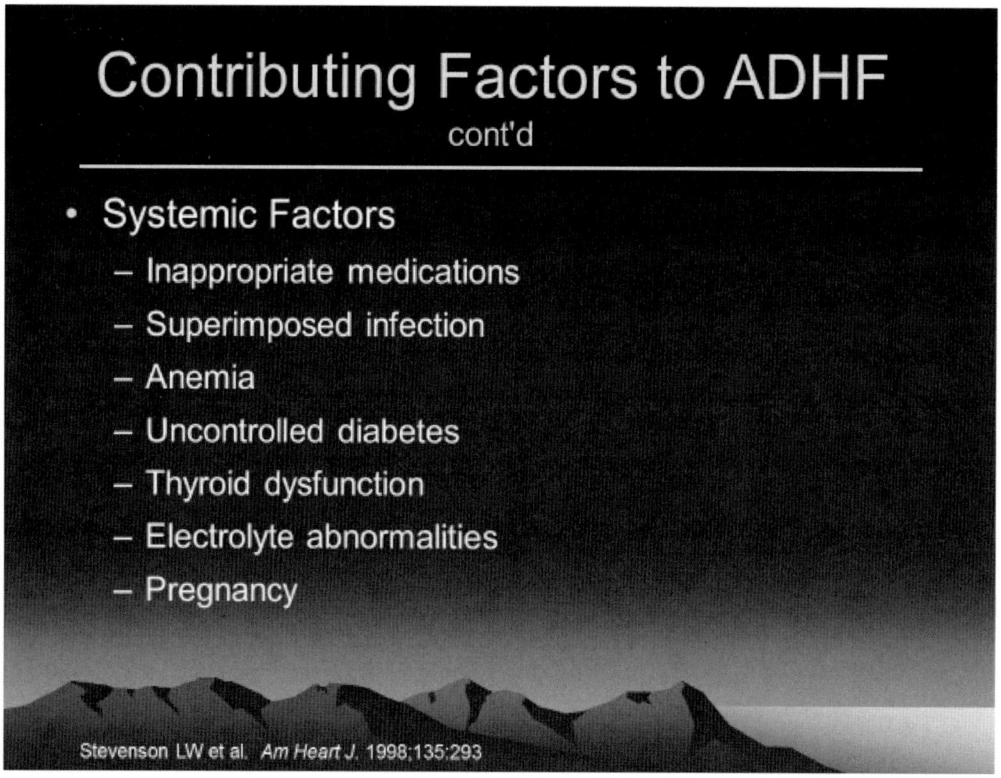
Contributing Factors to ADHF
cont'd
• Systemic Factors
– Inappropriate medications
– Superimposed infection
– Anemia
– Uncontrolled diabetes
– Thyroid dysfunction
– Electrolyte abnormalities
– Pregnancy
Stevenson LW et al. Am Heart J. 1998;135:293

Fig. 8

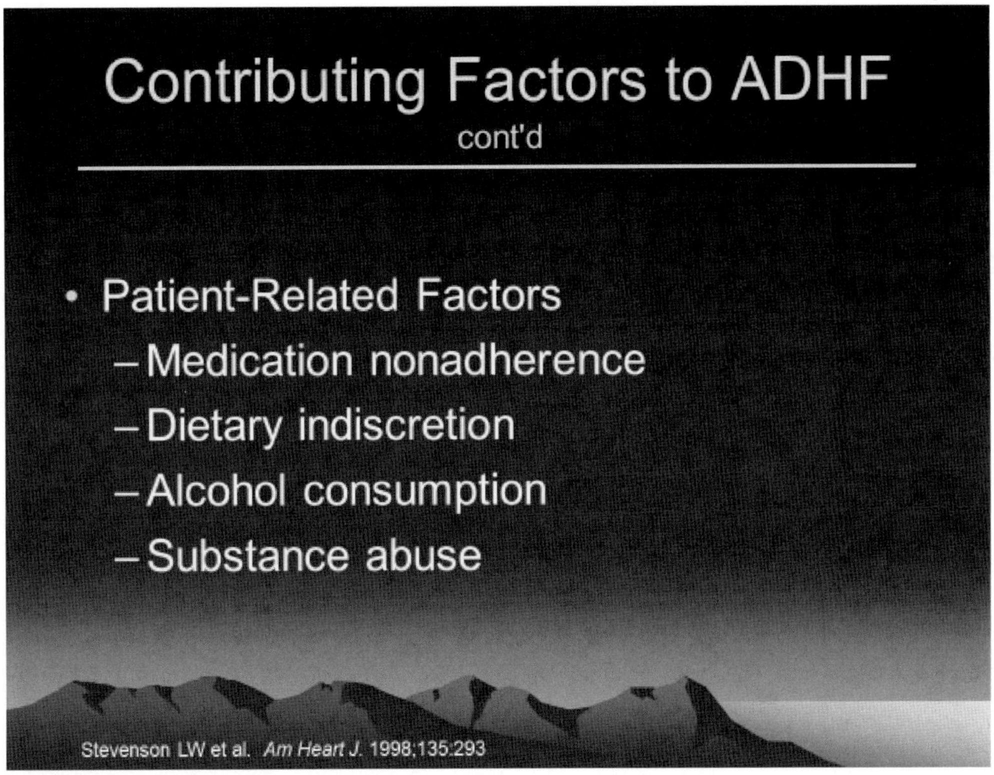
Contributing Factors to ADHF
cont'd
• Patient-Related Factors
– Medication nonadherence
– Dietary indiscretion
– Alcohol consumption
– Substance abuse
Stevenson LW et al. Am Heart J. 1998;135:293

Fig. 9

SECTION III

Risk factors and Co-Morbid Conditions

CHAPTER 8

Hypertension

WATCH NOW

Hypertension

Mr. JB is a 70-year-old male who has been seeing us for years for being grateful for the diagnosis we made when previous doctors had attempted to make him feel better by controlling his blood pressure but were unsuccessful. What had happened was that JB landed in the hospital with uncontrolled blood pressure, fluid retention in his lungs, and heart failure. We attempted to control his blood pressure and remove the fluid which did not correct his blood pressure for good. He kept getting hospitalized for the same symptoms. We tried to make sure there were no occlusions. He has a left heart catheterization that showed patent coronary arteries. His potassium levels were low, but this was attributed to his diuretic and was given supplements. He also has an intermittent weakness because of his potassium and was believed to be losing potassium from the kidneys.

He was then placed on spironolactone but later developed gynecomastia and stopped taking this medication. His blood pressure had gone up and the thought was that he could have Conn's Syndrome. His plasma renin and aldosterone were checked which revealed that he had high levels of plasma aldosterone and low levels of renin. This led us to believe that he had primary hyperaldosteronism. A CT scan of the abdomen also revealed a large adenoma of his adrenal gland and once laparoscopically removed, his blood pressure and potassium normalized, and he was placed on eplerenone instead of spironolactone which alleviated the side of effects of the gynecomastia. He is very thankful to us for digging a little deeper to assess if he had secondary hypertension and the reasoning behind his uncontrolled hypertension.

> The lessons learned from JB is that when blood pressure gets too high and when one gets hospitalized, then, one has to probe a little more and see if they have secondary hypertension from renal artery stenosis, sleep apnea, hyperaldosteronism, or other conditions that deviate from the original thinking process. Being open-minded and accepting flaws and making mistakes are part of life and while realizing that we commit errors, we should not give up hope but start to think outside the box to make patients feel better and live longer.

Hypertension

Hypertension is the leading cause of mortality and complications; the prevalence of hypertension globally is somewhere close to 40% above the age of 25. Worldwide, elevated blood pressure has accounted for more than 8 million deaths, and more than 60 million disability-adjusted lives. A total of more than 1.2 billion people in the world have high blood pressure. According to the WHO, it is estimated that the high prevalence of high blood pressure is in Africa, where it is 46% for both sexes combined.

The WHO has initiated extensive programs across the world and according to them about 1 in 4 men and 1 in 5 women are observed to have high blood pressure. Many of them may be aware of high blood pressure but not receiving the treatment or getting it under control to a target level. The WHO has the mandate to reduce the prevalence of hypertension by 25 percent by 2025. So, the questions that come up include the following: a. Who is at risk? Well, men seem to be at greater risk if they are above 55 years old and women seem to be at higher risk at over 75 years of age. b. Who are the people in the United States and around the world that are highly susceptible?

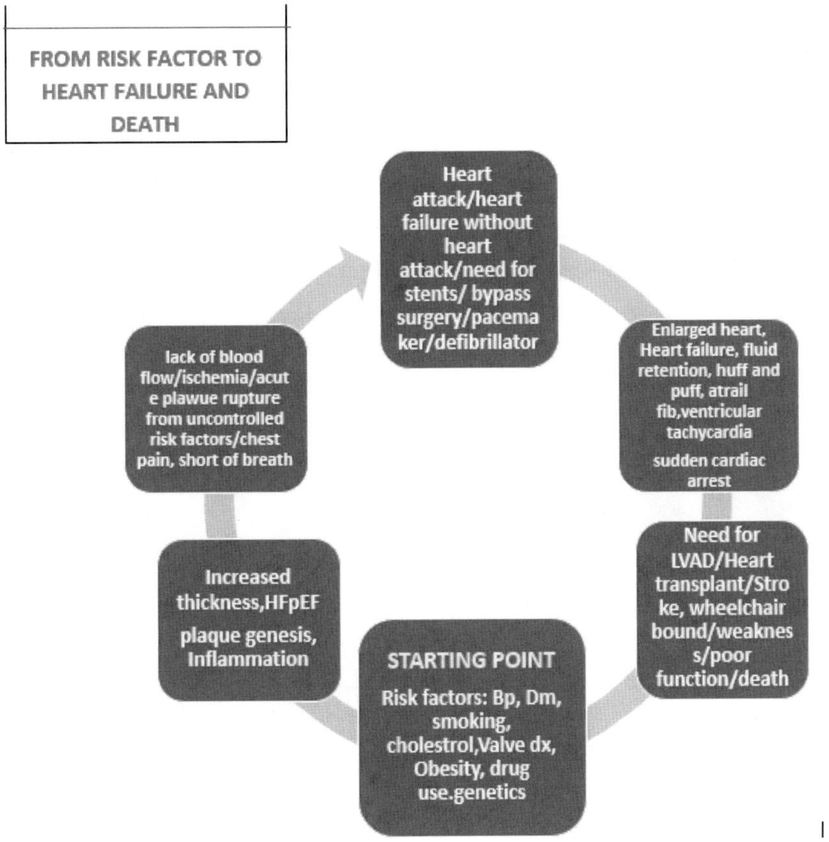

Fig. 10

African Americans seem to have a high prevalence of high blood pressure. Puerto Ricans, Cubans, Mexicans also develop high blood pressure more than the Asian population. A large survey that has been going on for more than 20 years called National Health and Nutrition Examination Survey (NHANES) states that ⅔ of the population are aware of high blood pressure, less than half are seeking adequate treatment and less than 30% have their blood pressure under control. So, clearly, there is a major opportunity to improve blood pressure with education, lifestyle modifications, and low-cost medications.

The reason why high blood pressure is important to control is because of the risk factors that are associated with high blood pressure. For one, high cholesterol, obesity, and diabetes are all related to high blood pressure. Another reason why high blood pressure needs to be controlled is because of the complications that may arise from this condition which include:

i. Cardiovascular: hypertensive emergencies with BP exceeding 220 systolic can lead to heart failure; heart failure can be slow or rapid, and, if rapid, then water can pour into the lungs or "pulmonary edema" ensues. This can lead to a medical emergency which will require respiratory support. If it is long term, then it can lead to congestive heart failure because of the thickening of the heart muscle which leads to heart failure with preserved ejection fraction (HFpEF) mainly from problems with relaxation. Also, thickening of the heart muscle can slowly lead to thinning of the heart muscle over time leading to dilated cardiomyopathy. In addition, other complications from a cardiac standpoint include acute heart attacks, dissection of the aorta, plaque buildup in coronary arteries which supply the heart muscle leading to angina and heart failure.

ii. Neurologic complications include strokes that can occur from plaque rupture in the brain artery called cerebral or cerebellar infarction or rupture in the small blood vessels which can lead to hemorrhage, hypertensive encephalopathy, subdural hemorrhage/hematoma.

iii. Kidney complications include end-stage renal failure when kidneys fail, and many patients can require dialysis.

iv. Electrolyte imbalance: low potassium is usually associated with uncontrolled hypertension which can lead to arrhythmias and sudden cardiac arrest or if they have kidney failure, they can present with high potassium levels which can also be life-threatening.

v. Other conditions that can complicate high blood pressure include blindness. The eyes are a very tenuous anatomical organ, the blood vessels in the eyes are very thin and if the pressures within these vessels are exceedingly high, then blood vessels in the eye can pop and lead to bleeding in the eye, retinal detachment, and blindness. Another complication can also be from papilledema or fluid retention at the level of the macula or optic nerve, which can lead to blindness.

What is normal blood pressure? Well, there are many societies and organizations that recommend a certain blood pressure threshold which can result in complications. The previous recommendation used to be below 160mm Hg systolic which has now lowered to 140mm Hg and even 130mm Hg in certain clinical co-morbid states. Diastolic or "the lower number", is currently expected to be less than 80mm Hg, and anything over 130/80 mmHg, one needs to be aware that complications can happen over longer periods of time. Hence, lifestyle medications with the target to keep blood pressure under control is extremely important.

The other reason why blood pressure needs to be under control is that an irregular heartbeat called atrial fibrillation can get precipitated. The other condition that can happen over time with uncontrolled high blood pressure is dementia where there is a gradual decrease in one's ability to think and remember, affecting activities of daily living. Microinfarcts can happen in the brain without knowledge of the patient and this can lead to reduced brain function, as well as emotional problems, difficulty with language, decreased motivation and decreased functionality overall. In terms of signs and symptoms, what can happen if blood pressure is uncontrolled? Most patients are asymptomatic while others can develop headaches, lightheadedness, vertigo, buzzing sensation in the ears, altered vision, or fainting episodes.

What are the causes of high blood pressure? Well, to answer this question, we will need to divide hypertension into two separate categories: primary and secondary hypertension. Primary hypertension is a complex interaction of environmental and genetic factors. There are quite a few genetic variants that have been identified in Genome-Wide Association Studies (GWAS). There are more than 35 genetic loci (location on the chromosome) related to blood pressure. Primary hypertension seems to be mostly genetically mediated but can also be controlled with lifestyle modifications because aging itself is a risk factor for high blood pressure.

Most subjects would become hypertensive above the age of 65 and following orthodox treatment strategies such as low salt intake, keeping weight under control, reducing stimulants such as caffeine can lead to postponement of high blood pressure even as we age. Smoking is also associated with high blood pressure because this can lead to plaque buildup in the blood vessels from head to the toe and will narrow the blood vessels over time which will increase blood pressure.

What are the causes of secondary hypertension? Renal vascular hypertension which is secondary to a blocked artery in the kidneys, atherosclerotic disease, fibromuscular disease, pheochromocytoma which is a tumor of the adrenal gland, hyperaldosteronism, Cushing syndrome, coarctation of the aorta is all some of the causes. There are also medications that can lead to high blood pressure such as nasal decongestants which include phenylephrine, and pseudoephedrine, cocaine, nonsteroidal anti-inflammatory drugs, ibuprofen, prednisone, and high licorice consumption.

In addition, antirejection medications used after kidney or heart transplants such as cyclosporine and tacrolimus can lead to hypertension as well. Some antidepressants, excessive alcohol, sleep apnea, preeclampsia, or eclampsia during pregnancy are all causes of secondary hypertension. Controlling the root cause will usually eliminate hypertension. Endocrine issues such as low thyroid function or hyperthyroidism can lead to high blood pressure as well. Many of these secondary hypertensive conditions are discovered usually after failure of the standard of care medications that the health care provider will use. Hence, one needs to be aware of other possible conditions if they are resistant to many of the garden variety of medications. In addition, if blood pressure does not remain controlled, one possibility includes intolerance/side effects and at times cost is an issue. If one is using a medication 2-3 times a day, then the cost can add up quickly and non-compliance becomes a matter to be addressed. Instruction errors, inadequate education about diet and salt intake and the complications of uncontrolled BP, inadequate support, organic brain syndrome, dementia are all potential causes for therapeutic failure.

There is a condition called "white coat hypertension" which usually occurs when there is underlying anxiety when visiting a healthcare provider and the patient is usually given a cushion of 15-20 mmHg. Therefore, monitoring blood pressure at home becomes more important as it is more accurate and consistent. Sometimes inadequate blood pressure measuring techniques or calibration issues with blood pressure machines can be a factor as well. It is always a good idea to get an accurate measurement of blood pressure at home with proper calibration of equipment and remove discrepancies with doctor's measurement and measurement at home. Other associated conditions include weight gain, excessive alcohol use, anxiety, hyperactive states.

Despite complications from elevated blood pressure, it is possible to avoid all the detrimental scenarios if patients follow an empowered lifestyle modification program. The basic simple philosophy of body weight maintenance with target BMI between 21 and 25, reduced salt intake to less than 5 g per (less than 2 g of salt per day if CHF), engaging in daily aerobic activity such as walking, jogging, bicycling, swimming, rowing, treadmill, etc., will allow for a better blood pressure control. Alcohol cessation, consuming large amounts of fruits and vegetables has also proven to reduce the risk of heart attack/heart failure in the INTERHEART study. Approximately 5 portions of vegetables a day are highly recommended.

The combination of alcohol and smoking exponentially increases the risk of heart disease and strokes. Preventing the onset of diabetes can also be especially important with the avoidance of simple sugars or carbohydrates. Reducing trans-fat is crucial to avoiding high blood pressure. Reducing stress is beneficial to avoid this condition as well. From a diet perspective, there are multiple diets practiced in the United States but a great diet to avoid hypertension is called the DASH diet which is essentially a low salt diet. Vegetarian or vegan diets have also proven to make an impact on reducing high blood pressure and high cholesterol, diabetes, and weight. Some people recommend green tea consumption and increasing dietary potassium consumption with fruits and vegetables lowers the risk of increased blood pressure.

> Stress-reducing techniques such as biofeedback therapy, transcendental meditation, yoga, tai chi is beneficial in maintaining good blood pressure. There are specific medications that one could use to control blood pressure based on genotype or risk factors, physical appearance or phenotype, and ethnic background. The health care provider will make a specific decision to use precise medications to control blood pressure.

For the most part, a greater number of people require 2-3 types of antihypertensive medications to get blood pressure under control. The common medications usually prescribed include diuretics (water pills), calcium channel blockers, angiotensin II receptor blockers, angiotensin-converting enzyme inhibitors, beta-blockers, vasodilators, isosorbide, hydrazine, aldosterone inhibitors and/or clonidine and minoxidil.

Factors to consider when Blood Pressure is not controlled

Incorrect measurement	Physician inertia	Whitecoat syndrome
Incorrect therapy	Insufficient dose	Patient non-adherence
Complicated regimen	Financial issues	High salt intake
High alcohol intake	Obstructive sleep apnea	Side effects of medications
Entrenched belief about target blood pressure goals	Patient's lack of disease perception	Morbid obesity
Medication-induced high BP e.g. Licorice, ephedra, NSAIDs, steroids, Oral contraceptives, decongestants OTC, cancer medication, tacrolimus, cyclosporin, cocaine	Secondary HTN such as Kidney disease, kidney artery stenosis, Thyroid disease, Adrenal gland disease such as Primary hyperaldosteronism or Cushing's syndrome, Pheochromocytoma, Coarctation of the Aorta	

Ongoing Research in Blood Pressure

Uncontrolled blood pressure can lead to complications such as blindness, heart attacks, strokes, heart failure, and renal failure. The WHO has set a goal to control blood pressure worldwide by 2025. In addition, the World Hypertension League is an organization of 85 national societies that are addressing this problem through wellness campaigns. May 17 is widely known across the world as hypertension day. The burden from an economic standpoint is huge as the cost of blood pressure management, according to the American Heart Association, is more than $80 billion.

Hence, there is a significant challenge for us to make sure that we are vested from an individual and societal standpoint to take care of ourselves and each other. As we set goals to improve our health and seek ways to pursue cost-saving techniques to control hypertension, there are research studies occurring on a continuum. New techniques are being studied to see whether blood pressure will be better controlled with ablation of nerves around the kidneys and many other newer therapies pharmaceutically as well as devices are currently under research.

I've had the immeasurable pleasure of knowing Dr. Kris Vijay for the past two years, as he is an esteemed physician that works with the Abrazo Arizona Heart Hospital.

When I first met Dr. Vijay, I was in awe of his enthusiasm and energy when it came to patient care. To him patient care goes far beyond a hospital bed or clinic visit and extends into his patients and their family's homes. His genuine care for people is a light that inspires us all; he is the definition of a true patient advocate. He lives out his work, has a servant heart, and is a natural born teacher. Dr. Vijay is always there as a mentor, resource, and support to his colleagues, while elevating our hospital teams with the very passion that drives him to be a pioneer and leader in his field.

Dr. Vijay opened the first Cardiorenal Center in the Southwest and has served as the Congestive Heart Failure Medical Director at the Abrazo Arizona Heart Hospital while working diligently to keep patients with cardiorenal syndromes out of the hospital and home with their loved ones. In addition to the countless hours he dedicates to his patients, Dr. Vijay continuously strives to empower our communities by "serving the underserved"-a mantra he wholeheartedly embodies.

I'm proud to know Dr. Vijay for the legacy he has created within our hospital system, the respect he's earned from his peers and community leaders, but most importantly for the friendship we've cultivated over the years.

Nelson Mandela stated, "It always seems impossible until it's done." Dr. Vijay's accomplishments are a testament to the heart and soul he puts into everything he sets his mind to. We are all better people because of who he is and what he continues to do.

Phil Fitzgerald MBA, RN
President, Abrazo Arizona Heart Hospital
Phoenix, Arizona

CHAPTER 9

Diabetes

"Do not judge me by my successes, judge me by how many times I fell down, and got up again."

— Nelson Mandela

WATCH NOW

Patient Story

Ms. TP is a 63-year-old female who has had issues with complications from diabetes and was diagnosed with type 2 diabetes at age 41 with an A1C of 13.5 and kidney failure where she was on dialysis. Despite her visual impairment, she needed to get a kidney transplant. Her family was supportive, and she decided to pursue a kidney transplant and was followed by nephrology, endocrinology, podiatry, ophthalmologist, urology, and psychiatrist.

She had attempted to lose weight but was unable to. After her transplant, she was placed on a healthy eating program which eventually lowered her A1C to 7.2. GFR improved to 58, she was placed on a GLP1 agonist and healthy lifestyle and was losing muscle bulk. She enrolled in cardiac rehab and specialized program where her muscle strength returned. This seemed to improve her kidney function and a1c levels which she was thrilled about. The patient was still having visual issues, despite laser surgery, hence, her mobility was restricted.

> There is an accumulation of fatty tissue intramuscularly which reduces muscle strength and function. However, the evidence is mounting on the relationship between sarcopenia and diabetes. Does sarcopenia accelerate the onset of diabetes in susceptible individuals or do diabetics get sarcopenia later and start performing poorly due to muscle loss of function? Both these statements may be true.

She was doing a lot of sand work as she was Native American and despite her disability from the visual challenges, she continued to work with sandstone and has been resilient in spite of her challenges with diabetes and its complications. The patient did not have any strokes, heart attacks, or other vascular diseases. She has been aggressively watching her feet with podiatry to rule out foot ulcers. TP has been a success story, but what she taught us was about the muscle bulk that she developed with a lot of physical activity and rehab programs. One of the things that happen with diabetes is the loss of muscle strength and muscle bulk called sarcopenia. This can also be due to an age-related muscle loss. In this condition, an enzyme called cyclic AMP kinase activity gets suppressed.

Whether increasing muscle mass will improve type 2 diabetes and prevent complications is another question that is commonly asked. In terms of anecdotal evidence, we have TP who has shown us that with persistence and buoyancy of spirit, she could protect herself notwithstanding all the different challenges that she had to overcome.

The **cyclic AMP kinase** is another biomarker that we measured which seems to have been suppressed before her physical activity was initiated. Following physical activity, and increasing muscle bulk, she seems to have improved her cyclic AMP protein kinase activity. AMP protein kinase activity seems to be a target to improve diabetes and protect diabetic-related complications. A lot of things have been taught by Ms. TP to start engaging in new research concepts and will hopefully bring up new therapeutic agents in diabetes and its comorbidities to help so many other patients with similar problems.

Diabetes Mellitus and Heart Disease

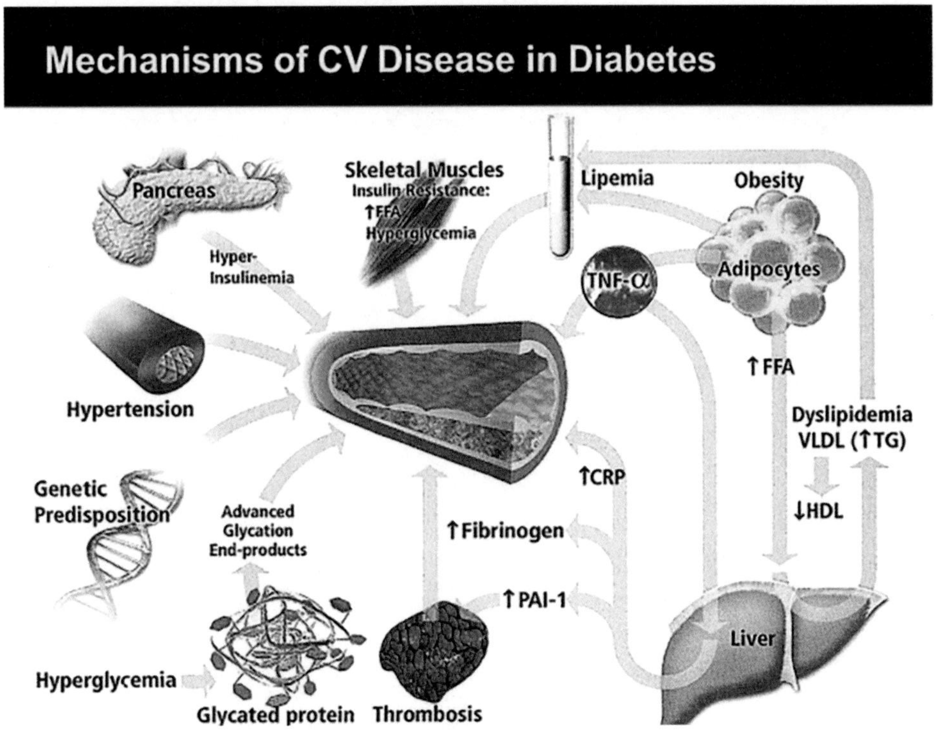

Fig. 11

Diabetes is a common metabolic disease that is characterized by high sugar levels in the blood. There are different types of diabetes such as type 1, type 2 diabetes mellitus, and gestational diabetes. Type 1 diabetes is secondary to the failure of the pancreas because beta cells in the pancreas have lost their ability to produce insulin. This used to be called "insulin-dependent diabetes or juvenile diabetes" and the loss of beta-cell function was thought to be secondary to autoimmune conditions. At present, a genetic basis has been identified but there is still uncertainty as to why diabetes starts at a noticeably young age.

Type 2 diabetes or "insulin-resistant diabetes" is characterized by the proper function of the pancreas but the cells are inadequately able to respond to insulin endogenously. As a result, there is a lack of insulin in the bloodstream and poor insulin function; hence the cells will not be able to control the blood sugar in the bloodstream leading to elevated glucose levels. This form of diabetes is usually associated with obesity and those with sedentary lifestyles. Gestational diabetes occurs with pregnant women who may or may not have a history of diabetes and have abnormally high blood sugar levels. This form of diabetes may eventually lead to type 2 diabetes when they get older. Gestational diabetes is diagnosed through prenatal screening as opposed to symptoms identification as this condition does not usually cause symptoms.

Why is getting blood sugar controlled important? Regardless of which form of diabetes mellitus one person has, it is important to control the blood sugar levels to prevent complications in the long-term. On a short-term basis, high blood sugar can lead to associated high levels of lipids which can acutely block the coronary arteries and lead to a sudden heart attack. In addition, this can lead to vision loss, increased blood viscosity, increased stroke risk, nerve damage, worsening feet ulcers on previous injuries, and possible limb amputation in the long run and possible kidney failure. Chronic high levels of high blood sugar can lead to complications such as:

a. Microvascular disease (those in the eyes, kidneys, nerves). This condition can erode the inner lining of the blood vessels called the endothelium and affecting the blood vessels. When this occurs in the blood vessels in the eye, it can cause damage to the retina, and lead to retinal detachment, and blindness. When this occurs in the blood vessels of the kidneys or a structure in kidneys called the glomerulus, the body's filtration system takes a toll. One starts to spill protein or "albumin" in the urine. When this happens, the kidneys fail which may lead to end-stage renal disease with a need for dialysis. When one is on dialysis, the mortality risk is extremely high. The small vessel disease affecting the nerves is particularly important because it affects the functional capacity or quality of life. A microvascular disease affecting the nerves is known as "neuropathy, which can occur acutely or chronically.
b. Macrovascular disease is a condition that affects the large blood vessels. The large blood vessels that supply the brain or carotid arteries can get damaged and plaque can build up in these arteries. If one has high blood pressure as well, which is common in 75% of diabetics, they are then at high risk for stroke. This combination of risk factors can also lead to dementia. A macrovascular disease of the coronary arteries consist of disease in any of the following four arteries: right coronary arteries which supply the right side of the heart left main artery, left anterior descending which supplies to 60-70% of the heart in the front portion and between the two sides of the heart and circumflex artery which supplies to the left side and back of the heart.

   Plaque accumulates outside the lumen of the arteries in the wall of the blood vessel. The inner lining called "endothelium" is dysfunctional if diabetes is out of control, so the small dense LDL and cholesterol can seep underneath and accumulate in the wall, slowly encroaching into the cavity of the blood vessel. When 70% of the circumference of the blood vessel is occupied, there is a lack of blood flow and the patient becomes symptomatic. When 30 or 40% of the circumference is occupied by the plaque, but the plaque itself becomes unstable due to high BP or other uncontrolled risk factors, there is a high level of inflammation that triggers plaque rupture leading to complete occlusion of the blood vessel with clot formation. This can be life-threatening. In addition, other macrovascular diseases involve the carotid arteries and brain which can lead to stroke. If it involves the peripheral arteries or arteries that supply the legs, one can have a macrovascular disease of the lower extremities with blockages over time. Smoking adds to the risk of amputation in diabetes due to the propensity for blocked peripheral arterial systems. The risk of leg amputation is almost 8-fold compared to someone who does not smoke or have diabetes. Endothelium (inner lining of the blood vessel) plays a major role in the expression of the mechanistic behavior of vascular disease in diabetes. See Fig. 11 above – Mechanisms of CV Disease in Diabetes

Epidemiology and Burden of Diabetes Mellitus

Did you know that the number of people with diabetes mellitus in 1980 was 100 million in the world and by 2014 the number had increased to 422 million? Indeed type 2 diabetes is a global epidemic and will affect 592 million people worldwide in 2035. This is a significant increase and the prevalence may be widely underestimated. In the United States alone, there are more than 30 million adults with type 2 diabetes which is 12-13% of the population with type 2 diabetes mellitus. Interesting enough, more than a quarter of these individuals are not aware that they have diabetes. Type 1 and 2 diabetes are different with respect to the etiology; hence, the disease progression can also vary significantly. However, type 2 accounts for more than 90% of all cases, hence, the focus has been more to control this form of diabetes.

> Patients with type 2 diabetes have twice the risk of developing heart failure than those who do not have this condition. The Framingham Heart Study estimates that diabetes independently increases the risk of heart failure 2-fold in men and 5-fold in women. Although this discrepancy is not clearly understood, the increased incidence of heart failure and diabetes persist even after controlling for risk factors such as age, high blood pressure, high cholesterol, and coronary artery disease. While we have noted the prevalence of diabetes is 10-15%, the prevalence of heart failure in patients who have diabetes and hospitalized is about 44%.

Heart Failure and Diabetes Mellitus

As mentioned above, diabetes when uncontrolled can lead to microvascular and macrovascular complications. However, an area that has not been explored includes the link between diabetes and heart failure.

The association between mortality and A1c levels (a form of hemoglobin which is linked to sugar) appears to be a U-shaped curve with a lower risk of death among patients with A1C under 7%. Many other studies suggest the persistence of death and hospitalization despite better blood sugar levels. In addition, when blood sugar is better controlled, one would want to believe that the complications of macrovascular disease will be reduced, however, this is not always the case. In multiple large clinical trials such as ACCORD trial, United Kingdom Prospective Diabetes Study (UKPDS), ADVANCE trial, Veterans Affairs Diabetes Trial (VADT), we have found that intensive control of blood sugar levels reduces microvascular complications such as retinopathy, nephropathy, and neuropathy, but did not show evidence of a reduction in cardiovascular mortality such as heart attacks or strokes.

Although in many of these trials, heart failure was not a primary endpoint, we have learned that intensive blood sugar control did not reduce heart failure or heart failure hospitalizations. The effects of diabetes treatment on the risk of HF has been sparse. The agents that we use commonly for management of diabetes include metformin, sulfonylureas, glinides, DPP4 inhibitors, glitazones, acarbose, and insulin. None of these agents have had an impact on reducing cardiovascular events.

However, newer agents such as SGLT2 inhibitors and GLP-1 receptor agonists are proving to be effective in the reduction of cardiovascular mortality and hospitalizations from heart failure. These are new agents and there is still active research being done to further assess the efficacy of these treatments for changing the outcomes and dynamics for those with or without heart failure, and with or without diabetes or any form of heart disease.

At present, there is a new indication for an SGLT2 inhibitor as a treatment to reduce the risk of heart failure hospitalization or dying from heart disease even in the absence of diabetes, but in those with a reduced ejection fraction of 40% or less. As we move forward in the next couple of years, we will notice more clinical trials possibly revealing more benefits in patients with prediabetes to prevent or manage heart failure or any other cardiovascular events and hopefully slowing the progression of kidney disease as well. Figure in pharmacology section depicts some of the commonly used pharmaceutical agents used to control blood sugar.

The organs that play a significant role in blood sugar control include the pancreas, liver, kidneys, fatty tissue, and skeletal muscle. The commonly used agents to decrease blood sugar levels in the bloodstream include metformin, sulfonylureas, GLP-1 receptor agonist, dpp4 inhibitors, SGLT2 inhibitors, and insulin. The mechanism of their blood sugar control differs from each other. For example, metformin acts on the liver and improves peripheral utilization of blood sugar levels to reduce blood sugar levels as the liver takes up most of the burden and transmits it to the skeletal muscle; whereas sulfonylureas and glitazones act on the pancreas. The GLP-1 receptor agonist acts on the beta cells of the pancreas and is favorable to the kidneys, as well as impact intraepithelial lymphocytes thereby reducing inflammation and controlling plaque inside the blood vessels.

DPP4 inhibitors work by inhibiting the enzyme that degrades the glucagon peptide and improving blood sugar levels. This has a neutral effect on the kidneys or heart. Whereas the SGLT2 inhibitors tend to dump the sugar in the urine by blocking a receptor in the kidneys. These receptors continuously reabsorb sugar that comes into the kidneys back into circulation and increasing blood sugar levels. Blocking the SGLT 2 receptors in the kidneys leads to excretion of sugar, sodium, and water in the urine. This, in turn, likely has a benefit that impacts the heart favorably by improving preload to the heart, afterload from the heart by excreting sodium and water, and reduces neurohormones and sympathetic activity.

This may be the mechanism by which there are cardiovascular mortality benefits and benefits in the reduction of heart failure hospitalization. Using lipids as an alternative fuel source instead of glucose may be a lot more efficient in subjects with heart failure. It is like using a 91 octane rather than an 85 octane, hence, your car has got more of a turbo effect which helps it run more efficiently. Whether this analogy can be translated to the heart muscle is not clear, but it is one of the mechanisms touted. There is other bioenergetics located in the mitochondria level which may be influenced favorably. There are reduced oxygen free radicals that reduce stress-induced reactive oxygen species that may influence the heart favorably.

Inflammation is reduced and less bad cholesterol present if blood sugar is low. Hence, toxicity imposed by lipids called lipotoxicity is also reduced. There is a reduction of the mitochondrial stress levels and better signaling of insulin pathways at the molecular level. In addition, there is a probable reduction of advanced glycation end products (AGEs) which are toxic agents that harm the eyes, kidneys, peripheral nerves, heart, brain, and peripheral vasculature. Hence, reducing AGE may be another mechanism of these two agents called SGLT2 inhibitors and GLP-1 receptor agonists that may be contributing to beneficial effects of the heart.

Insulin is also an important agent that endogenously increases the effect on the beta cells and reduces blood sugar levels but is also proven to be an inflammatory agent that can harm in the long run and one needs to be cautious of overuse as it can also worsen metabolic health and increase weight gain or cause hypoglycemia. Both sulphonylureas and Insulin can cause hypoglycemia and weight gain. Hypoglycemia can be detrimental to brain function and one must be cautious in using these medications in combination with SGLT2 inhibitors.

CHAPTER 10

ASCVD Calcium Score

"I love the man that can smile in trouble, that can gather strength from distress, and grow brave by reflection. 'Tis the business of little minds to shrink, but he whose heart is firm, and whose conscience approves his conduct, will pursue his principles unto death."

—Thomas Paine

WATCH NOW

Patient Story

Mr. AR is a 40-year-old male who was very distraught when he came to see me for the first time as his father had passed away at age 46, his brother recently passed away at age 37. His older brother also had multivessel coronary artery disease and also had bypass surgery at a younger age. He was told that his cholesterol was within normal range and he did not need therapy such as statins. He was very worried about the recent death of his younger brother who experienced cardiac arrest. It was not noticeably clear if his cholesterol was elevated as he did not take care of himself in regard to protecting himself from the progression of diabetes, vascular disease, or cancer.

Nobody was a smoker; his mother is still alive, but he wanted to make sure that he was not a candidate for blocked arteries and a cardiac arrest. When we did an exercise stress test, it was normal, and he walked for about 9 minutes and did not have any major abnormalities. His echocardiogram had shown normal heart function. His LDL was 72mg/dL which is decent. Due to the strong family history of sudden cardiac arrests, I ordered a lipoprotein (a) level and recommended that although his LDL cholesterol was 72, he could be in the intermediate-risk and may benefit from a coronary artery calcium score assessment. Hence, he underwent calcium score and lipoprotein (a) test which showed a calcium score of 1440 and his lipoprotein (a) was 245.

Both of them were extremely elevated. A calcium score of 0 indicates no plaque buildup, 1-100 indicates mild disease, 101-300 is a moderate disease and over 300 is an extensive vascular disease with calcification with or without occlusions. A normal lipoprotein (a) is a level of less than 75 ml/deciliter, hence, he had almost a 4-fold increase from the upper limit of normal. When we figured this out, he was placed on a statin, niacin, and recommended that he undergo a coronary angiogram. He was having vague, nonspecific chest tightness intermittently and was not clear if this was exercise-induced muscle pain or he had small vessel disease.

The stress test may have been falsely negative or maybe it was just about 70% sensitive to detect occlusive disease. Once he had the angiography, his left main artery was found to be extensively calcified and 70% blocked, his left anterior descending had 80% narrowing and more than 60-70% narrowing in the circumflex artery, as well as a right coronary artery, showed extensive calcification. He was given a choice of undergoing bypass surgery or stent procedure but told that the stent would be risky as opening up the left main artery with a balloon could have cardiac arrest if we did not protect his left ventricle with an Impella catheter device and is a high-risk procedure. He decided to undergo bypass surgery and he did well without any complications. He now feels much improved regarding his energy and has a drive for contributing to society. He feels recharged and determined to talk about his condition in the community to educate the people who may have a strong family history and maybe at risk for something that happened to his immediate family members. Clearly, the mastery of his own condition with a personal compass to be his own driving force has been a great example for us to emulate. He clearly demonstrates gratitude as well as having some sort of a rekindled source of energy to make an impact on other people's lives.

Very few times in life does one have the opportunity to encounter a person that you immediately know was placed here to change lives—a lot of them. Dr. Kris Vijay embodies that gift in his soul, and you feel it in this book. His passion and compassion shines through each page as he shares his experiences and learnings of his life's work in heart failure and impacting people. This book opens a door inside the mind of a global leader in his space to fill the many misconceptions and misunderstandings around heart failure. Dr. Vijay is a master at connecting with any audience and simplifying complexities to the basic form. This book is a true contribution to those wanting or needing to understand how to best navigate modern heart failure.

Michael Gratch
President & Founder
Legacy Heart Care

CHAPTER 11

Cholesterol

WATCH NOW

A lot of bad publicity about cholesterol makes one's head spin and you start to wonder what is fake and what is science. The Internet has been a major source of negative advertising and cholesterol has been one of the prime targets over the years. Knowledge about the topic with scientific evidence has busted a lot of myths about this risk factor for heart disease. As we learn more, we will update the evidence as it is indeed a dynamic and evolving field. In this chapter, we will look at the evidence from a cardiac perspective and how it may relate to heart failure.

What is Cholesterol?

Cholesterol is a waxy substance found in many of the foods that we eat and in every cell of our body. Our body needs some cholesterol to function normally and can make all the cholesterol it needs. Cholesterol is needed to generate enzymes, hormones, vitamins, some minerals, and combines with proteins to form lipoproteins. They play a major role in digestion as well. There are 3 types from a simplistic point of view: HDL, Triglycerides, and LDL (The GOOD, The BAD and THE UGLY!!). High-density lipoprotein, or HDL, often called the good cholesterol, helps to remove excess cholesterol from your body. Very low-density lipoprotein, or VLDL (Bad Cholesterol) which is 1/5th of the total Triglycerides also tends to promote plaque buildup. The most important and atherogenic cholesterol is the Low-Density Lipoprotein cholesterol (LDL or the Ugly Cholesterol).

TC= HDL+LDL+1/5 TG

High triglycerides may be a sign that you have excess body fat or maybe at an increased risk for Type 2 diabetes. They also may be a signal that you are consuming too many calories, especially from refined grains or foods and beverages with added sugars. Triglycerides also can be elevated in people who smoke or drink too much alcohol. Low-density lipoprotein or LDL is the bad or "lousy" cholesterol that can build up plaque in the arteries.

Am I at Risk?

Many things may increase your risk for high cholesterol, including:

- **Genetics:** High cholesterol runs in some families.
- **Age:** As we age, our cholesterol levels rise.
- **Medicines:** Certain drugs can elevate cholesterol levels.
- **Obesity:** Individuals that are overweight or obese body mass indices are at a greater risk for high cholesterol.
- **Diet**: Consuming high quantities of saturated and trans fats can raise LDL cholesterol levels.
- **Inactivity**: Activity helps to elevate HDL cholesterol. Lack of activity has the reverse effect — it increases LDL cholesterol.
- **Smoking**: Tobacco products decrease HDL and increase LDL. The link between smoking and high cholesterol is greater for women.

LDL Story:

We will make a few points from all the research that has been done in this space.

- Evidence from controlled clinical trials has confirmed a causal role for LDL-C in plaque genesis inside the arteries. Lowering LDL-C levels is associated with reduced risk of cardiovascular disease (CVD) mortality, heart attacks, and stroke rates that is directly proportional to the magnitude of LDL-C reduction.

- Epidemiological and interventional studies show that a 50 mg/dL decrease in LDL-C results in a 32% reduction in heart attack and 20% reduction in stroke
- The optimum LDL-C level is currently standardized at 40 mg/dL.
- The guideline recommendation is less than 130 for most. Less than 100 for moderate-risk and less than 70 for high risk. Many individuals are at extremely high risk and do not even know it. LDL level less than 55 is recommended for extremely high risk by most societies. Fetal LDL is around 30-35 mg/dL. We develop increasing levels as we age. Scientists have demonstrated a linear relationship between increased serum LDL-C levels and increased risk for coronary artery disease. For every 1 mg/dL increase in LDL-C, the relative risk increases by 1%. Thus, an individual with an LDL-C of 70 mg/dL has a 30% higher risk than one with an LDL-C of 40 mg/dL
- Intense LDL-C lowering yields superior benefits than moderate lowering; the absolute benefit is related to the persons baseline absolute risk and the degree of LDL-C lowering but not the initial LDL-C level.
- The Cholesterol Treatment Trialists' (CTT) Collaborators have made recommendations based on all trials reducing LDL with lifestyle and medication. It has been demonstrated that more-intensive therapy produces further reductions in each category of major CVD events (coronary death, heart attack, coronary angioplasty/stent/bypass, and stroke).
- An 80 mg/dL reduction in LDL-C and/or non-HDL-C confers a 60-80% reduction in CVD after 5 years of treatment
- Although LDL-C goal attainment rates have overall improved during the past decade, only about one-third of high-risk patients with CVD attain levels of LDL-C < 70 mg/dL. Some patients who do not attain LDL-C goals may be unwilling to take or intolerant of high dose statin therapy or physicians may be reluctant to use high-dose statins.
- Combinations therapy (with niacin, fibrates, ezetimibe, or resin) may help to limit the need for higher statin doses in those patients requiring more intensive LDL-C reductions (e.g. > 50%) and provide greater drug adherence as well. While the lipid-lowering efficacies of these combination therapies are known, randomized clinical trials assessing the effects of these therapies on CVD outcomes are still awaited.
- Much of the progress in reducing CVD and mortality, is largely attributed to improved cholesterol management, especially the use of higher efficacy LDL-C lowering agents.
- Although statins have become the mainstay of lowering LDL-C, weight reduction of 10 kg can decrease LDL-C by 8mg/dl and dietary modification can reduce LDL-C by 7-10% and up to 40 mg/dl
- In patients with heart failure due to ischemic etiology (previous heart attack or blocked arteries), it is recommended that their LDL goal is set < 70 mg/dL

- New agents beyond statin are available for LDL reduction if they are statin intolerant and not at goal. These include ezetimibe, PCSK9 antibody, and Bempedoic acid. Two other agents are awaiting FDA approval.
- Myalgias with a statin can occur in 20-25% of subjects. This side effect is genetically mediated by a few genes such as OATP1B1, CYP, SLCO1B1, ABCB1, GATM, COQ2, etc.

Recently approved agent Bempedoic acid reduces LDL by 18% and when ezetimibe is added, LDL reduction is as much as 36%. This seems to be a good agent when statins are not tolerated or at maximally tolerated dose, target goal is not achieved. One has to watch for uric acid levels and onset of gout as one of the side effects.

Triglycerides

- Triglycerides (or blood fats) are an important barometer of metabolic health; high levels may be associated with CAD (coronary artery disease), diabetes, and fatty liver. Recommended optimal fasting triglyceride levels are less than 150 mg/dL. Subjects who reach a target less than 100 mg/dL seem to be at a lesser risk
- According to NHANES data, the mean triglycerides are 144 mg/dl and 13% of the US population has high triglycerides. Mexican Americans have the highest rates of triglycerides (35.5%), followed by non-Hispanic whites (33.2%), and African Americans (15.9%).
- Blacks have lower triglycerides than whites, in both men (127 vs 158) and women (102 vs 135 mg/dl), despite higher rates of obesity.
- Non-fasting blood can now be used to screen for high triglyceride levels. A non-fasting level of <200 mg/dL is commensurate with a normal (<150 mg/dL) or optimal (<100 mg/dL) fasting triglyceride level and requires no further testing. In fact, non-fasting triglycerides predict CAD more strongly than fasting triglycerides.
- Simple sugars (high fructose syrup), saturated fats, and trans-fats raise triglyceride levels, whereas weight loss or use of unsaturated fats, especially those containing marine omega-3 fatty acids, lower triglyceride levels.
- Consuming too many simple sugars, refined grains, and alcohol will increase triglyceride levels for those who have not been diagnosed with triglycerides outside the normal range.
- Diabetes, hypothyroidism, kidney disease such as nephrotic syndrome, liver disease, excess alcohol, lack of physical activity, certain medications, and genetics are all causes of high TG levels.

- Alcohol intake has a major effect on triglycerides, especially when consumption is in excess of 1-2 drinks per day
- Consumption of 15-20% of energy from fructose, especially soft drinks or table sugar, results in a 30-40% increase in triglycerides. Conversely, regular exercise and weight reduction can cause a 20-30% decrease in TG levels
- People with high triglycerides (≥ 150 mg/dL) should limit their intake of fructose that is mainly found in soda and fruits, and instead, emphasize a healthy diet including an increase in consumption of vegetables and low fructose fruits.
- The American Heart Association recommends limiting added sugars to fewer than 100 calories daily (6 tsp) for women and 150 calories (9 tsp) for men (≈5% of total energy). The lowest triglyceride levels were observed when added sugar represented <10% of total energy. Conversely, higher triglyceride levels (5% to 10%) were observed when added sugar represented a greater proportion of energy intake.
- In general, most refined starchy foods in the diet have a high glycemic index, whereas non-starchy vegetables, fruits, and legumes typically have a low glycemic index.
- The glycemic index is defined as the ratio of the blood glucose response to specific food and the glucose response to standard food (e.g. white bread).
- Americans consume fructose in large quantities (up to 150 g/d) but a dose >50 g increases triglycerides. The major sources of fructose include soda and other soft drinks with high fructose syrup (14-23 g per oz), honey (17 g per 2 tbsp). Fruits like apple and pear are low in fructose (4-10 g).
- A diet that produces significant and sustained weight loss offers the most favorable reduction in triglyceride levels, regardless of the carbohydrate, protein, or fat intake. For everyone, adopting and maintaining a healthy lifestyle (i.e. diet and physical activity) is highly effective and can lower triglyceride levels by up to 50%.
- Overall, the treatment of elevated triglyceride levels focuses on an intensive therapeutic lifestyle change that can bring about a total reduction of 50%. Triglyceride levels can be reduced by weight reduction (5% to 10% reduction in body weight anticipates a triglyceride-lowering response of 20%). Reducing carbohydrates particularly added sugars and fructose while increasing unsaturated fat intake may contribute an additional 10% to 20% reduction in triglyceride levels. Elimination of trans fats, restriction of saturated fats, and increasing consumption of marine-based omega-3 products, coupled with aerobic activity, will further optimize triglyceride-lowering efforts.
- In patients with high triglycerides, potent statins such as rosuvastatin 20 mg/d or atorvastatin 40-80 mg/d can lower triglycerides 40-50% (similar magnitude as LDL-C reduction).
- Triglycerides >500-1000 mg/dl are associated with acute pacreatitis, the former accounting for 10% of the latter. Such patients require a restriction of fats to 10-15%

of energy, abstinence from alcohol, along with fibrates, omega-3 fatty acids 3-4g/day, and prescription niacin. Insulin therapy may be required in those with high blood sugar. While fenofibric acid is safe in reducing TG levels, there is no evidence in reducing CVD

Recent studies on higher doses of omega-3 ethyl esters (EEC) (2 to 4 g of Eicosapentaenoic acid [EPA] lower plasma triglycerides by 30-35% with little effect on plasma levels of LDL or HDL cholesterol and also reduce cardiovascular events by 25-30%

HDL — High-density lipoprotein

- High blood levels of HDL-C and apo A-I (a precursor of HDL) are inversely related to the risk of CAD (coronary artery disease) and CVD (cardiovascular disease) events in both men and women. High levels of this lipoprotein are associated with reduced risk for atherosclerosis. Low levels of HDL are also associated with worse prognosis after a heart attack.
- A 1% increase in HDL-C confers a 2% decrease in CVD risk and a 1 mg/dL decrease confers a 4% decrease in CVD risk.
- Almost one-fifth of patients with a heart attack in a hospital setting have extremely low HDL levels (10-29 mg/dl) — a finding that adds incrementally to a greater burden of atherosclerosis and a higher risk of mortality

HDL Subclasses

- HDL particles can be categorized into 12 subclasses. The largest α-1 particle is the most cardioprotective and 1 mg/dl increase confers a 26% decrease in CAD risk compared to a 4% decreased risk with I mg/dL increase in HDL-C.
- **Is Very High HDL good for you? HDL functionality has been researched recently. Increasing HDL with medications has not led to a cardiovascular benefit. One study showed harm. It is not clear if the HDL number or function is important**
- Epidemiologic, pathologic, and experimental studies have demonstrated a role for HDL in protection from CAD (coronary artery disease). HDL has been demonstrated to reduce the risk of atherosclerosis and CVD (cardiovascular disease) by multiple pathophysiological mechanisms.

Whether high HDL-C level (greater than 85 mg/dL) can be regarded as protective in all people has recently been debated. High concentrations of **dysfunctional HDL** may be more dangerous for cardiovascular health than having low levels of functional HDL.

It is like garbage trucks in New York City. If we have 100 of them, but they are not running properly, to clear the garbage, to get to Hoboken New Jersey to the landfill, because of faulty tires/transmission/drivers being drunk/roads are closed for whatever reason, then garbage will accumulate. If HDL were like garbage trucks and if you just had a few that are functional, one can still get the job done in clearing the garbage. This analogy is hopefully beneficial in understanding the concept of HDL number and function.

In this light, research studies are ongoing to address the relationship between HDL functionality and arterial disease.

Lipoprotein(a)

- Lp(a) concentrations are largely genetically determined through the autosomal-dominant transmission. Lp(a) levels are high in people with a family history of early heart disease or personal history of premature heart disease, stroke or repeat coronary angioplasty, stent, or bypass surgery
- Lp(a) is therefore strongly associated with premature, severe cardiovascular disease that often leads to massive heart attacks and strokes at a noticeably young age.
- High levels of Lp(a) are often found in people with family history.
- Lp(a) is a strong independent risk factor for premature CAD in many populations including Europids, Chinese, Japanese, French Canadians, Afro Americans, and South Asians
- Lp(a) levels >30 mg/dL is an independent risk factor for premature CAD with risk comparable in magnitude to a total cholesterol level of >240 mg/dL or an HDL-C level of <35 mg/dL. The risk increases to 25-fold in those who have all three of these lipid abnormalities.
- High Lp(a) is associated with early onset of Aortic stenosis in some susceptible individuals

Lipoprotein(a) (pronounced Lp-little-a) is a strong, putative, and causal risk factor for heart attack and stroke. Lp(a) is a genetic variant of LDL (low-density lipoprotein) particle with one molecule of apolipoprotein B100 (apoB) and an additional protein, apo(a), attached to LDL. Research has revealed a 2-fold risk of CAD (coronary artery disease) independent of all modifiable risk factors.

Cholesterol-lowering statins do not lower Lp(a) directly, but they help reduce the risk since Lp(a) is more harmful when working in concert with high LDL-C. PCSK 9 antibody lowers Lp(a) by 25-30%, but data on risk prevention of CVD is lacking. Most recently, apheresis has been approved as a treatment in high-risk individuals with exceedingly high Lp(a)

Nutritional advice regarding cholesterol

If your cholesterol is high because of genetics, you might need to take a cholesterol-lowering drug. However, everyone with high cholesterol can benefit from a heart-healthy lifestyle. And, if you are at risk, simple lifestyle changes can help reduce that risk. These include eating a heart-healthy diet, being physically active, and achieving or maintaining healthy body weight. While dietary intervention with low fat diet will drop LDL cholesterol by 7-10%, overall, following a heart-healthy diet will reduce the global burden of risk. Obesity, diabetes, lack of activity, high-stress level, high blood pressure, increased alcohol intake, and smoking can all add to the risk of heart attacks and stroke. Hence it is important to have a comprehensive balanced meal plan to reduce the global burden off risk and not just that of the bad and ugly cholesterol.

When it comes to a healthy eating plan, four dietary changes may help keep your cholesterol in check:

Replenish Foods with Plant Sterols and Stanols

Some foods — vegetable oils, nuts, seeds, and whole grains — contain substances called plant sterols and stanols. Eating foods rich in these substances may help combat rising total and LDL cholesterol levels. To increase your daily intake, also look for foods fortified with plant sterols and stanols. For example, some orange juice, cereals, and breakfast bars may be fortified.

Limit Your Intake of Saturated Fat

Saturated fats are mostly found in animal-based foods such as meats and whole-fat dairy products. Higher intakes of saturated fat have been found to elevate LDL cholesterol.

Studies have also shown that replacing sources of saturated fat with unsaturated fats can help decrease your total and LDL cholesterol levels. To help reduce your intake of saturated fat:

- Cook with vegetable oils, such as avocado oil or canola oil. They have a high "smoke point" and do not get oxidized easily. Olive oil should be used raw in salads, pasta, etc. The next best oils to use include sunflower and safflower. Avoid palm oil at all costs.
- Eat foods rich in omega-3 fatty acids such as salmon, walnuts, and ground flaxseed.
- Choose low-fat or fat-free dairy products, such as 1% or skim milk and non-fat yogurt or low-fat cheeses, such as reduced-fat feta and part-skim mozzarella.
- Swap out butter and lard for healthier vegetable oil options.
- Avoid trans fats — they have been found to increase LDL levels and are found in highly processed foods. In the ingredients, if it says the food contains hydrogenated fat, put it back.

Select Lean Proteins

Lean proteins provide fewer calories from fat. To choose lean cuts:

- Check the package for the words "loin or round".
- Strip the skin off your chicken and turkey to get a healthier option.
- Bake, broil, roast, stew or stir-fry lean meats, fish, and poultry.
- After you cook ground meat, carefully drain off any excess fat.
- Limit fatty, marbled meats, fried or deep-fried foods and other foods that are high in saturated fat, such as organ meats
- Choose healthier options when eating out by selecting foods that are baked, broiled, or grilled.
- If you can substitute vegetable proteins for proteins from meat, that is even healthier.
- *Seafood with high Omega 3s:* Salmon (Atlantic, Chinook, Coho), Arctic char, Anchovies, Herring, Mackerel, Oysters (Pacific), Sablefish/Black Cod, Sardines, Pomfrets, Trout, Tuna, Snapper, Seabass, Rockfish, Mussels. Avoid Tilapia due to its high-fat content and Swordfish due to high mercury content

Add Soluble Fiber: Dietary fiber is found in fruits, vegetables, beans, lentils, and whole grains. These nutrient-dense foods provide two types of fiber, soluble and insoluble. Both types are important for good health. Getting adequate amounts of dietary fiber from a variety of foods is important for everyone.

Research has shown that soluble fiber from fruits, vegetables, beans, lentils, and whole grains, may help to lower LDL cholesterol. In the stomach, soluble fiber forms a thick, jelly-like substance, which helps bind dietary cholesterol from foods you are eating. So, load up on vegetables and fruits:

- Select fruits and vegetables that are good sources of soluble fiber. For example, asparagus, Brussels sprouts, sweet potatoes, turnips, apricots, mangoes, and oranges.
- Eat a variety of different colored fruits and veggies.
- Shift to more plant-based or vegetarian meals by including beans, lentils, and soy foods.
- Focus on whole forms of produce, which includes fresh or frozen
- Choose low-sodium canned veggies or varieties with no added salt.

Whole grains also are a great way to get the benefits of fiber:

- Eat barley, oats, and oat bran — all are good sources of soluble fiber.
- Make sure the food label on your bread says 100 percent whole-grain or lists a whole grain as one of the first ingredients.
- Limit refined carbohydrates, especially sources of added sugars, such as sweets and sugar-sweetened beverages.

One note of caution: as you increase your fiber intake, also increase your intake of water. This will help to reduce your risk of becoming constipated. If you find it difficult to get enough fiber in your diet, ask your health care provider before considering a fiber supplement.

If you have heart failure, you will need to restrict fluid intake to 50 ounces or so daily.

High vegetarian proteins:

Grains and pasta: Oats, buckwheat, oat bran, spelt, sorghum flour, cornmeal, teff, amaranth, quinoa, wheat pasta, Japanese somen, brown rice, millet, couscous, oatmeal, bulgur, white rice, ragi, barley, hominy

Fruits high in protein: guava, avocado, apricots, kiwi, blackberries, oranges, banana, cantaloupe, raspberry, strawberry, peaches, plums

Vegetables high in proteins: Soybean, lima bean, pea sprouts, succotash, lentil sprouts, peas, kidney beans, straw mushrooms, spirulina, taro, peapods, spinach, broccoli, artichokes, asparagus, arrowroot, collard greens, sweet potatoes, yellow corn, fiddlehead ferns, red potatoes, Brussel sprouts, bamboo shoot, kale, palm hearts, green beans, mustard greens, beet greens, swiss chard, mung sprouts, okra, kohlrabi, casava bean, pumpkin, bok choy, cauliflower, garden cress, squash, zucchini, lotus root, banana pepper, bell pepper

Dairy: cheese, butter, milk, buttermilk, yogurt, eggs

Nuts high in protein: Hemp, pumpkin, peanut, walnut, almonds, pistachio, sunflower, roasted squash, flaxseed, cashew, sesame seeds, chia, safflower, hazelnut, brazil nut, pine nut, coconut, pecan, chestnut, macadamia

Beans high in proteins: Tofu, soybean, lupin bean, navy bean, edamame, lentils, white bean, red kidney beans, cranberry beans, split peas, black beans, great northern beans, lima bean, chickpeas, mung bean, baked bean, pinto beans, black-eyed peas, cowpea, fava bean, veggie burger, peanut butter, soymilk, hummus

When a patient and their loved ones hear a diagnosis of heart failure it arrests your breathing and sucks all the air out of the room. I know this because on two occasions my husband Raymond has been given a diagnosis of congestive heart failure in connection to his kidney failure.

Once when his kidneys first failed, and he had to start dialysis. The second time was years later when Raymond thought he was having a heart attack. The ER doctor delivered the good news that Raymond did not have a heart attack but shocked us when he casually said that the symptoms were caused by congestive heart failure.

Thankfully, we determined that a few months earlier he stopped eating after 7pm and didn't realize that he had lost 10 LBS, therefore he had not adjusted his dry weight for dialysis and was carrying the excess fluid. Once Raymond had a few dialysis treatments to adjust him down to his new target dry weight he was fine.

It is clear that the personal story Dr. Vijay shares fuels his passion and compassion to make a difference in the lives of patients and their families.

Dr. Vijay does a masterful job to bring greater awareness to all aspects of heart failure by intertwining clinical information and patient stories that bring an enlightened perspective together that encourage and empower readers from the non-medical community and medical community alike.

Analyn Scott
Founder & CEO of 1in9

CHAPTER 12

Endothelial Function, Atherosclerosis, and Heart Failure

Endothelium, that lines the 50,000 miles of arteries and 50,000 miles of veins that course through our bodies.

WATCH NOW

The endothelium is an interesting organ which lines inner portion of all the blood vessels in the body. If entire endothelium is put side to side, it can occupy the distance of this entire earth almost 3-4 times. Hence, injury to this inner lining can lead to complications which is important because the role of this inner lining has 5-fold functions:

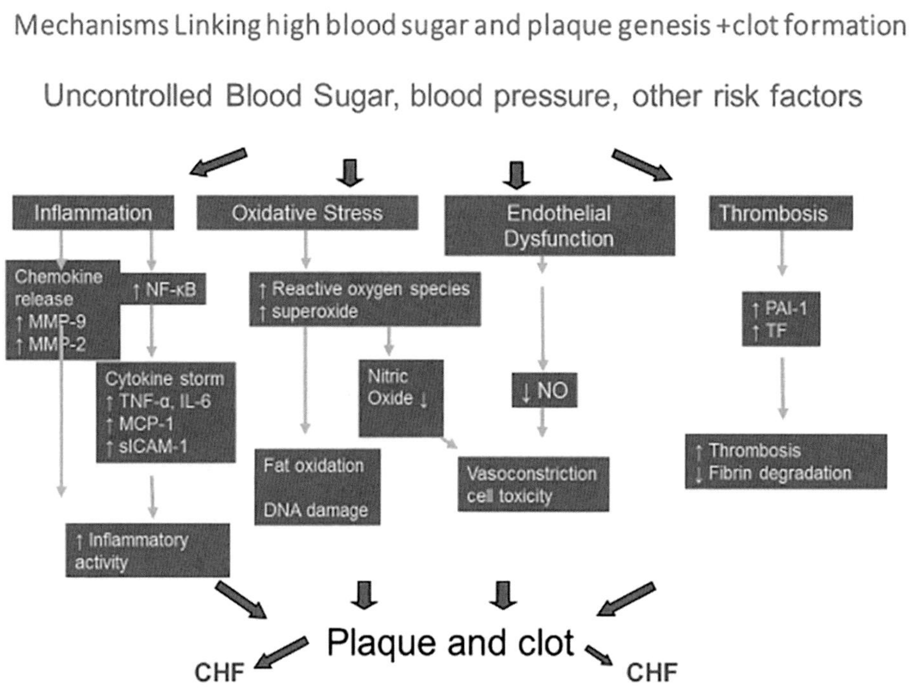

Fig. 12

1. **It acts as a permeability barrier in preventing deleterious plaque developing** agents like small dense cholesterol called sdLDL and apo B from seeping underneath the cells of the endothelium into the tissue of the subendothelial layer which is where the accumulation of plaque begins.
2. **It acts as an organ that balances clotting and bleeding.** The most important clotting factor is made by the endothelium and is called the Plasminogen Activator Inhibitor or PAI-1. There are other clotting factors that are called the Von Willebrand factor which is also produced by the endothelium. These clotting properties are offset by other proteins produced by the endothelium that cause bleeding and do the intricate stabilizing act. These include tPA (Tissue Plasminogen Activator), APC (Activated

Protein C), EPCR (Endothelial Protein C receptor), PAR (Protease-activated receptor) and TF (Tissue Factor)

3. **The endothelium also balances the narrowing and dilatation of the blood vessels.** Narrowing also called "vasoconstriction" is also caused by an agent called angiotensin. Endothelin is also another vasoconstrictor produced by the endothelium and balanced by the release of vasodilating agents to maintain its integrity. As for vasodilators, the most important one in the body is called endothelium-derived nitric oxide which maintains stability.
4. Another function is **the balancing act of blood force within the blood vessels** called transduction or buffering. The endothelium acts a transducer of the biomechanical forces inside the blood vessel to prevent shear stress from rupturing the plaque that develops inside the blood vessels.
5. Another function is **the production of cytokines and neurohormones which maintains balance.** There are good and bad cytokines which are constantly in a state of flux. This dynamic activity needs a steady poise and equilibrium that is maintained by the endothelium.

Overall, the main function of the endothelium is to protect the main organs in the body from injury as endothelial vascular injury can lead to the accumulation of lipids, inflammatory markers, the proliferation of fibrous tissue, and smooth muscle, all of which can be harmful in the long run. The initial lesion of atherosclerosis is called a fatty streak which is found in all ages and sexes and found in the same location in arteries in children where the plaque is found in adults. The fatty streak is predominantly found in one cell type called lipid-laden macrophages which contains cholesterol droplets. The microscopic appearance looks like a foam cell. Smooth muscles are dispersed around these macrophages. The fatty streak will expand slowly, and smooth muscle can accumulate at the side of the streak and slowly increase lymphocytes which are part of the defense mechanism called white blood cells. As the plaque develops, there is an increase in the amount of fatty tissue around the connective tissue forming fiber cap which is usually thin and vulnerable to rupture.

Coronary thrombosis or clotting occurs due to rupture of the plaque and it is indeed platelet-rich which can quickly block off blood vessels. The endothelium plays a role in defense and prevention of acute and chronic communicable and non-communicable diseases in the body. Even in subjects with an infection such as pneumonia, urinary tract infection or sepsis or even any form of cancer, endothelium becomes precipitously dysfunctional. So, anything that causes endothelial dysfunction can lead to disease state and complications thereof. CVD risk factors such as high cholesterol, uncontrolled blood pressure or diabetes, smoking, obesity, stress, genetic predisposition, lack of physical activity, unhealthy eating habits with high fat and carbohydrate consumption can lead to inflammation, release oxidized free radicals, cause vasoconstriction, increase clotting tendency, release bad cytokines and increase shear forces to cause plaque instability and plaque rupture causing heart attacks/ strokes and other complications.

In patients with blocked arteries, there is a significant reduction of blood flow to multiple portions of the heart muscle. In subjects with atherosclerotic plaque, which may build over time, sometimes in the large arteries and many times in the small arteries supplying the myocardium. These small arteries are not visible in a coronary angiogram. Large coronary arteries may not be blocked but small vessels may have atherosclerotic plaque which may decrease blood flow to the heart muscle causing the cardiac myocytes to decrease in number and density. The surrounding area will be taken over by collagen or smooth muscle tissue which will not have any contractile reserve. These effects can translate to a reduction in ejection fraction and congestive heart failure will ensue. This is specifically called ischemic cardiomyopathy.

If large coronaries are affected with blockage more than 70% of the circumference of the blood vessels, then they may need angioplasty and stent placement, or bypass surgery to increase blood flow, and to increase the quality of life, functional capacity, and survival. If small vessels are narrowed, medical management is the best option along with lifestyle modifications. Hence knowledge about the endothelium is extremely important. When the above message is taken in the context of all disease states, we now believe that a functional endothelium is essential to maintain homeostasis, hemostasis and prevent thrombosis. Thus, a greater understanding of the role of the endothelium can provide new avenues for exploration and novel therapies for the management of both communicable and non-communicable risks and disease states.

CHAPTER 13

Obesity and Heart Failure

WATCH NOW

Obesity is becoming a global health problem. The association of obesity with high blood pressure, diabetes, metabolic syndrome, and sleep apnea is increasing cardiovascular risk. Obesity plays a significant role in the development of blocked arteries, atrial fibrillation, cardiac arrest. Data from WHO reveals a grave picture of the prevalence and morbidity of this disease. About 39% of the global population above the age of 18 seem to be overweight of which 13% seem to be obese. The definition of obesity is a body mass index of over 30. The relationship between atherosclerosis and obesity is significantly increasing.

The relationship between obesity and heart failure is a major cause of death globally with the prevalence being 3% in developed countries and correlation can be seen between heart failure and obesity in the Framingham Study as well.

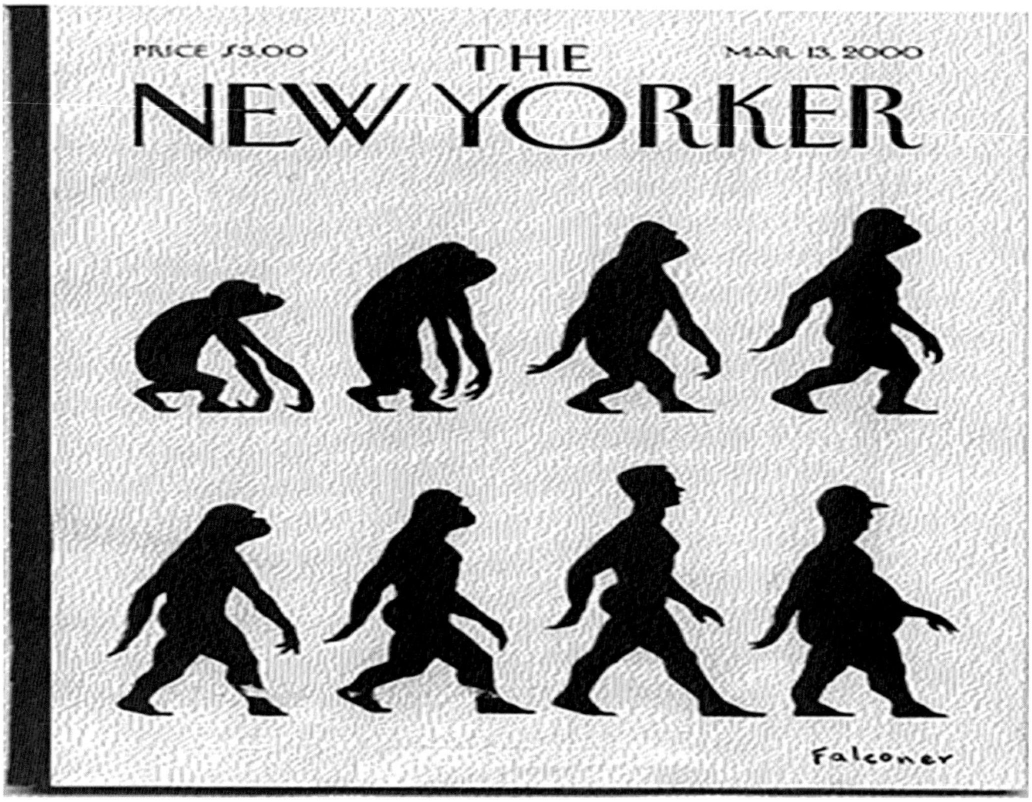

Fig. 13

Evolution of the origins of man started with Ramapethicus to Dryopithecus to Australopithecus, Homo Habilis, Homo Erectus, Homo Neanderthal and Homo Sapiens. Now it looks like we are on our way to a new species, probably apt to name it Homo-Obesiens!!!

Obesity leads to heart failure in both direct and indirect mechanisms. Excess weight leads to alterations in hemodynamics, an increase in blood pressure leading to an increase in neurohormone activation and thickening of the heart muscle. This, in turn, leads to problems with the relaxation of the heart muscle and heart failure follows. HFpEF seems to be a major player in patients with obesity.

Multiple clinical trials have shown alterations in neurohormones which lead to an increase in cardiac fibrosis, aggregation of platelets, and an increase in plaque genesis which may eventually cause occlusion. Endothelial dysfunction present in obese individuals can also lead to significant cardiac conditions and heart failure. Inflammation with an increase in interleukins, TFN-alpha, inflammatory mediators, toxic metabolites such as ceramides, diacylglycerol can render risk for the development of cardiomyopathy. Obesity can lead to cardiac arrhythmias with an increased risk of atrial fibrillation between ages 40-50.

Obese patients have over 1.5% more risk of developing atrial fibrillation as opposed to non-obese people. Structural and electrical remodeling of the heart occurs with obesity with alteration of the pulmonary venous system at the cellular level, myocyte level, and lipid accumulation. Obesity is linked to the development of type 2 diabetes and all the complications that occur with it. Newer treatment options are now available for obesity, hypertension, diabetes, beyond lifestyle modifications. Bariatric surgery significantly improves cardiac geometry, function, and symptoms related to obesity-related cardiomyopathy.

There is a consistently positive impact of bariatric surgery on diastolic function (relaxation problems/HFpEF) with the potential to significantly improve systolic function as well as measured by ejection fraction in patients with advanced heart failure. For end-stage heart failure patients, including those requiring mechanical circulatory support who are ineligible for organ transplant due to morbid obesity, bariatric surgery has been successfully used for weight loss as a bridge to cardiac transplantation.

I have known Dr. Vijay for more than 20 years as a colleague and friend. He is an exceptionally gifted physician who truly treats people, not diseases. He understands that treating body mind and soul with medical therapies that touch every facet of the human condition leads to the best possible outcomes. His medical life has been a relentless pursuit of both knowledge and wisdom that improves the lives of everyone he touches.

This book on heart disease and heart failure is a comprehensive approach to medicine that only Dr. Vijay has mastered. In lay terms it creates an awareness of an under recognized medical malady, while providing a rare insight into the multiple manifestations of this disease and its impact upon society.

I hope every physician who cares for patients, and every patient with a heart reads this book!

Joseph L Lillo, DO, FNLA, FAPCR, CPI
Board Certified in Family Practice
Board Certified in Clinical Lipidology
Immediate Past President,
Southwest Chapter, National Lipid Association

CHAPTER 14

Sleep Apnea

"All the adversity I've had in my life, all my troubles and obstacles, have strengthened me… You may not realize it when it happens, but a kick in the teeth may be the best thing in the world for you."

— Walt Disney

WATCH NOW

Patient Story

Mr. BG is a 62-year-old male who had problems with alcohol and hypertension. He continued to have uncontrolled hypertension despite multiple different medications. We felt alcohol was playing a role and he cut back on this. Yet, when BP was persistently high, we resorted to addressing possible sleep apnea as his underlying condition that was responsible for lack of BP control. He also had mild to moderate obesity, neck thickness, fatigue, and inability to lose weight, and was struggling to tolerate these medications. His ejection fraction was normal, the right side of the heart was moderately enlarged.

Other than that, he did not have any blocked arteries which pointed to sleep apnea as the possible cause of symptoms. He told me that he wanted to die as he was so distraught with sleep disturbance emotional distress. He was an engineer in Arizona for many years and now single, with no job, he was a mess. We decided to work on the core root cause of all of his problems: his weight. He was willing to work closely with frequent follow up to keep him engaged and not lose control of himself. He said he would put all his eggs in one basket and work closely with me and his PCP and pulmonologist. He then went through a weight loss program by being a vegan and lost weight with the supervision of a physician-driven and monitored weight loss program.

He developed a philosophy of improving his diet and performed exercise at a specialized physical therapy unit where he started getting better from his spondylolisthesis on his back. He did get some shots in his back which helped the pain. He started feeling better with weight reduction with his new diet that gave him more strength. He followed up with sleep apnea specialists and surgeons where he underwent adenoidectomy, CPAP and BiPAP, drugs, devices which he did not tolerate or help him. He was then sent to an ENT surgeon for a pacemaker-like device with a wire that connects to the glossopharyngeal nerve which attaches to the hypoglossal muscle and with more contraction of this muscle, more air opens up.

> Sleep apnea is an important topic that is not discussed enough with patients who have heart disease or heart failure. There is a significant amount of comorbidity associated with sleep apnea in subjects with heart failure. There is a huge economic cost associated with this due to increased morbidity and mortality as well as increased hospitalizations. Hence, identifying sleep apnea patients with heart failure is important.

He started to feel better and sleep better. With vegan diets, alcohol cessation, and medications, he was getting stimulated to live. He was not overwhelmed anymore and found a balance and drive to keep his mind occupied despite being stressed at first. BG is also a success story, although he did not have florid heart failure. He did have some right-sided dilatation because of sleep apnea. The treatment for the underlying root cause seemed to help his diminished functional capacity. Hence the lesson that we learned is that the heart is not always the issue and we as healthcare providers have to open our minds to unravel other underlying reasons. I believe that multimodality treatment strategies with coordinated care can make a huge difference in our patient's lives

Sleep Apnea and Heart Failure

Sleep apnea is an important topic that is not discussed enough with patients who have heart disease or heart failure. There is a significant amount of comorbidity associated with sleep apnea in subjects with heart failure. There is a huge economic cost associated with this due to increased morbidity and mortality as well as increased hospitalizations. Hence, identifying sleep apnea patients with heart failure is important. This chapter will discuss the type of sleep apnea, overlapping symptoms of heart failure and sleep apnea, neurohormonal and pathophysiological basis, impact, and treatment strategy.

Did you know that 50% of patients with heart failure (either heart failure with reduced ejection fraction or heart failure with preserved ejection fraction) have sleep apnea? There are two types of sleep apnea: central sleep apnea and obstructive sleep apnea. a) In Central sleep apnea, there is a temporary failure of an area in the brain between the pons and the medulla which is the pacemaker for the brain that dictates breathing patterns. Hence, with this form of sleep apnea, the brain activity is impaired and the nerves which innervate the diaphragm and intercostal muscles that arise out of this brain stem area are not active. This triggers the absence of nasal oral airflow and affects the normal excursion of breathing between the chest and the abdomen causing abnormal thoracoabdominal breathing.

This condition can lead to the retention of carbon dioxide and low oxygenation. Central sleep apnea is rare but can be present in some people with a stroke in the brainstem as well. b) Obstructive sleep apnea is due to obstruction of oral airways. Hypoglossal nerve and genioglossus muscles are controlling the activities of the tongue. Normally during sleep, this muscle activity is reduced and during inspiration, negative airway pressure is created, and the tongue falls backward and results in normal breathing. In patients who are susceptible to sleep apnea, tongue falling backward can result in airway closure which leads to obstructive sleep apnea. Obesity is a major risk factor due to high-fat deposits in the pharynx. Heart failure patients with obstructive sleep apnea are usually obese and have excessive snoring.

Many times, it is difficult to tease out who has sleep apnea and who has heart failure if they have not been diagnosed with heart failure, to begin with. Many of the patients with sleep apnea usually have nocturia, orthopnea, paroxysmal nocturnal dyspnea, or wake up in the middle of the night with shortness of breath. Similarly, patients with sleep apnea without heart failure also have frequent waking and symptoms similar to heart failure. Hence, it is important to specifically identify which condition they have. Due to lack of sleep, they have a lack of energy during the day and functional capacity diminishes as well.

Because of a lack of oxygenation, the partial pressure of oxygen called PO2 decreases, and the reduction of oxygen to tissues can lead to organ failure. Due to this lack of oxygen, there is an alteration of the inner lining of the blood vessel which leads to vasoconstriction of the blood vessels and increases the potential for clotting and inflammation. Due to the decrease in oxygen levels, there is an increase in carbon dioxide levels that can trigger vasoconstriction of the blood vessel leading to pulmonary hypertension. This can cause increased right ventricular load and right-sided heart failure. There is a sympathetic nervous system activation that leads to adrenaline or catecholamine release which instigates an increase in blood pressure and heart rate. There is parasympathetic withdrawal which leads to increased heart rate as well. Also, the increase in pressure in the ventricles and pulmonary vascular bed can lead to alteration in the shape and geometry of the right ventricle producing RV volume overload and heart failure. Sleep apnea is also associated with daytime sleepiness, which increases the risk of motor vehicle accidents and depression. Other complications include high blood pressure (hypertension), stroke, heart attack, diabetes, gastroesophageal reflux disease, nocturnal angina, hypothyroidism, atrial fibrillation, rhythm abnormalities secondary to increased catecholamine drive, heart rate variability, increased sympathetic activities which lead to decreased functional capacity.

Mechanism of Heart failure and complications in sleep apnea:

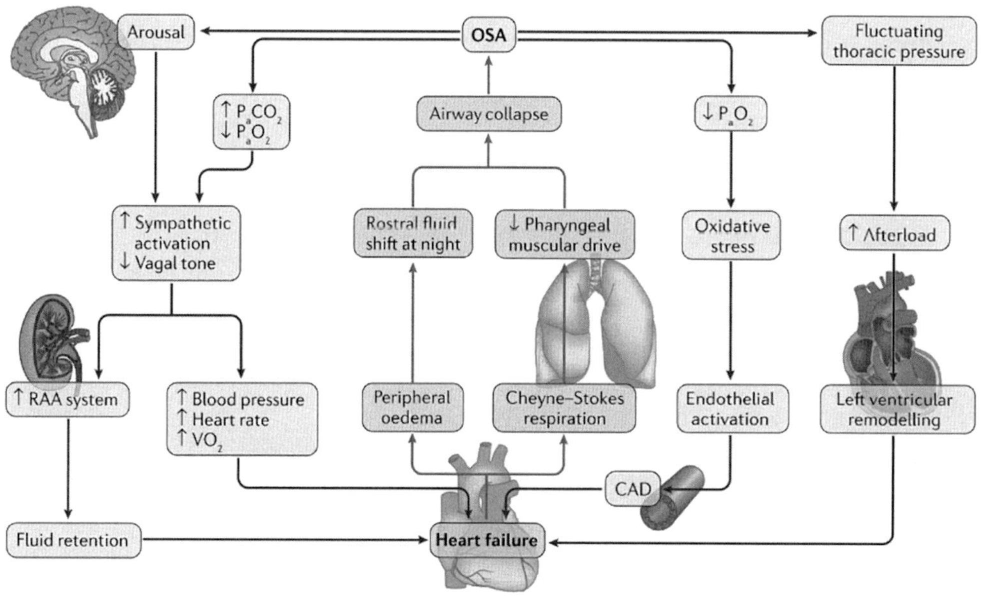

Fig. 14

Latest Treatments for OSA:
Standard treatments for OSA: Positive Airway Pressure Therapy

Positive airway pressure machines, used with a variety of breathing masks, are the most widely used treatment for moderate and severe sleep apnea. The mask, worn snugly over the nose, or sometimes nose and mouth, during sleep, supplies pressurized air that flows continuously or intermittently into the sleeper's throat. The increased air pressure prevents the sleeper's airway from collapsing. The pressurized air is supplied through a flexible tube from one of several types of machines: CPAP (continuous positive airway pressure), BiPAP (bilevel positive airway pressure), VPAP (variable positive airway pressure), and so on.

Studies of the effect of PAP therapy show that people with sleep apnea who consistently use their machines feel better and, as a result of the reduction of apnea and hypopnea episodes during sleep, (Apnea-Hypopnea Index: AHI) encounter fewer complications of the disease. Although PAP devices are not used to treat snoring alone, they do eliminate snoring in addition to treating obstructive sleep apnea.

Oral Appliances

Oral appliances for the treatment of sleep apnea continue to increase in popularity as awareness grows amongst the public that oral appliances are an effective first-line treatment for many sleep apnea sufferers. Over 100 different oral appliances are FDA approved for the treatment of snoring and obstructive sleep apnea. These appliances are worn in the mouth while you sleep. They are just like a sports mouthguard or an orthodontic appliance that holds the lower jaw forward just enough to keep the airway open and prevent the tongue and muscles in the upper airway from collapsing and blocking the airway.

The American Academy of Sleep Medicine (AASM) has approved oral appliance therapy (OAT) as a first-line treatment for patients diagnosed with mild to moderate OSA. The AASM also recommends oral appliances for patients with severe OSA, who are unable to tolerate or cannot wear CPAP devices. Another option for people with severe OSA is combination therapy (wearing CPAP and an oral appliance together) to help reduce the pressure on a CPAP machine, making it more comfortable to use. Some of the oral appliances include MyTAP, TAP 3 Elite, ApneaRx, OASYS Hinge Appliance, and OASYS with Option for Combination Therapy.

Oral appliance therapy is an effective, non-invasive treatment that fits easily into a patient's lifestyle. They are more comfortable, easy to wear, quiet, portable, convenient for travel, and easy to care for. Although there are a few over-the-counter appliances one can purchase at drug stores or even online, remember that these oral appliances are not FDA approved for sleep apnea. When they are not fitted properly, these OTC over-the-counter devices can cause unwanted side effects, such as jaw problems or tooth movement, or can even have the opposite effect and worsen sleep apnea. If a patient has symptoms of shortness of breath, fatigue when waking up, snoring at night and fluid retention, they could have heart failure, and sleep apnea may be the underlying cause. They should contact their primary care physician to refer to a sleep study center and perhaps to a cardiologist to determine if they have OSA or heart failure or both.

Behavioral Treatments

For milder forms of OSA, changes to lifestyle and sleep habits can help. For example, losing weight is known to improve OSA, as is limiting the consumption of alcohol and sedatives. If someone experiences snoring when sleeping on their back, some positioners will help maintain a side sleeping position, to improve breathing and promote continuous, healthy sleep.

Hypoglossal Nerve Stimulation: A relatively new advancement (approved by the FDA in 2014), hypoglossus nerve stimulation (HNS) is a small device, surgically implanted in the chest, and can be turned on and off by the patient. While the patient sleeps, the device monitors the breathing and stimulates a nerve that keeps the upper airway open. Initial research has shown that HNS improved patients' sleep apnea symptoms, and had few side effects and good compliance. This therapy is indicated in moderate to severe obstructive sleep apnea who are not helped by CPAP or BIPAP therapy.

Expiratory Positive Airway Pressure (EPAP): The EPAP system uses disposable adhesive valves that are placed over the nose when patients sleep. During inhalation, the valve opens and helps the airway to remain unobstructed. When one exhales, the airflow is directed into small channels, which creates pressure and, again, keeps the airways open. Open airways mean fewer incidences of obstructed breathing and interruptions in sleep. Initial research has shown EPAP therapy has a high level of adherence.

Medications:

Sometimes individuals with treated sleep apnea still experience excessive daytime sleepiness (EDS), a chronic condition, and need help with improving wakefulness. A new generation of medications more specifically targeted to treat EDS cases may be available. Nasal decongestants are more likely to be effective in cases of snoring or mild sleep apnea. More recent medications such as acetazolamide may reduce carbon dioxide retention, beta-blockers may reduce catecholamine drive and improve function/longevity, if heart failure is present concomitantly, management of fluid retention, and neurohormonal blockage for improvement in survival, reduction of fluid/sodium intake is beneficial.

Abstinence from alcohol before bedtime is an important part of treating sleep apnea. The presence of sleep apnea presents special challenges to the administration of anesthesia and pain medications that may affect respiration or relax muscles. Since most people who have sleep apnea do not know it, the anesthesiologist or pain clinician is well advised to screen the patient for OSA before proceeding. Should it be determined there is a likelihood that OSA is present, the next move is to order a sleep study to make sure or, at a minimum, to take the precautionary steps that should be taken with a patient whose sleep apnea has been diagnosed.

Surgical interventions: Surgery may be indicated if one has facial abnormalities that contribute to OSA and the anatomy of each person's upper airway and the type of surgery may need to be discussed. For severely overweight or obese patients, bariatric surgery may be considered as part of the treatment strategy for weight loss, which is tied to OSA symptoms Some patients benefit from pacemaker implantation if they have AV node dysfunction. Surgical treatment such as relieving the anatomical obstruction such as septoplasty, tonsillectomy, turbinate modification, correction of hypoglossal nerve (pacemaker of hypoglossal muscles), Uvulopalatopharyngoplasty (UPPP), and phrenic nerve stimulation have shown variable success.

Heart failure patients will feel better, happier, and safer after reading this book. Dr. Kris Vijay has shared his 40 years of clinical experience in an elegant but easy language. This book will take patient's fear away by clearing a lot of misconceptions about heart failure and will help in prevention and recovery from heart diseases. An invaluable comprehensive guide for the patients with heart failure. This book is a must read for all the heart failure patients and non-medical community.

Dr. Perminder Sanghera MD, FACP
Associate Program Director, Abrazo Internal Medicine Residency Program
Clinical Assistant Professor of Medicine,
University of Arizona, College of Medicine – Phoenix

CHAPTER 15

Cardiorenal Syndrome

> *"You may not be able to change the direction of the wind,*
> *but you can adjust the sails to always reach your destination."*
>
> **– Jimmy Dean**

WATCH NOW

Patient Story

RK is a 52-year-old male who had presented with kidney failure and his creatinine was 5.6 and eGFR had gone down to 15 with a normal level being over 90. He was not passing enough urine which he attributed to worsening diabetes management as he was unable to tolerate many medications and had side effects to which his a1c was 11. He clearly had diabetic kidney disease with worsening kidney disease. However, when we saw him in the hospital, he was dehydrated and we gave him fluid and tried to see if we could salvage his kidneys without dialysis, however, his renal function did not improve. His potassium went up to 6.8 (normal is less than 5) which warranted nephrology evaluation and he was placed on dialysis. What has been interesting was that after undergoing dialysis for 3 days, his kidneys began to open up and started to have decent urine output. Hence, dialysis was stopped, and we began to hydrate him and administer diabetic medications and insulin in the hospital.

In addition, he had heart failure and was symptomatic of diastolic heart failure (HFpEF). His left ventricular cavity was smaller, and his cardiac output was low despite normal ejection fraction which goes to show that heart and kidneys were connected and the cardiometabolic renal syndrome he was facing was real. One system is interconnected with the other in a vicious cycle. Once we started correcting his fluid status, diabetes status, heart failure, blood pressure, and renal function, he started to improve. He also has sleep apnea and morbid obesity at 280 pounds. His uric acid levels were high, and his blood acid levels were high as his sodium bicarbonate levels were low. When we saw all of this, we knew that RK was in deep trouble although he was young and did not qualify for a heart transplant because his heart pump was normal or kidney transplants because his renal function improved with his eGFR going up to 34 and 46 within a short period of time.

> We were humbled and grateful for the patient to follow the recommended therapies and the ability to use newer therapies. Hence, the patient decided to change the perception of the cardiorenal syndrome and become a pioneer in blazing a trail in managing this disease.
>
> He had a longing to heal, and with his monumental wherewithal and drive for finding his own calling, he started to heal. The lesson we can learn from RK is that the trifecta between the heart, diabetes, and kidneys are real and that we were cognizant of the agents used to impact the kidneys favorably. He has allowed us to research on therapies that help in this triple threat disease state.

His blood sugar levels were better controlled with SGLT2 inhibitors and GLP1 agonists. These are 2 groups of agents for diabetes and now approved to reduce the risk of cardiovascular events.

We have learned that even with low GFR, we can manage fluids, acidosis, bone metabolism, uric acid elevation, inflammatory response, and with judicious use of antidiabetic agents and heart failure agents with close monitoring, we can have a successful outcome. We are thankful to RK for helping us study this condition with his drive and passion.

Cardiorenal Syndrome

More than 10 years ago, the cardiorenal syndrome was coined by Dr. Claudio Ronco who hails from a small town in Italy called Vicenza more than 10 years ago. Since then more people have identified connections between the kidneys and heart more thoroughly. This chapter will discuss the relationship, risk factors, classification, epidemiology, physiology, the biology of the disease process, mediators, diagnostics, and therapeutics of cardiorenal syndrome.

The heart and kidneys are responsible for maintaining hemodynamic stability. Perfusion of organs, cardiac output, volume status, and tone of blood vessels are important in ascertaining such stability. Connections between these two organs show that physiological change of one system is tempered by compensation of the other organs. Hence, hemodynamic control, neurohormonal activity, vascular tone, cardiac output, and cardiac contractile reserve are all some of the important factors in improving heart and kidney health.

The cardiorenal syndrome itself is a terminology used where acute or chronic dysfunction of one organ can affect the function of the other. Since the two organs are connected at multiple levels, a definition of the cardiorenal syndrome was described by Dr. Ronco more than 10 years ago. The following is a classification that serves to identify the interaction. Type 1 is a condition called "acute cardiorenal syndrome" or abrupt worsening of heart function leading to acute kidney injury.

An example of this condition is acute decompensation of heart failure leading to acute cardiogenic shock. Type 2 cardiorenal syndrome is a chronic abnormality of heart function leading to the progression of kidney damage. An example would be chronic heart failure leading to chronic kidney damage. Type 3 cardiorenal is called acute renal cardiac syndrome where abrupt worsening of kidney function is an inciting event that leads to acute disorders such as heart failure, abnormal heart rhythm, pulmonary edema. An example of this would be acute kidney failure for different reasons such as hypertension, dye overload, toxic agents, kidney infection, renal artery blockage, blockage in the bladder in a retrograde fashion leading to heart failure.

Type 4 cardiorenal syndrome is chronic kidney disease such as glomerulonephritis/nephrotic syndrome, CKD and ESRD as an inciting event leading to decreased function, thickening of the heart muscle called hypertrophy or other adverse cardiovascular events. Type 5 cardiorenal syndrome is when the inciting event is a systemic condition such as lupus, an autoimmune condition or diabetes, or sepsis affecting kidneys and heart simultaneously. Risk factors for cardiorenal syndrome include older age, diabetes, uncontrolled hypertension, anemia, medications such as non-steroidal anti-inflammatory agents, chronic use of diuretics, heart failure with impaired ejection fraction, history of heart attack, cardiomyopathy, increased cardiac troponin, amyloidosis, sarcoidosis, kidney disease, and genetic disorders.

I have had 4 patients so far who have a genetic condition called Alport's syndrome. This is characterized by dilated cardiomyopathy, congenital deafness, and kidney failure. Two of them are on dialysis now and have heart failure. One of them is awaiting a dual organ transplant of heart and kidney at the same time. When heart and kidneys fail in a young person, Alport's syndrome may be a potential underlying genetic abnormality. At present there are no genetic manipulation or gene therapy available, but genetic counseling is particularly important in this setting.

Heart failure affects about 2-3% of the population resulting in more than a million annual admissions in the United States. We do not have enough data around the world in terms of the prevalence of heart failure, but we know that more than $77 billion are spent in the United States for heart failure alone. If we add kidney injury to this complication, now the readmission rate to the hospital is significantly increased as well as mortality. There is clearly an opportunity to prevent kidney injury, end-stage renal disease, the onset of heart disease by preventing the onset of high blood pressure, diabetes, high cholesterol, obesity, smoking, and metabolic syndrome. There is also an opportunity to prevent heart attack and stroke and by preventing these, we can prevent heart failure, kidney disease, and heart disease as well as a cardiorenal syndrome.

If we are able to prevent worsening heart failure and kidney failure, we may be reducing the need for devices such as LVADs, Bi VADS, Heart Transplant, Dialysis as well as kidney transplant. This is indeed a great thing from a patient and family perspective. It will also reduce the overall cost of care and a societal financial burden since the taxpayer dollars are at work when Medicare and Medicaid are the payers for many of these patients. All these conditions are aligned in a linear fashion and from the perspective of management, there will be an opportunity to curb the inciting event itself.

The Underlying Physiology and Pathophysiology of Cardiorenal Axis

There are multiple different reasons behind the activation of the cardiorenal axis and the worsening of disease states leading to the cardiorenal syndrome. The first one includes low ejection fraction or reduced relaxation of the heart leading to under perfusion of the heart. This condition can result in reduced effective filling and when the perfusion pressure is reduced, then the tissues are not receiving an adequate supply of oxygen delivered to itself. One of the major organs that need to receive blood flow is the kidneys which are sensed by a tissue called macula densa and juxtaglomerular apparatus. These are the tissues inside the kidney that activates the renin-angiotensin-aldosterone system which is important in sodium and water regulation. Hence, if this system is affected negatively then improper sodium and water balance contribute to fluid overload. When this happens, other neurohormones such as norepinephrine gets stimulated which causes the heart rate to increase and blood pressure drops.

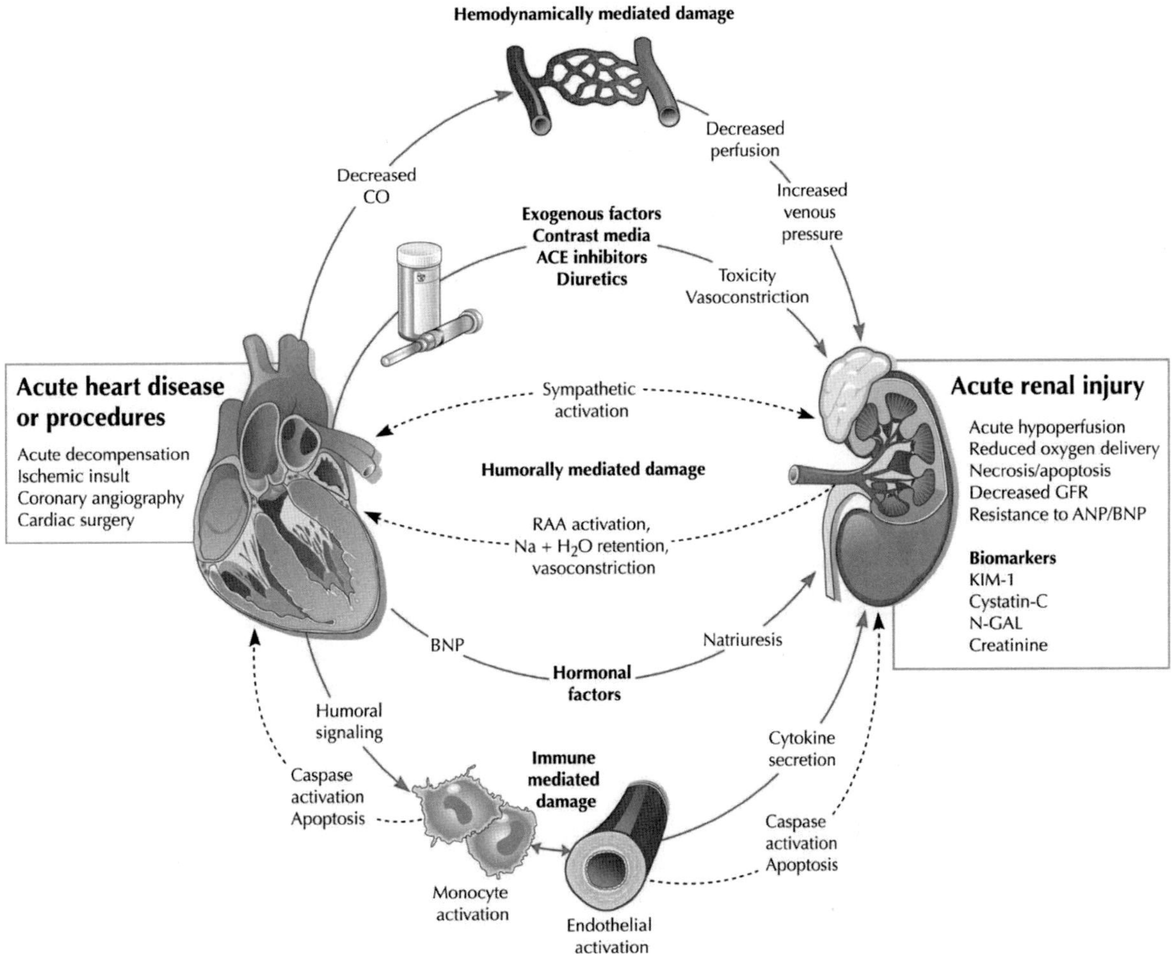

Fig. 15

There is a compensation mechanism of nitric oxide, prostaglandins, bradykinin but they may not be able to maintain adequate filtration in the kidney. This leads to progressive worsening of renal function. The reduced forward flow due to reduced pump function of the heart leads to a high-pressure system in the atrium which is connected to the pulmonic venous system and pulmonary capillary system. This pressure increase is transmitted to the right ventricle, right atrium, inferior vena cava. When the inferior vena cava pressure is high, the venous congestion increases, and the liver enlarges because of liver venous congestion.

The same thing happens in the kidneys with increased renal venous pressure leading to reduce function, filtration, and reduction in glomerular filtration rate (eGFR). The kidneys begin to choke with the high-pressure system, thus, distention of venules leading to compression of the tubules inside the kidney. This leads to a back leak of the filtrate outside of the tissues which translates to a significant amount of leg swelling, abdominal distention, shortness of breath, and fluid accumulation outside the lungs called pleural effusion. Intra-Abdominal Hypertension is another reason why the cardiorenal syndrome can get activated. The decline in kidney function due to increased intraabdominal pressure is related to venous congestion. Other mediators of the cardiorenal syndrome include neurohormones such as renin, angiotensin, aldosterone, and inhibition of nitric oxides, and natriuretic peptides.

The vicious cycle of decreased glomerular filtration with increasing spilling of the proteins increased venous congestion and decreased cardiac output can lead to impaired renal perfusion which in effect causes altered glomerular and tubular pressure system. This leads to injury to the inner lining of the blood vessels and reduced oxygen to the tissues and inflammation and a hyperactive healing process called fibrosis. This generates worsening fibrous tissue in the kidney and worsening kidney function, increased protein loss, and progressive damage to the kidney. In patients with acute decompensated heart failure in CRS type 1, management is particularly challenging.

The therapies that need to be used include diuretics, which may reduce fluid retention. The water has to be let out of the body through urine and if the kidneys are not working adequately, then this can lead to a vicious cycle of worsening kidney function. Hence, optimizing therapy using monitoring regularly in the ICU or hospital setting is incredibly important. Treatment with natriuretic peptides seems to have benefitted the kidney to some extent while protecting the heart pump function. Vasopressin antagonists have been utilized to protect the kidney. Inotropic support of the heart by pumping the heart better and utilizing diuretics to remove water may result in a reversal of cardiorenal syndrome in the short term. This can enable the use of life-saving medications in the long run. Ultrafiltration is another modality of therapy that can remove the fluid without affecting the electrolytes Newer therapies such as GLP-1 receptor agonists and SGLT2 inhibitors are showing benefits among patients with cardiorenal syndrome. More data will become available in the next year or two with use of these newer classes of agents in the cardiorenal space.

CHAPTER 16

Cardiomyopathy

"Champions realize that defeat – and learning from it even more than winning – is part of the path to mastery."

— Rasheed Ogunlaru

WATCH NOW

Patient Story

Mr. MQ is a 34-year-old male who had severe nonischemic cardiomyopathy with multiple hospitalizations, meth abuse with a low ejection fraction of 10%. He was told he had 6 months to live and have up in life. He had abused smoking, drugs, alcohol, and substances over his life and had more recently resorted to meth use. His story is that of so many patients in our community who have gotten lost in their quest for life's meaning and purpose. They have resorted to personal happiness as the main goal in the bargain, not realizing that the agents they use to make themselves happy have also contributed to significant physical damage.

The mechanics behind the surface of our bodies is fascinating. When we have mental or physical trauma as a child we suddenly have to deal with that suffering. Either we must put up with it or escape it. The fragmented mind cannot be put together because it is now more like Humpty dumpty. When these patients put up with it or fix it, they resort to various nutritional interventions and eastern philosophical concepts such as yoga, which may succeed or fail. Then, they will realize that the physical contortionist construct is not a normal way of respecting your body. The mind is truly a phenomenal organ that can allow the consciousness to meet the body where the mind, body, and spirit can be aligned on a continuum.

The brain can empower one to reach their own inner healer who understands the hidden meaning, and the value of their existence. The destination of happiness is not just a pleasure principle but an experience of their own essential being and to be in harmony with their own inner therapist. Once this concept is instilled in somebody's mind, they are educated in what this substance abuse can do to their physical structure. Once the body starts to hurt and reacts to a weakened heart in ways one has not experienced before, then they realize that perhaps there is a different way, a different path out of this jungle, and seek a light source for guidance to get out of the darkness.

> At the outset of the treatment program, he was told by other doctors and ER physicians that he had 6 months to live. And now, 2 years later to believe he has normalized his heart function is a blessing from above and he realizes how fortunate he is to have had this extra time. He has now started a new company that is successfully growing with energized employees who are amazed at his resilience and positive attitude about life.

One has to feel that there is hope and that their heart will get stronger and they will start to feel better. However, this can only be done with a support system including a team of healers from the healthcare team and family and friends. There is an opportunity for the care team to empathize with patients who have gone through a lot of trauma and have gotten lost in this maze. Once the patient and the care team are willing to participate, then improvement will come. MQ was a patient who also allowed himself to open up by quitting meth and followed a set of self-styled rules involving compliance with therapy. He needed short term medications to get his blood pressure up to enable the use of life-saving medications. He promised to not abuse his PICC line and comply with his oral therapy to improve his ejection fraction.

After 3 months, it was possible to initiate cardiac rehab when gradually exercise and muscle building was physically possible.

Ischemic cardiomyopathy is a type of disease affecting the heart muscle caused by a narrowing of the coronary arteries which supply blood to the heart. Typically, patients with ischemic cardiomyopathy have a history of acute heart attack however, it may occur in patients with coronary artery disease, but without a past history of acute heart attack, but partially blocked blood vessels. This cardiomyopathy is one of the leading causes of sudden cardiac death. When there is too little blood flow and lack of oxygen reaching the muscular layer of the heart due to a narrowing of coronary arteries, it can lead to cell death. This can cause different levels of tissue injury and affect large and intermediate arteries alike. Diagnosis is made by non-invasive tests like nuclear stress test, echocardiogram, and cardiac MRI. Treatment is to revascularize the heart muscle by angioplasty/ stents or bypass surgery.

Restoring adequate blood flow to the heart muscle in people with heart failure and significant coronary artery disease is strongly associated with improved survival, some research showing up to 75% survival rates over 5 years. A stem cell study indicated that using autologous cardiac stem cells as a regenerative approach for the human heart (after a heart attack) has great potential.

American Heart Association practice guidelines recommend implantable cardioverter-defibrillator (ICD) use in those with ischemic cardiomyopathy (40 days post-MI) that are (NYHA) New York Heart Association functional class I. A LVEF measurement of less than 35% is often used as indication for a defibrillator.

Dilated cardiomyopathy is defined as a disease of the heart muscle secondary to many conditions without having any blocked arteries. A few of the conditions include dilated cardiomyopathy secondary to chemotherapeutic agents, HIV, viral, fungal, or bacterial infections or pneumonia which can cause the heart muscle to become damaged. In addition, alcohol or other substance abuse with methamphetamines, cocaine, heroin, and other combination of street drugs can be contributors. Dilated cardiomyopathy can be a contributor for ventricular arrhythmias which is usually secondary to multiple conditions.

Infiltrative diseases causing cardiomyopathy include amyloidosis, sarcoidosis, and hemochromatosis (deposition of iron in the heart muscle), which is associated with diabetes and liver dysfunction with extra iron deposits in the liver and heart muscle. Ferritin levels are high in this condition. Infiltrative cardiomyopathy later can become dilated over time if not adequately treated. If cardiomyopathy occurs around pregnancy, it is called peripartum cardiomyopathy. Dilated cardiomyopathy also can occur in other conditions such as muscular dystrophy, and atrial fibrillation.

Hypertrophic cardiomyopathy is a unique condition believed to be genetically mediated. It manifests as an increased atypical septal thickness on the left side of the ventricle or apical thickness. The thickening of the heart muscle itself can lead to obstruction of the flow of the left ventricle into the aorta. Left ventricular outflow tract obstruction becomes narrowed and the suction forces the mitral leaflet to be pulled into the left ventricular outflow tract and obstructing flow when the heart is trying to contract and send blood into the aorta. This obstructs the blood flow to all parts of the body including the brain. Because the door is closed while the blood is trying to get out, there can be a lack of blood flow to the brain which can cause someone to faint. Fainting can be associated with sudden cardiac arrest from ventricular tachycardia or fibrillation. In addition, there is abnormal relaxation of the ventricle and with the mitral valve open during systole or contraction of the left ventricle, blood gets regurgitated across this valve into the left atrium. An increase in left atrial pressure transmits to the pulmonic vein and fluid gets poured into the lungs causing flash pulmonary edema and acute heart failure. Treatment strategies for this condition include medical management with beta-blockers, sometimes pacemaker implantation, alcohol ablation of the septum to reduce the thickness, and create more opening of the LVOT, myomectomy, and at times implantable defibrillator to prevent sudden cardiac arrest.

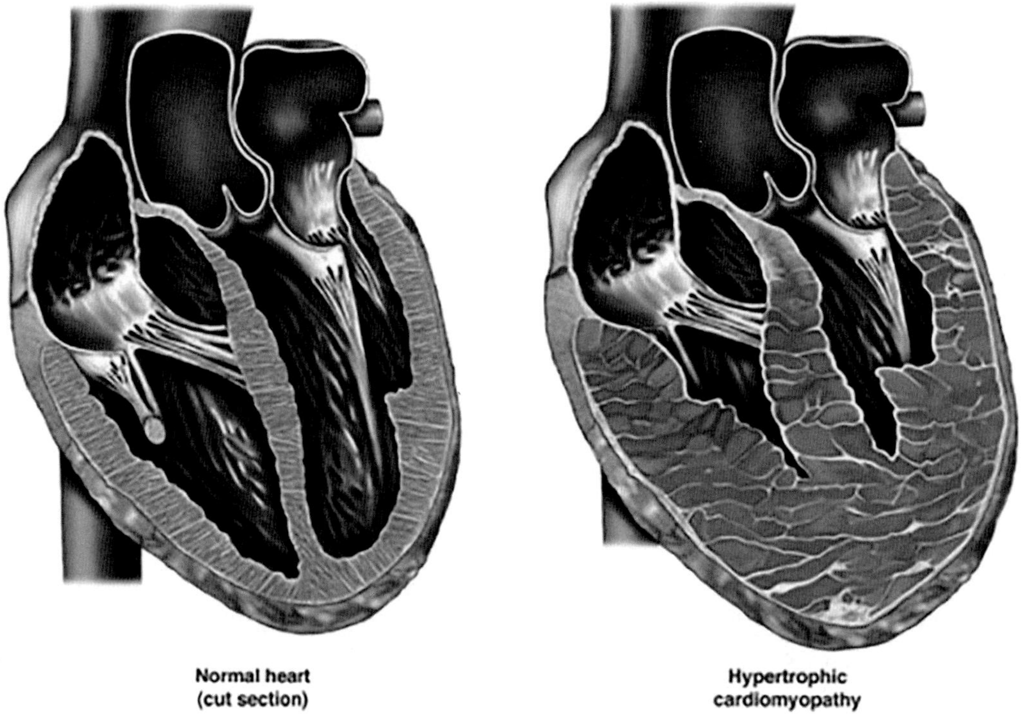

Fig. 16

Chemotherapy-induced cardiomyopathy is a common condition with the use of toxic agents such as doxorubicin or Adriamycin for breast cancer which is chemotherapy dose-dependent and one needs to be closely monitoring ejection fraction with echocardiography to ascertain if this medication is taking a toll on the heart. Treatment strategies for dilated cardiomyopathy are like any other condition that leads to heart failure with neurohormonal blocking agents, lifestyle modifications, fluid management, sodium control, dietary modifications. Sometimes, patients may need a Biventricular pacemaker, ventricular assist device, or even heart transplant.

This book is hard to put down! Engaging! A true gift to humanity! This book explores the connection between mind and body, health, and disease. It examines the power of our attitudes and outlook on healing. Dr. Vijay shares stories of growth and the journey to better health, which many of his patients have experienced. As a practicing cardiologist, he has impacted countless lives by treating the heart AND the mind! I am truly blessed to call Kris a colleague, mentor, and friend.

Kari Uusinarkaus, MD, FAAFP, FNLA, FASPC
Specialist in clinical hypertension and obesity medicine
Medical Director – Centura Health Physician Group, Pikes Peak Region, CO.

CHAPTER 17

Pericardial Effusion

WATCH NOW

Patient Story

A 22-year-old South Asian male was hospitalized when I saw him for the first time with fluid retention, shortness of breath, leg swelling, and was believed to have congestive heart failure. Hence, a cardiology consultation was requested. He mentioned that he was having low-grade temperatures at home with sweating daily over the past 6 months and unexplained weight loss. These symptoms made me believe that he could have tuberculosis. He had come to Arizona to study at Arizona State University. He mentioned that he had no family here and only a few friends since joining the school. The story itself was very classic from a tuberculosis standpoint, however, the fact that he was hospitalized for a cardiac condition did not make sense.

Hence, when we did an echocardiogram and he was found to have a large pericardial effusion and had to undergo pericardiocentesis and sent the fluid for testing. One of the important testing that we do includes the QuantiFERON Gold blood test assessment which came out positive and gave us a hint that he probably had tuberculous pericarditis. The fluid after a week or so came back positive for tuberculosis and we started treating him with multiple different anti-tuberculosis therapies. While we had to treat him for tuberculosis and wait, it was clear that in 8 weeks when he showed recurrence of his pericardial effusion, we had to perform more testing for this recurrence. We found something interesting when we dug deeper with Left and right heart invasive catheterization to assess pressures inside the heart.

We discovered he had equalization of pressures between the right and left side of the heart and a restrictive pattern of relaxation on the echo. This made us suspect constrictive pericarditis. Once we found that out and stabilized, a few weeks later he underwent pericardial resection or pericardiectomy. After anti-tuberculosis medications, he has improved markedly. His fluid retention in the legs and abdomen were a result of the venous return being impeded returning to the right side of the heart due to the compression from the pericardial fluid itself. His left side of the heart was normal and was making a full recovery with weight gain and performing well in school. He is very thankful for the treatment but we in turn are thankful for him allowing us to think outside the box.

A message from this experience is that when someone comes from another country, there are different variations to the theme in terms of the genetic basis for disease and environmental basis for disease. If someone comes in from Africa, one needs to think about some infectious diseases. If one comes from South Asia, one needs to think about tuberculosis as a potential etiology. Even in Africa, tuberculosis is increasing due to the higher prevalence of HIV and immunocompromised states are triggering other fungal, bacterial, and viral infections. Hence, he has taught us to be wary of infectious etiology, even from a heart failure perspective. So, we thank him for that.

Pericardial Disease

The pericardium is an organ that envelops the heart and contains two components: the visceral component which is the lining that surrounds the inner lining of the heart and the other is the parietal component which is the outer fibrous layer. In between the two, there is a certain amount of clear fluid which is about 25-50 cc which is believed to be a source of normal pericardial fluid and needed for the following two reasons: it protects the heart when the heart is in excessive motion with body position/exercise and it lubricates the heart and prevents friction between the heart and surrounding tissues and spread of infection and cancer. It has a significant hemodynamic impact on the atrium and ventricle on both sides of the heart but mostly on the right side. The normal pressure inside the pericardium is equal to the pressure in the pleural space which is also a space that is between the inner lining of the lungs. There are other functions of the pericardium which is about maintaining synchrony between the two ventricles. This interdependence is important when the pressure inside the heart muscle increases.

Acute pericarditis can occur with inflammation of the pericardium itself from possible virus infection, cancer, inflammation post-heart attack, inflammation after bypass surgery, autoimmune diseases like Dressler's syndrome, and post-cardiotomy syndrome. Sometimes fluid accumulates in the pericardial space leading to increased pressure and compression on the right side of the heart called tamponade which raises a need to remove fluid with catheter or other surgical techniques. Pericarditis can happen with infections, inflammation, virus infection, tuberculosis, HIV which may cause restrictive flow to the right side of the heart leading to heart failure. Respiratory variations occur frequently in this condition. Other diseases of the pericardium include radiation induce trauma to the pericardium causing pericarditis. Symptoms consist of chest pain with position and many times there are EKG changes in which the healthcare provider will be able to detect if there is possible pericarditis; however, this can sometimes be confused with a heart attack.

In terms of treatment for acute pericarditis, they include nonsteroidal anti-inflammatory agents or colchicine and rest. Sometimes steroids may be needed. Treatment for pericardial tamponade includes fluid removal, surgical intervention of stripping pericardium for constrictive pericarditis may alleviate symptoms and worsening of heart failure.

CHAPTER 18

Valvular Heart Disease

WATCH NOW

The most common valvular heart diseases include aortic valve stenosis, mitral valve stenosis, aortic valve regurgitation, mitral valve regurgitation, tricuspid valve regurgitation, and pulmonic valve regurgitation.

Aortic Stenosis

Aortic Stenosis is a disease where there is progressive calcification of the aortic valve leading to obstruction of the flow of blood from the left ventricle to the aorta cross a narrowed aortic valve. There are three different leaflets in the aortic valve. The most common reason

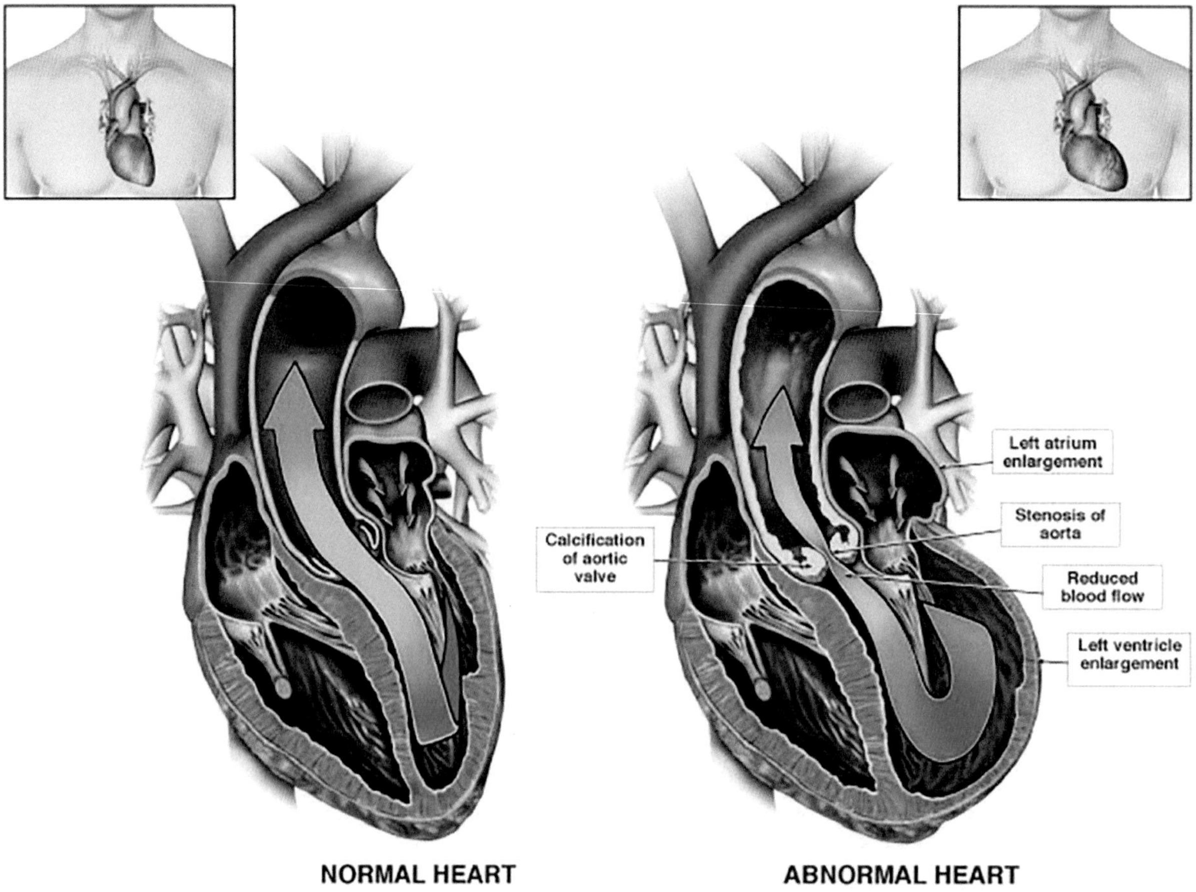

Fig. 17

why an aortic valve becomes stenosed is due to rheumatic valve disease or degenerative disease. There are 3 different types of aortic valve stenosis:

a. Supravalvular or above the area of the aortic valve which gets calcified and narrowed. This is usually a congenital abnormality and is associated with a congenital deformity when the child is born. Manifestations of this disease include elfin like facial appearance, high calcium level, and pulmonic valve stenosis in association with this type of supravalvular stenosis.
b. Sub valvular stenosis which is just below the valve. This is usually accompanied by an aortic valve leak or regurgitation. The most common cause of this stenosis usually is due to another genetic abnormality that should be differentiated between a dynamic outflow tract obstruction with hypertrophic obstructive cardiomyopathy.
c. The third type of stenosis is called valvular aortic stenosis which is caused by older age, rheumatic fever, and degenerative changes. Sometimes, severe aortic stenosis at a younger age is associated with high levels of Lp(a).

Due to the narrowing of the valve, the left ventricle must function harder, hence, the left ventricle becomes thicker and is called left ventricular hypertrophy. Because of this thickening, the pressure inside the left ventricle becomes higher. Because of the narrowing of the aortic valve, the blood pressure beyond the area of obstruction is lower. The differential pressure between the area above and below the aortic valve in the left ventricle can be significantly elevated. The more the gradient increases, the more symptoms are present. The more the narrowing of the valve, the higher the gradient. Hence, since the valvular narrowing and gradient are directly proportional, one needs to be aware of the symptoms that can develop because of narrowing.

These symptoms usually consist of shortness of breath, anginal symptoms, or passing out (syncope). One is at risk of ventricular tachycardia leading to cardiac arrest. Other complications occur because of abnormal relaxation of heart due to thickening called diastolic dysfunction which can lead to heart failure with preserved ejection fraction. Many patients have concomitant narrowing of coronary arteries and may cause a decreased supply of blood and an increase in demand and may also have reduced ejection fraction.

The way to diagnose aortic valve stenosis is to do testing if the patient has symptoms or a loud murmur is heard during a physical exam. The most common testing includes electrocardiograms and echo. The echocardiogram reveals the valve area and if the gradient is more than 50 mmHg across the aortic valve. If the valve area is less than 0.8 cm^2, it is deemed as critical and recommendations for valve replacement are usually made. Although some patients may be asymptomatic and may still have severe aortic valve stenosis, the healthcare provider may suggest valve replacement through surgical or transcatheter aortic valve replacement (TAVR). The reason for this is that when the aortic valve stenosis is severe, it is associated with a risk of ventricular tachycardia and sudden cardiac arrest. Hence, most cardiologists will recommend valve replacement.

Mitral Valve Stenosis

Mitral Stenosis is the narrowing of the mitral valve due to the thickening of the leaflets and the fusion of the commissures that are holding the mitral valve in position. The calcification can be seen in patients with a history of rheumatic valve disease, but most of the time in older people, the calcification can be due to degenerative changes. When the mitral valve area is less than 1 cm^2 it is severe, 1-1.5 is moderate, more than 1.5 is mild and more than 2 cm^2 is normal. When the gradient (difference in pressure) across the mitral valve increases to more than 10 mm, then it is severe, and patients become symptomatic.

These symptoms can be associated with heart failure symptoms because valve narrowing translates to an increase in the size of the left atrium. The left atrium is attached to the pulmonary veins and with increased pulmonary venous pressure one can pour fluid into the lungs and cause pulmonary edema. Hence, the treatment strategy for mitral valve stenosis

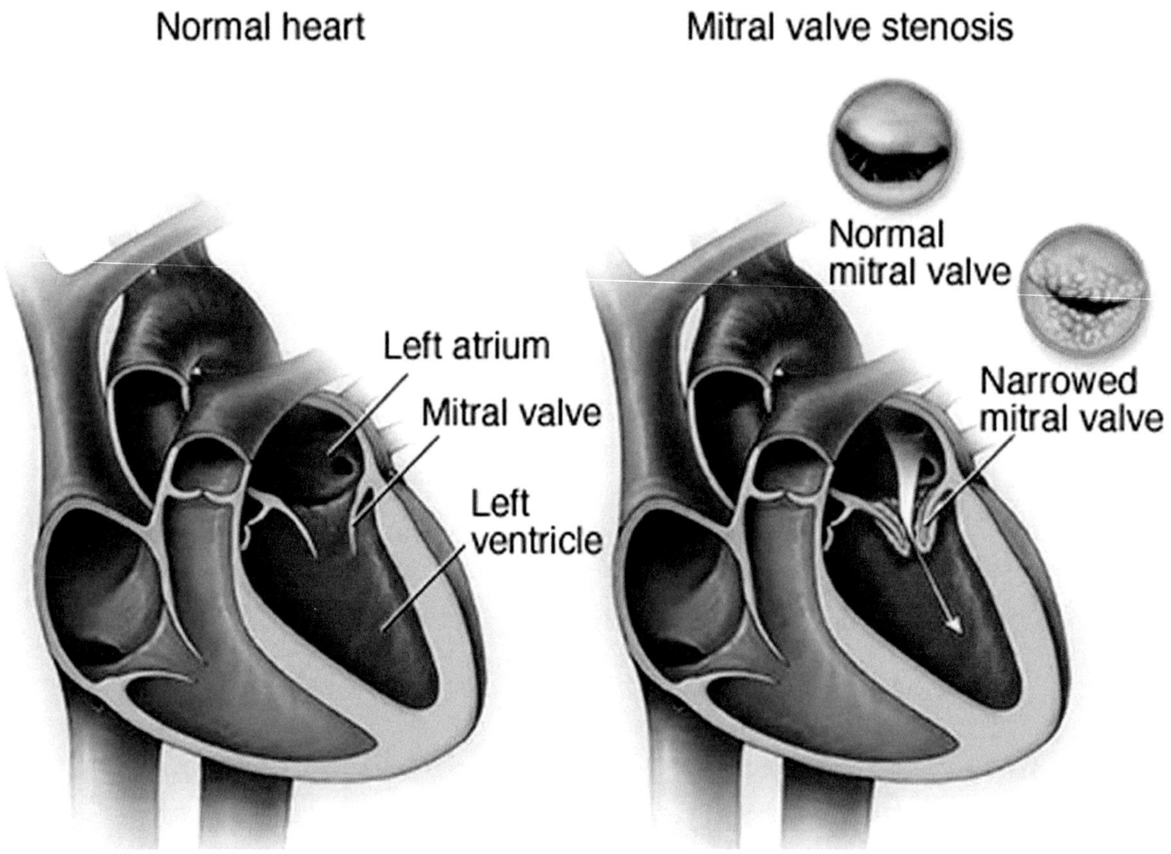

Fig. 18

is surgical intervention. At present, there is a mitral valve replacement that is being studied with a transcatheter approach. There are transcatheter approaches to opening the mitral valves called balloon valvuloplasty which seems to be successful in a subset of patients to suppress symptoms. Most of the time they will need surgical intervention.

Mitral Valvular Regurgitation

Mitral Regurgitation is the leakiness of the valve with blood flowing into the left atrium from the left ventricle when the valve is closed when all the blood ought to be squeezed into the aorta across the aortic valve. There are 3 different mechanisms of mitral valve regurgitation. The first one alters the anatomy of the leaflet itself or the ring of the mitral valve becomes abnormal and calcified. The apposition of the valve leaflets may not be adequate and there is leakiness of the mitral valve. Also, in some patients who have dilated cardiomyopathy with enlargement of the left ventricle the valve can get pulled apart and lead to malposition of the valve leaflets leading to valvular regurgitation. Another reason for mitral regurgitation is degeneration, or infection of the leaflets called endocarditis, rupture of the infrastructure of the valve called chordae which are holding the mitral valve

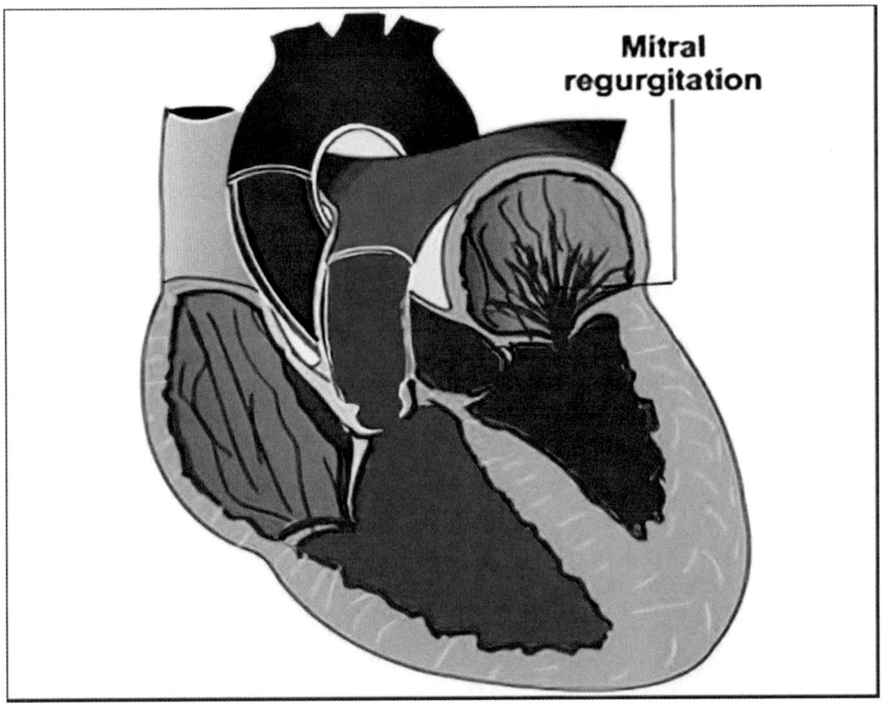

Fig. 19

in position. Any rupture secondary to a heart attack or lack of blood flow can also lead to defective apparatus and cause leakiness.

The leakiness is not outside the heart, but it is in between two chambers of the heart. This mitral regurgitation, if severe, can cause shortness of breath due to increased volume and pressure in the left atrium, pulmonic veins, and into the lung tissue triggering pulmonary edema. Other patients develop enlargement of left atrium and ventricle as well as right ventricle and right atrium gradually, thereby become fatigued, winded, get pulmonary hypertension, and other heart failure symptoms. Treatment for this condition is surgical requiring repair of the mitral leaflets, or mitral valve ring or replacement of the mitral valve. More recently, transcatheter approaches are now approved for mitral clip placement without opening the chest cavity. There is a clinical trial called TMVR or transcatheter mitral valve replacement that is currently being evaluated to replace procedures that include opening the sternum.

Aortic Regurgitation:

Leakiness of the aortic valve happens when this valve is closed and the blood from the aorta goes back into the left ventricle during relaxation of the heart. During relaxation of the heart, the aortic valve remains closed and blood from the left atrium is pouring into the left ventricle with the mitral valve being open. The reasons for aortic valve leak include endocarditis, rheumatic fever, collagen vascular disease, Marfan's syndrome, congenital aortic valve

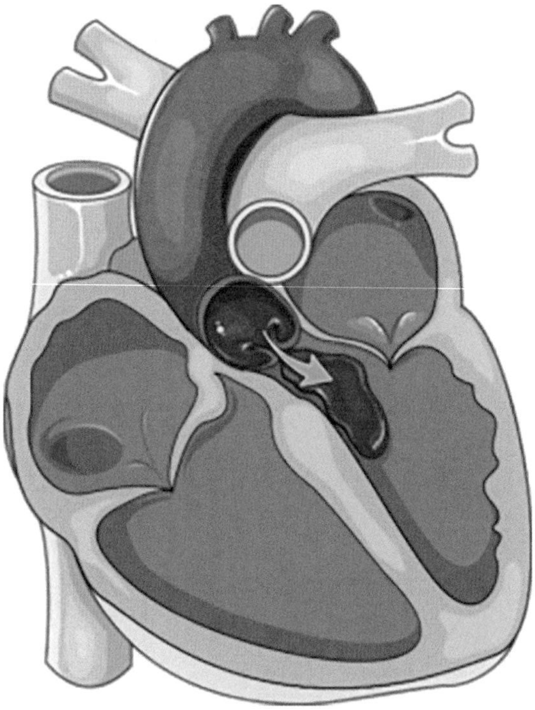

Fig. 20

leak, and diseases of the ascending aorta such as an aneurysm or dissection of the aorta. Acutely, if aortic regurgitant murmur is heard in someone with chest pain/mid back pain stabbing in nature, one must suspect aortic dissection. It may need urgent surgical intervention. In chronic aortic regurgitation, the symptoms are usually secondary to heart failure because of increased volume and pressure load of the left ventricle. This can lead to dilatation of the left ventricle and the pump can get weaker as well. Patients present with increased shortness of breath and progressively can have decreased functional capacity with reduced exercise time.

There are a few parameters that can be assessed with echocardiography which can help the cardiologist determine the severity of leakiness. This is based on regurgitant volume, regurgitant fraction, aortic valve Doppler assessment, assessment of the volume of the left ventricle at the end of relaxation/contraction. If the diameter increases, then it can indicate that the aortic valve is becoming abnormal. Treatment for aortic valve regurgitation is usually surgical such as aortic valve replacement which is a procedure that is commonly used today as the transcatheter option is not used for regurgitation; it is only used for stenosis. Maybe with the advancement of science, we may be able to predict that even transcatheter aortic valve replacement for leakiness may be available over the next few years.

Tricuspid valve regurgitation is not an uncommon condition where the blood is leaking back into the right atrium from the right ventricle when the tricuspid valve is closed when all the blood ought to be squeezed into the pulmonary artery across the open pulmonic valve. It can happen due to the dilation of the right ventricle and tricuspid annulus. Right heart failure is a common cause of TR and RHF is most likely due to left heart failure. Most of the time, we believe that is a defensive mechanism of right-sided heart failure that the leakiness can be a good thing if mild or moderate. Hence, we usually leave it alone and assume that tricuspid regurgitation is more of a functional etiology rather than an anatomical deformity that needs correction. In the past, we have not corrected this condition surgically or via a transcatheter approach. Other reasons for acquired tricuspid valve regurgitation include rheumatic fever, endocarditis, carcinoid syndrome, pacemaker wire, lupus, rheumatoid arthritis, tumors, and trauma. The symptoms of tricuspid regurgitation are shortness of breath, fatigue, abdominal distention, and leg swelling. If severe and symptoms are not controllable with medical management, then surgical intervention may be needed. More recently, a clinical trial called "TRILUMINATE" is evaluating transcatheter valve replacement in severe tricuspid regurgitation.

Pulmonary regurgitation is leakiness across the pulmonic valve from the pulmonary artery into the right ventricle when the pulmonic valve is closed. It is usually present on doppler echo when recognized but does not usually cause symptoms. It is due to a high-pressure system in the pulmonary artery called pulmonary hypertension. It is rarely secondary to rheumatic heart disease, endocarditis, an infection of the pulmonic valve, trauma, or carcinoid disease. Treatments for pulmonic valve regurgitation include medical optimization to reduce pulmonary hypertension.

I would like to extend heartiest congratulations to Dr. Kris Vijay for bringing a masterpiece, "Invoking your Inner Therapist in Heart Failure."

Dr. Vijay's extensive experience as a clinician and works at the grass roots across geographies places him in a unique position to pen this book. How complex heart conditions are intertwined with the real-life stories, is engrossing and provides an interesting perspective. The text is interspersed with numerous illustrations to help explain the different heart conditions. I am sure the book will serve as a milestone in enhancing knowledge and removing apprehensions in the community at large about heart disease.

All the best.
With warm regards
Yours sincerely

Prof. Anupam Sibal, MD, FIMSA, FIAP, FRCP (Glasg), FRCP (Lon), FRCPCH, FAAP
President, Global Association of Physicians of Indian Origin (GAPIO)
Group Medical Director, Apollo Hospitals Group
Senior Consultant Pediatric Gastroenterologist and Hepatologist, Indraprastha Apollo Hospitals; Clinical Professor, Faculty of Medicine and Health Sciences Macquarie University, Sydney, Australia |Member, Asia – Pacific Advisory Council of Joint Commission International (JCI)
Author of The National Best Seller *"Is Your Child Ready to face the World?"*

CHAPTER 19

Congenital Heart Defects

In this chapter, we will discuss the five most common types of congenital heart defects which include: **atrial septal defect, ventricular septal defect, patent ductus arteriosus, Eisenmenger syndrome, and tetralogy of Fallot.** All these conditions, if left untreated, can lead to congestive heart failure and death.

There are two types of **atrial septal defect**: Secundum vs primum. **Secundum ASD** is the most common. The defect is in the central portion of the atrial septum and there is shunting of the blood from left to right, hence the volume on the right side of the heart increases. Most of these people are asymptomatic, however, a physician may find a heart murmur upon physical examination. This leads to an assessment with an electrocardiogram and echocardiogram, This, then, leads to the diagnosis of this condition. The management of this condition is usually to leave it alone if the patient is asymptomatic or if the hole in the heart is minuscule.

However, if there is an increased volume on the right side of the heart, then patient can go into heart failure. Also, a clot can travel from the venous circulation, cross over to the left atrium and then left ventricle. This can get pumped out into the brain causing a stroke. If this happens or one is at risk for stroke, the defect should be closed. The closure can occur nowadays with a device called the Amplatzer which closes the hole in the atrial septum percutaneously without open-heart surgery. If the hole is too big and the device is unable to be deployed to be secured in position, then they may need open-heart surgery. This may also be done with a minimally invasive technique which can make the patient recover quickly.

I remember seeing a patient close to 18 years ago admitted with a heart attack. The patient had right coronary artery occlusion that led to a right ventricular infarct. Since BP was low, he was getting IV fluids in the ER and patient suddenly started to drop his oxygen levels. He urgently needed 100% oxygen and by the time he had a coronary angiogram, he had to be supported on a ventilator. In the Cath lab, he was noted to have a total occlusion of the right coronary artery and also the atrial septum had a large hole and an ASD was noted. This would have happened after the heart attack due to high right atrial pressure that had to open a door. Patient was taken to the operating room by the surgeon, but since the right ventricle had failed, he was too far gone even after one vessel bypass and repair of the ASD. He passed away during that admission.

> This taught me a lesson and every time a right coronary artery occlusion is suspected, one has to keep a close eye on the right sided hemodynamic pressures and keep an open mind about suspecting ASD, as it can be lifesaving if detected early. I have had 3 more cases since then, and all of them have made it, God willing!

Primum ASD is not that common and is in the bottom portion of the atrial septum. Hence, there is a defect between the atrium and the ventricle called the atrioventricular septum and these valves are also abnormal. Classically, the mitral valve is a cleft, but about 40% of the defect may be associated with a double orifice mitral valve and there may be a leakiness or stenosis with this valve. The leaflet that is closer to the septum of the tricuspid valve is also affected. Many times, a heart murmur is the first manifestation of a physical exam. Management again is patch closure or surgical intervention as seen with the secundum ASD.

Ventricular Septal Defect (VSD) is a defect between the left and right ventricle which is the bottom portion of the heart. Usually, a loud murmur is present during the physical exam and confirmed through an echocardiogram. If large, it may lead to what is called Eisenmenger syndrome. This syndrome is caused by an increase in pressure on the right side of the heart which leads to the right to left shunt which can decrease the survival in patients significantly because it can lead to pulmonary hypertension. This may need surgical correction.

Patent ductus arteriosus is a congenital defect with a connection between the pulmonary artery and aorta. This is supposed to close early in life, but sometimes remains patent and leads to shunting of deoxygenated blood to aorta and all parts of the body. This condition is at times associated with maternal rubella, which causes a small ductus with no consequence and is consistent with normal life span. However, when sustained during adulthood, it can become calcified and cause Eisenmenger syndrome. When this happens, surgical intervention may be required.

Eisenmenger syndrome is usually secondary to a large VSD, or PDA which usually starts off with a left to right shunting in early childhood, and with increased pressure, on the right side of the heart, it can result in pulmonary hypertension. This pulmonary hypertension can slowly lead to a reversal of the shunt. Many times, when we mention a blue baby, it is because of this Eisenmenger syndrome. The deoxygenated blood from the right side of the heart now goes to the left side of the heart to pass through the aorta and is not well oxygenated. Hence, the deoxygenated blood gives rise to cyanosis. which leads to the blue baby syndrome. Most are detected early in life and present with mild to moderate to severe symptoms. Electrocardiography usually reveals enlargement of the right side of the heart and the chest x-ray will have prominent pulmonary arteries and the right ventricle may be enlarged. Management of patients with Eisenmenger syndrome is complex due to poor long-term survival. They may need heart-lung transplantation or single transplantation with a closure of the defect.

Tetralogy of Fallot is a common congenital heart defect that consists of four abnormalities such as large VSD, obstruction of the pulmonary outflow tract, right ventricular hypertrophy, and overriding of the aorta. The pressure on the right ventricle is the same as that of the left ventricle because of the large VSD. The obstruction of blood flow to the lung causes blue blood to be diverted to the enlarged aorta. Most patients have this repaired during childhood but occasionally they reach adulthood without surgical intervention. These adult patients do not have right ventricular failure until they reach about 40 years of age. This can be discovered with a physical examination, EKG, and chest x-ray. Similar abnormalities are present as in Eisenmenger syndrome, but the patient with tetralogy may survive because of earlier shunts that improve the pulmonary flow and have pulmonary arteries grow. They have different types of surgical interventions creating shunts They are called the Blalock Taussig, Waterston, or Potts shunt.

Surgical interventions may be needed in some patients.

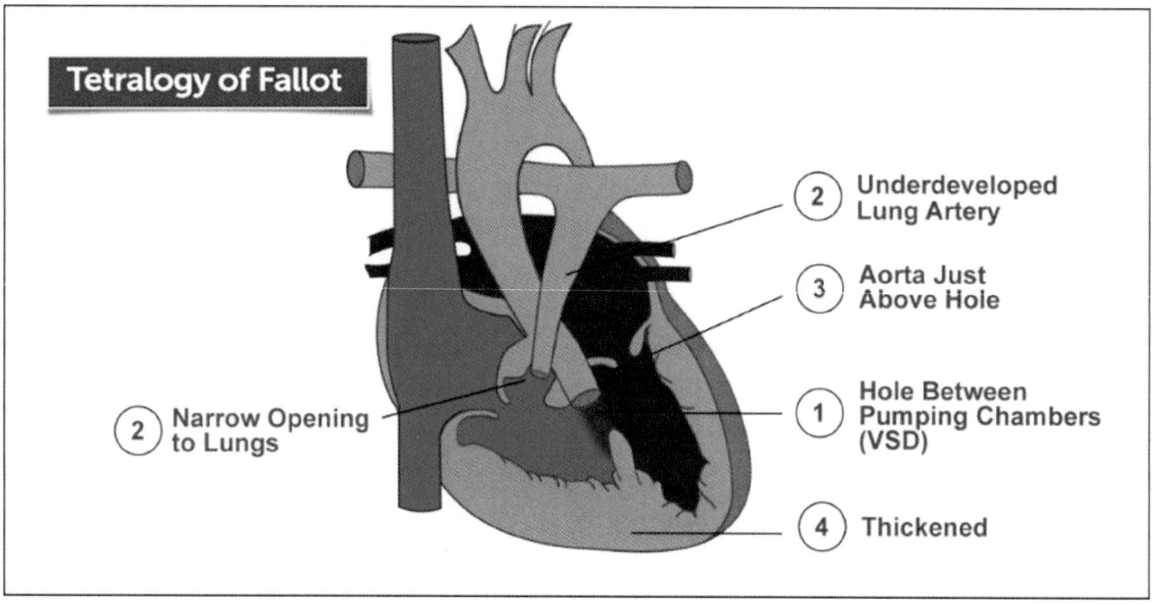
Tetralogy of Fallot
2 Underdeveloped Lung Artery
3 Aorta Just Above Hole
2 Narrow Opening to Lungs
1 Hole Between Pumping Chambers (VSD)
4 Thickened

Fig. 21

CHAPTER 20

Arrhythmias and Heart Failure

WATCH NOW

Arrhythmias essentially means an abnormal rhythm. There are multiple types of abnormal rhythms of the heart which include: supraventricular and ventricular arrhythmias. Ventricular beats come from the bottom of the heart and supraventricular come from the top. Other kinds of SV arrhythmias include supraventricular tachycardia which can be broken down into sinus tachycardia, atrial tachycardia, AV nodal reentry tachycardia, multifocal atrial tachycardia, junctional tachycardia, atrial flutter, and atrial fibrillation. Of all the supraventricular tachycardias, the most common one is the AV nodal reentry tachycardia which is also referred to as SVT. AV nodal tachycardia is a common one that occurs in young people which is usually secondary to a slow pathway which causes short circuits in AV nodes. We talked about the anatomy of the electrical pathway in the first chapter when we discussed the sinus and AV node.

Anything arriving from the sinus node is referred to as **sinus tachycardia.** If the heart rate is faster than 110 beats per minute and rising from the sinus node, this refers to sinus tachycardia. The reason for sinus tachycardia includes many noncardiac issues such as infection, dehydration, medications, stimulants, pulmonary embolism, or anxiety. There is also a condition called inappropriate sinus tachycardia which can be secondary to the automatic enhancement of the normal sinus node function, probably secondary to an abnormal automatic electrical trigger. This can be triggered by increased sympathetic tone or increased catecholamine. Sometimes, low oxygen levels, acidosis, or electrical abnormalities can also lead to sinus tachycardia.

Supraventricular tachycardia can be secondary to **AV nodal reentry tachycardia** which is most common in young people. It occurs through two pathways: slow or fast. This can be because of a short circuit that occurs in the AV node. Many times, this is secondary to an abrupt onset and offset as well with fast and slow fluctuations before sudden termination. Many times, the rate can range from 100-280 BPM. Sometimes the patient may experience near-syncope, lightheadedness, or dizziness. The treatment for this arrhythmia is through catheter ablation which usually works more than 95% of the time.

Often, to sustain the gain, they may need to be on medications such as calcium channel blockers, diltiazem, verapamil, or beta-blockers. **AV reciprocating tachycardia** is a different kind of arrhythmias, that initiate because of an accessory pathway in its circuit. The electrical complex can sometimes be narrowed or be wide. Another accessory pathway called the Wolf Parkinson White (WPW)syndrome can lead to SVT or AFIB. Agents like adenosine or verapamil can be effective in terminating this type of tachycardia. Obviously, acute therapy if someone comes to the emergency room is medications to block the AV node but once a patient has been stabilized, they may benefit from catheter ablation.

Multifocal atrial tachycardia (MAT) is a poorly organized rhythm coming from the top chamber of the heart with predominance in the right atrium. This occurs secondary to lung disease such as chronic obstructive pulmonary disease. Many of the COPD patients have enlarged right atrium and right ventricle which gets stretched and triggers MAT. The most common way to fix this problem is to stabilize lung disease and use oxygen.

Paroxysmal atrial tachycardia is a kind of abnormal rhythm from the right atrium or left atrium. The origin is usually secondary to the P wave being abnormal because of the stretching of the atrium itself. Sometimes medication such as digoxin can lead to paroxysmal atrial tachycardia and eventually lead to a conduction system block. Treatments include ablation with success in 75-80% of the subjects.

Atrial flutter: These are arrhythmias that occur because of AV nodal dysfunction. There is a triangle called the Koch triangle which is where the origin of this atrial flutter is. It is formed by the coronary sinus on one side and tricuspid valve on the other, connected by a tendon called the tendon of Todaro. The origin of atrial flutter is in this triangle. The diagnosis is easily made when a sawtooth pattern is noted on the EKG and the ventricular rate is over 150 beats per minute. Sometimes when the ventricular rate is over 110 beats per minute, the atrium can be beating twice as fast and the ventricle will be beating at 220 beats or more with a sawtooth pattern.

This can clearly be missed in the ER as it can be hidden, hence, when the HR is 110 BPM and someone comes into the ER with symptoms of palpitations, it can be mistaken for sinus tachycardia. One needs to make sure that it is not secondary to atrial flutter with underlying hidden flutter waves. The reason to detect this is that more than 90% of the time, catheter ablation will cure the atrial flutter rhythm and sustain the gain over the lifetime. The risk of pulmonary embolism is present in atrial flutter but much less than in atrial fibrillation. Many times, atrial flutter patients will also require blood thinners to protect strokes.

"People are much more than their diseases;
Doctors are much more than technicians.
And treatments are much more than commodities on a menu."

This is what I frequently say that as practitioners in this corporate world sometimes we tend to forget.

The essence of the book brought out by Dr Kris Vijay clearly conveys this message and in a way creates an opportunity to democratize cardiac care. The tremendous experience, multidimensional thought process and hard work brings out a true innovative approach that is so simple and accessible to everyone. Having a heart of gold himself and a true passion to not just provide the best of care to his patients but to serve them with compassion, Dr Vijay's message in the form of this book is a must read for both doctors and patients alike. "

Dr Dayaprasad G Kulkarni
Founder and Director AarogyaSeva
Assistant Professor
Dept of Biomedical and Chemical Engineering
Syracuse University

CHAPTER 21

Atrial Fibrillation

She was buried. The ritual noises were made.
The earth was smoothed. The day ended.
The sun rose. The day ended.
Day, day, day, and then no more days.
Now the weeks came, now a month.
Time was a shattered window into the void.
And into the void, his tears fell.
Into the blackness, the mouthing blackness, the tears fell, never stop,
I swear it, never, never, never. And then they stopped.
And one day one week of one month after the breast had healed after the jags were lonely palisades peering the unknown, one day the glass was whole again.
And time was a window. And beyond the window was Ouida, dead.
Beyond the window.
Not gone.
But gone, all the same.

— Morton Thompson in "Not as a Stranger"

Patient Story

Rita was a 32-year-old female whose story is blood draining and yet has somehow transitioned from Grief to Wholeness. She had presented with severe shortness of breath more than decades ago. At the time, we had done some diagnostic testing which revealed that she a pulmonary artery pressure that was 120 mmHg. We did not know whether there was another underlying reasoning behind her pulmonary hypertension. We did all kinds of workup and concluded that she had primary pulmonary hypertension. She had invasive procedures which revealed that the left side of her heart was completely normal. The right side of the heart had issues; she had presented to the hospital within a few weeks with atrial fibrillation.

She was going rapid and we had to control the heart back into a rhythm although she kept failing to maintain sinus rhythm and was placed on medications after cardioversion. She was followed by a pulmonologist who was aggressive with medical management, but she could not tolerate many of these due to low blood pressure. In the meantime, she slowly deteriorated with right-sided heart failure and fluid retention and was placed on medications. At the time, almost 20 years ago, there was no major treatment for primary pulmonary hypertension, and one had to resort to lung and heart transplants. There were no medications such as sildenafil which is now commonly used for patients with this condition. In higher doses, it is used for men with erectile dysfunction. However, in lower doses, 2-3 times a day both men and women seem to find improvement with this medication in primary pulmonary hypertension a as it drops the pulmonary artery pressure and makes it easier to breathe.

Now we have other medications that are being used such as prostacyclin and endothelin receptor antagonists. I have had a few patients who are on some of the newer medications and doing better, however, Rita did not have the advantage of all of these therapies at the time and subsequently passed away. She did teach us to explore causes of underlying AF, one of which is PPH. Hence, I created a mnemonic on why someone would go into atrial fibrillation.

> Since Rita had primary pulmonary hypertension, I created a mnemonic which is explained in the atrial fibrillation section called RITA HAS PPH, which includes the etiology of why someone can go into heart failure.

But the lessons learned from Rita's condition has been humbling. Rita taught us about the perspective of mortality at a young age. Rita taught us about why we have to have a meaning, purpose, and value to our existence and why we should maintain the perfection of postural, physical, intellectual, and spiritual to transform our lives and other's lives. This has to be done with contemplation, clarity of mind, compassion and once you add empathy and kindness, there is a certain level of internal satisfaction that makes you feel at peace. Rita's message is powerful because she was young and had all the incredible values growing up and yet had a strong impact on other people's lives.

Atrial Fibrillation

Atrial fibrillation is one of the most common arrhythmias present in adults. It is usually age-dependent with over 10% of the people aged 75 years having this condition and more commonly those over the age of 60 who are admitted to the hospital have this condition over 30% of the time. With atrial fibrillation, the atrial impulses are running at a rate of 350-600 beats per minute, hence, the atrial wave itself becomes small and creates a fibrillatory wave that truly does not have any contractile reserve. Hence, the atrium is quivering as opposed to contracting. The AV node is unable to conduct this atrial quiver rapidly, hence, the ventricular response in the absence of any therapy can be between 150-180 complexes per minute with an irregularly irregular pattern. The underlying reasons for atrial fibrillation are many. There is a mnemonic that I developed in our clinic from a patient named Rita who had primary pulmonary hypertension and atrial fibrillation. The causes are as follows from the mnemonic: **RITA HAS PPH.**

R stands for rheumatic heart disease in someone who has had rheumatic fever, as a child and developed rheumatic valve disease in adult life. Rheumatic fever can affect the heart and cause valvular heart disease such as mitral valve stenosis/regurgitation, aortic stenosis/regurgitation. These are the most common valves affected. These conditions can lead to the stretching of the left atrium and trigger atrial fibrillation.

I stands for ischemic heart disease which is due to coronary occlusions in the LAD or circumflex or commonly the RCA which supplies the AV node.

T stands for thyroid disease which includes thyrotoxicosis or hypothyroid disease which can lead to abnormal rhythms.

A stands for atrial septal defect or acute infectious etiology such as pneumonia or sepsis or alcoholism.

H stands for hypertrophic cardiomyopathy.

A stands for amyloidosis

S stands for sarcoidosis. These are all the infiltrative diseases that contribute to cardiomyopathy and can lead to atrial fibrillation.

P stands for primary pulmonary heart disease which can be secondary to COPD or pulmonary embolism. If someone comes in with chest pain and is tachycardic with a history of atrial fibrillation, one needs to wonder if they could have a pulmonary embolism or a clot in the pulmonary artery if they are predisposed to having this condition. One may need to rule this out as a potential possibility because it can be life-threatening.

P stands for a pericardial disease which is due to inflammation of pericardium called pericarditis, pericardial effusion, or other autoimmune disease or cancer. More commonly, lung cancer or breast cancer can lead to metastasis in the pericardium causing pericardial disease and atrial fibrillation.

H stands for hypertension which increases a propensity for atrial fibrillation. This occurs because the increased pressure system in the aorta causes thickening of the heart muscle which leads to altered relaxation of the heart. This causes left atrial enlargement leading to atrial fibrillation.

In addition to knowing the underlying cause of atrial fibrillation and ruling out potential reasoning to treat it, one needs to know how to control the rapid ventricular response and how to prevent the occurrence and minimize the risk of stroke. The three major things in terms of management include stroke prevention, rate control, and rhythm control. The patient is at high risk for stroke is because the atrium has lost its contractile function. The origin of atrial fibrillation is at the mouth of the pulmonary vein which drains into the left atrium.

When the left atrium is quivering and not contracting, it acts more like a pond rather than a river that is flowing. Hence, the blood flow from the atrium to the left ventricle across the mitral valve is significantly decreased and hence the amount of cardiac output is also decreased. There are pockets in the left atrium called the appendages where clots can easily accumulate. Due to the lack of contractile function of the atrium and quivering nature, left atrial appendage (Figure 22) specifically is at high risk for clots because of the stagnation of blood in the atrium. These clots can eventually be dislodged into the LV across the mitral valve if there is a strong quiver. This can then lead to the clot pumped across the aorta and into to the carotid arteries to the brain. Clot can embolize into the brain leading to a stroke. The first thing to do is to prevent a stroke from happening. Numerous studies have shown blood thinners to be effective at preventing stroke. However, one needs to be cautious when prescribing these blood thinners because they are only indicated for a patient at high risk for clot formation The risk for a stroke or thromboembolism occurs in the following subjects by utilizing a common mnemonic to assess if the patient is a candidate for blood thinners such as warfarin or other newer anticoagulants. The mnemonic is called CHADS2VASC score.

C stands for congestive heart failure, H for hypertension, A for age (over 74 years), D for diabetes, S for stroke, or TIA. The VASC is the European addition to this mnemonic and important to increase the efficacy of this tool. The V stands for vascular disease (carotids, legs, arms, aorta), A for age for women as women have a higher risk (over 65) of stroke. If the score is over two, then the increased risk of stroke is significantly higher and they may qualify for a blood thinner such as warfarin, apixaban, dabigatran, or rivaroxaban.

There is another mnemonic called HASBLED which stands for risk factors that can increase the chances of bleeding. Hence, we weigh the risk between bleeding and clot formation;

based on these, the cardiologist will recommend anticoagulation weighing the risk and benefit. In patients who are at high risk for bleeding or have had serious bleeding issues, a device called Watchman may help close off the Left atrial appendage which is where the clot forms for the most part. See Figure 23.

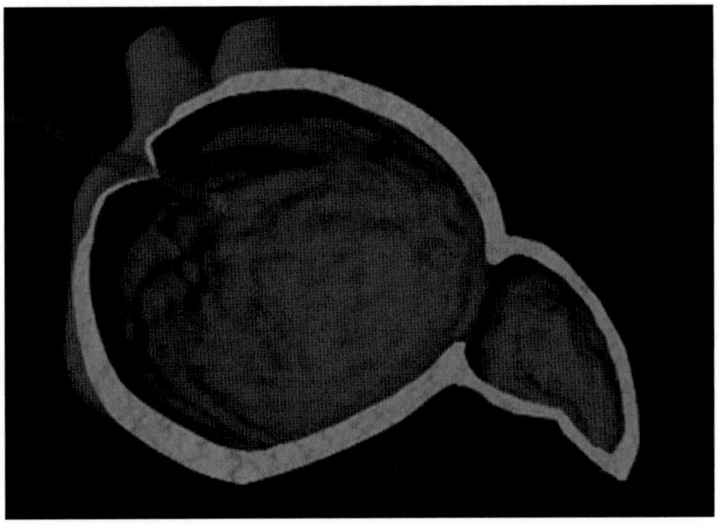

Fig. 22

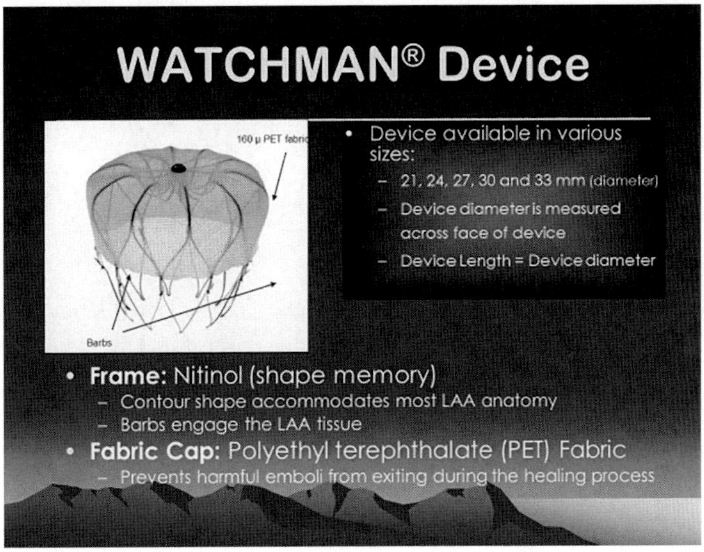

Fig. 23

The second treatment strategy is to rate control. The rate of the ventricle from 150-180 can be because of an abnormal conduction system. This rate itself can lead to low blood pressure, dizziness, and lightheadedness. This rate can reduce the filling of the left ventricle which will increase the left atrial pressure which is next to the pulmonary vein and fluid can get trapped inside the lungs which can lead to congestive heart failure. In the long run, if the patient continues to live with an increased heart rate, then the heart can get fatigued and fail. It is called tachycardia-induced cardiomyopathy and one needs to be aware of this as well which can lead to heart failure. Hence, it is important to control the ventricular rate. Agents that can be used to control the heart rate include beta-blockers, calcium channel blockers, digoxin, or Ibutilide (given intravenously). Adenosine does not seem to have a role in atrial fibrillation but does work in supraventricular tachycardia secondary to AV nodal reentry tachycardia. Once the rate is controlled, the next step is to control the rhythm.

To control the rhythm, one needs to make sure that the patient is on anticoagulation. If atrial fibrillation is acute, they may need hospitalization. If it has been present for a while and the patient is hemodynamically stable, then they can be treated in the outpatient setting. Acutely, the patient will be started on heparin or enoxaparin which will keep the blood thin. Once the blood is thin, it is worthwhile to convert them back into a rhythm because maintaining an abnormal rhythm on a continuum can lead to heart failure and may lead to a significant drop in quality of life. Rhythm control is important and in an acute setting patient may need a transesophageal echocardiogram (TEE) to assess for the presence or absence of clot in the left atrial appendage. If there is no clot, then one can proceed to shock the heart to get back in rhythm.

TEE probe is like an endoscope that is sent through the esophagus after giving sedation (happy juice) to better visualize the heart or left atrial appendage specifically for clots. Hence, it is important to anti-coagulate the patient's blood to prevent a stroke and rule out a blood clot before shocking the heart back into a rhythm (DCCV). In addition to cardioversion, there are two other categories of therapy commonly used called ablation or antiarrhythmic agents. The ablation is performed by inserting a catheter to the vein in the groin and directed towards the left atrium and identify the origin of the atrial fibrillation at the opening of the pulmonary vein. Once this is ablated, there is a 70-80% success rate and can be maintained for a long period of time.

Many times, they may need to stay on medications to maintain the normal rhythm. Medications that convert these patients into a rhythm can be found in another mnemonic called Every AM know your EF and mind your PQRST. A stands for amiodarone, M stands for Mutlaq, E stands for encainide, (withdrawn from market due to side effects and safety), F stands for flecainide, P for procainamide, Q for quinidine, R for Rythmol, S for sotalol and T for Tikosyn. This mnemonic is used to assess which medications are best for assessing the underlying profile of each patient and must be personalized because each medication has its own side effects. Sotalol and Tikosyn in particular have increased side effects of prolonging the QT interval (over 500ms) and patients may need to be hospitalized for 3 days to watch their EKGs for QT interval prolongation and early detection of ventricular tachycardia and possible cardiac arrest. Amiodarone is most commonly used agent. It also has side effects long term involving thyroid gland, liver, kidney, and lung. Toxicity to these organs need to be closely watched and monitored. Other agents are not so frequently used due to significant side effects.

WATCH NOW

Dr. Vijay is one of the rarest of physicians – he not only possesses an encyclopedic knowledge of the science and pathophysiology of illness, but he also intuitively understands the spiritual nature of our being. In today's world of high-tech Cardiology, we are paid to do things – tests, prescriptions, procedures – but there is little incentive to understand the impact that heart disease plays in our emotional health. In this short book you will gain insight into the ways that our cardiovascular system fails us and how we can work to repair the damage. But more importantly, you will see how a caring and skilled physician and educator can help integrate emotional and lifestyle changes with the medical therapies that are critical to living a more robust life. Dr. Vijay puts the high touch in high-tech, and we are all better for it.

Craig A. Hoover, MD, MBA, FACC, FSCAI
Assistant Professor of Clinical Medicine, University of Arizona College of Medicine
Director of Cardiovascular Quality, Carondelet Heart and Vascular Institute
Past President, Arizona Chapter of the American College of Cardiology

CHAPTER 22

Ventricular Tachycardia

WATCH NOW

Ventricular tachycardia is detected on the EKG which can be diagnosed with the use of a wide QRS complex. Also, many times the EKG can detect earlier if one is astute in identifying fusion beats, capture beats or AV dissociation, and axis deviation. These are all subtle changes that can be detected easily. If the patient has underlying heart disease, then the ventricular tachycardia prevalence increases significantly by more than 80%. If they have a normal structural heart, then the risk of ventricular tachycardia is exceedingly rare and if they have it in the absence of heart issues, then it is idiopathic ventricular tachycardia which occurs in less than 0.5% of the time. The ventricular tachycardia itself can develop after a heart attack. Causes of ventricular tachycardia include coronary artery disease, cardiomyopathy (ischemia, hypertrophic, dilated, arrhythmogenic right ventricular dysplasia, long QT syndrome, and polymorphic ventricular tachycardia.

These are the most common reasons why someone can have ventricular tachycardia. In patients who have had a heart attack in the first year after an event, the ventricular tachycardia can occur in about 2% of the patients, however more than 5% of the patients can experience sudden cardiac arrest during the same period of time. More than 80% of the patients who develop this during the first year have early complications after a heart attack. This includes conduction defects, congestive heart failure, hypotension, low EF with damage to the heart muscle, ventricular aneurysm, ventricular fibrillation, and cardiac arrest.

Hypertrophic cardiomyopathy can be a risk factor for ventricular tachycardia and cardiac arrest and the details are discussed in the separate section of cardiomyopathy.

Arrhythmogenic right ventricular dysplasia is another condition which can be familial and secondary to large amounts of infiltration in the right ventricle. The underlying reason for ventricular tachycardia is a short circuit with reentry and abnormal pathways leading to Arrhythmogenic right ventricular dysplasia induced ventricular tachycardia. Many of them may benefit from catheter ablation or defibrillators. Ventricular tachycardia in patients with normal structured hearts can occur because of substance abuse and right bundle branch ventricular tachycardia due to a catecholamine surge. Many of them recover without any major damage to the heart muscle but may need agents like beta-blocker or catheter ablations.

Long QT syndrome and polymorphic ventricular tachycardia can be a genetic or acquired condition. In genetic conditions, it may be secondary to abnormal electrolyte channels in the heart such as the sodium and potassium pump. Long QT syndromes can have many causes such as being on a special diet, medications, or lack of blood flow. The agents that can lead to this condition may consist of antiarrhythmic agents such as HIV agents, phenothiazines, psychiatric meditations, azithromycin, phenothiazines, or ketoconazole. The therapy for long QT syndrome includes beta-blockers, sympathectomy and/or Implantable defibrillators. Additional therapies for patients with ventricular tachycardia in the presence of blocked arteries are stent placement, bypass surgery and medical therapies. If there is damage to the heart muscle, then they may need medications such as amiodarone. Other patients may benefit from sotalol or Tikosyn if amiodarone is ineffective. Ablations and other surgeries may be used as well.

CHAPTER 23

Indications for Pacemaker Implantation

> *"When you walk to the edge of all the light you have and take that first step into the darkness of the unknown, you must believe that one of two things will happen. There will be something solid for you to stand upon or you will learn how to fly."*
>
> **Patrick Overton, in "Rebuilding the front porch of America"**

WATCH NOW

Patient Story

Ms. W.L. is probably one of the longest survivors of heart Failure that I have known. She had come from Midwest to relocate and was advised to follow up with a heart failure specialist. She was struggling with nonischemic cardiomyopathy probably triggered by a viral infection. She had difficulty with medications initially and when a research trial called SCD HeFT was approved for enrollment, she qualified. This was a trial where one could get randomly assigned to a defibrillator or amiodarone or placebo. From her point of view, fortuitously, she got randomized to the defibrillator arm. The trial after many years revealed that the defibrillator arm saved lives. By that time, she was already on her way to recovery while the ICD had provided her a certain feeling of security as a bodyguard in case of sudden cardiac arrest.

There was some comfort in knowing that you have someone watching over you. Be it Jesus or Mohammed or an ICD or any superpower you believe in, hovering above, giving you a sense of sanctuary, a refuge, so to speak, about life and death. This allowed her to be optimistic about her prognosis. She was optimized on her medical therapy and over time her Ejection fraction improved from 16% to 55%. She has sustained this gain over the years. When she was told she had 6 months to live, she was devastated. She, then, rekindled the flame within, and finding the mental energy to explore resources and medical professionals as well as specialists available to improve her cardiac status, she went on a limb to prove herself that she had more than 6 months to live, more than 6 years to live, and beyond.

Now more than 20 years later, she continues to thrive with a normalized heart function. She has had ups and downs in her relationships, financial security, and trusting many doctors along the way. I believe, that she made it through due to the availability of resources, such as a new clinical trial that allowed her to participate, a new technology that gave her the impetus and security, her ability to research into health care systems that would provide the care she needed and her own mental stamina to sustain the gain and overcoming the trials and burden of life stressors which made her only stronger.

Indications for Pacemaker Implantation

Indications include acquired complete heart block (third-degree) which is secondary to the electrical disconnect of the top and bottom chambers of the heart. Symptoms of this include syncope, seizures, dizziness, and limited exercise tolerance. Some may be asymptomatic and be exposed to danger from head injuries with exertional activity. If one is seen to have a complete heart block and heart rate is below 45 BPM, then it is an indication for a pacemaker. Some reasons for having an acquired complete heart block include RCA blockage which would normally supply the AV node and when there is no blood flow, then this can lead to a complete heart block and this can be an indication for pacemaker implantation.

Other indications include valvular heart disease, post-operative conditions, trauma, catheter procedures, radiation, infection disease (syphilis, diphtheria, Chagas disease, diverticulosis, Lyme disease, toxoplasmosis), other autoimmune conditions such as rheumatoid arthritis, lupus, scleroderma, Ankylosing spondylitis can affect the conduction system. Infiltrative cardiomyopathy, sarcoidosis, amyloidosis, lymphoma, cancer, tumors can lead to AV nodal block. Neuromuscular conditions such as muscular dystrophy, medications such as digoxin, beta-blockers, or calcium channel blockers can lead to conduction system abnormalities.

Congenital heart blocks may not be symptomatic at birth but may develop later on. Second degree AV block in symptomatic patients when the heart rate goes below 45 beats per minute is an indication for a pacemaker. Symptomatic sinus bradycardia when the heart rate goes below 40 beats per minute with syncope symptoms may need a pacemaker. Some patients with inappropriate sinus tachycardia will need ablation of the sinus node and may develop sinus node dysfunction requiring a pacemaker. Sometimes when a pause happens for more than 3 seconds with sinus node dysfunction or neuro cardiogenic syncope, one might need a pacemaker. Some patients that pass out because of a 3-second pause with a carotid sinus massage may require a pacemaker. Pacemaker implantation therapy itself is becoming easier as technology advances and operators have become experts in the procedure.

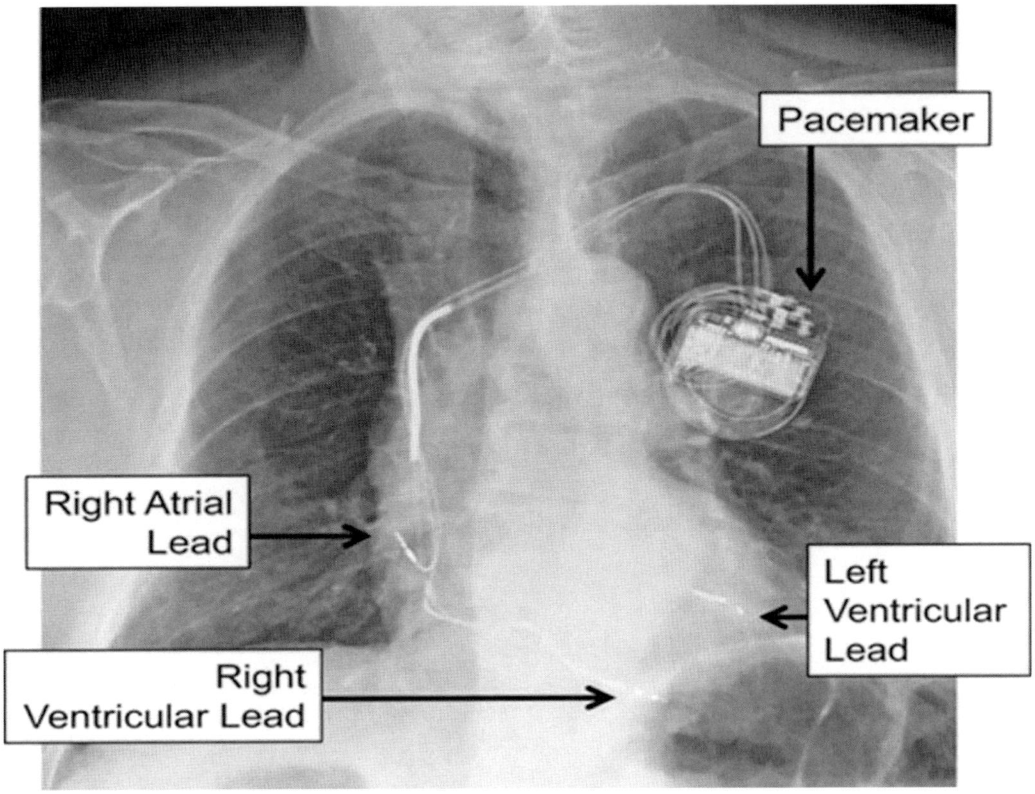

Fig. 24

Implantable cardioverter-defibrillator (ICD) indications include sustained ventricular tachycardia or fibrillation when in-home monitoring and guiding therapy is not feasible and antiarrhythmic agents contraindicated because of other comorbid indications or when sustained ventricular tachycardia itself is contributing to syncopal episodes. Patients with sustained ventricular tachycardia with no drug tolerance or failure of a drug proven to be effective are also indications for an ICD. In patients with Cardiomyopathy with ejection fraction under 35%, widened QRS (more 130 ms) with more than 90 days of medical therapy if dilated cardiomyopathy or more than 40 days after a heart attack/stent placement/bypass surgery, there is an indication for Biventricular pacemaker (3 leads) and ICD placement.

In the United States, there are 4 major companies that manufacture pacemakers: Medtronic, St. Jude, Biotronik and Boston Scientific. Vitatron is a major player in Europe. There are other smaller companies, but majority of market share is spread between these companies. Many of them have evolved in their technology and making smaller size pacemakers, leadless pacemakers, bionic ones, App based pacemakers, Pacemakers with multiple site pacing capabilities to allow for automatic capture of the electrical activity to sustain a synchronized pacing , Pacemaker with volume assessment capabilities in heart failure patients and beyond. An Electrophysiologist implanting a pacemaker will decide the right kind of pacemaker based on the needs of the individual patient.

This is a timely book on the important subject of heart failure. There are hundreds of books on coronary heart disease (CHD) prevention and treatment, but heart failure, which is usually a consequence of CHD is a relatively untouched subject.

In an extremely reader-friendly manner, the book explores the major gaps and misconceptions from understanding what heart failure is. It's a comprehensive review of all aspects of heart failure, ranging from prevention to the end-stage. It covers new modalities in diagnosis and therapies and also looks at what the future of heart failure therapy looks like.

The book is filled with real life patient stories, which Dr. Kris has gleaned from decades of clinical practice dedicated to heart failure. He covers all aspect of patient care, including the often-neglected psychological stressors, which have a huge impact on the patient's well-being. I would urge anyone with heart failure, caring for someone with heart failure or looking to just know more about the subject to pick up this book and read it in detail.

I have had the pleasure of knowing Dr. Kris Vijay for close to 15 years, and his superior clinical acumen is more than matched by his kindness and empathy as a human being. He has been involved in caring for the underprivileged in the remote areas of Ladakh in north India over the years, and one of my enduring regrets is that I have been unable to join him on any of these trips, as yet.

Dr. Aashish Contractor
Director: Rehabilitation and Sports Medicine
Sir HN Reliance Foundation Hospital, Mumbai, India
Vice-Chair International Council of Cardiovascular Prevention and Rehabilitation
Author: The Heart Truth: Prevention, Treatment and Reversal of Heart Disease

CHAPTER 24

Peripheral Vascular Disease Aortic Dissection

WATCH NOW

Patient Story

Mr. RP was a 64-year-old male who had a bicuspid aortic valve as a child which was not detected until later in his adult life and the valve was too tight and calcified that the patient started to experience symptoms of chest pain and dizziness. Hence, he underwent aortic valve replacement a couple of years prior. When we had seen him in the outpatient clinic, he was doing well on his beta-blocker and blood pressure was under control. His echocardiogram showed no major abnormality in the prosthetic valve and he had proper heart function. One night, he developed severe chest pain and landed up in the ED where he was found that his troponin levels were leaking and observed to have a heart attack. An XRAY there showed the mediastinum was a little wide and CT scan showed dissection of a proximal portion of his aorta.

Quickly, a heart surgeon was called who performed an aortic reconstruction. He had a type A aortic dissection which is very life-threatening and would have died if no operation were done. This procedure required multiple blood transfusion and he was in the hospital for about a month between the ICU and step-down care. He survived a major disaster and was doing well for a few years until he developed a prosthetic valvular infection that required long term antibiotics. His situation was complicated by a clot that developed on his valve and his anti-coagulation therapy was subsequently increased. He was incredibly happy about his life for being given multiple chances of survival and did not want his chest opened a third time.

Surgeons usually do not like to operate a third time around due to fibrous tissue that grows after previous surgeries and surgery becomes complex fraught with high risk. RP did well but developed a stroke as he was not very compliant with his anticoagulation medications. He followed up with a different provider who communicated with me that he was a DNR: "Do Not Resuscitate" patient and was shortly placed in hospice thereafter. After a few days, he died. From this story, it is important to realize that a bicuspid valve increases the risk of aortic stenosis and aortic dissection. Aortic dissection is a rare condition occurring in about 5-30 cases per 1 million people per year.

In 1-13% of autopsies, it is found that aortic dissection that usually occurs in patients with high blood pressure or history of the bicuspid aortic valve or aortic surgeries in general. The prognosis for this is not particularly good, Surgical mortality itself is about 30% and if they have type 1, then the mortality is much higher. Many patients present with neurological deficits and one must be cognizant of the atypical nature of the symptoms of aortic dissection. The underlying reasons for aortic dissection included high blood pressure, plaque buildup in the aortic arteries, connective tissue diseases such as Marfan's syndrome or Ehlers Danlos syndrome, and traumatic injuries. The lessons to be learned from RP include being aware of aortic dissection and that they frequently present atypically with or without the stabbing pain that is usually expected. One quickly must make sure to perform a CT scan to diagnose and act quickly. RP was very thankful for the extra time he had in his life and made the best use of it. We thank RP for giving us the knowledge throughout his life by his presence and we learned the complexity of his condition to impact other people's lives positively.

Peripheral Arterial Disease

> There is an increase in cumulative risk with diabetes and smoking history. The use of tobacco increases the risk of amputation by 10-fold in a diabetic.

There are multiple types of peripheral arterial or venous occlusive disease. Most of the time peripheral arterial disease includes blockages of the lower extremity arteries due to smoking, or diabetes which are the most common cause for these occlusions. Other categories include carotid artery disease, aortic aneurysm, aortic dissections, and autoimmune disease. Venous disease is the second category because of lower extremity thrombosis of the veins due to poor venous return from abnormal venous insufficiency (leg ulcers or lymphoedema). In diabetic subjects, the rate of above-knee amputation is 16.5 percent and below-knee amputations 5.7 percent.

The location also affects the prognosis overall. Patients with aortoiliac diseases have reduced survival rates as opposed to those with a disease in the femoral artery. Distally, if they have blocked arteries in the peroneal, popliteal, or Dorsalis pedis, then the risk is lower; but clearly diabetes in conjunction with femoral artery disease results in a decrease overall survival up to 38% over a 9-year period. Other arteries in the body such as the subclavian is also an area of interest and have a mildly increased risk of occlusions because of procedures done for other reasons.

The symptoms of these patients include intermittent claudication, leg pain, thigh pain, trouble with ambulation. This is usually diagnosed with an ankle-brachial index (ABI) which looks at the differences between the pressure in the brachial artery and posterior tibial artery. In addition, patients can be diagnosed with arterial ultrasounds or angiography. The treatment of these diseases can include walking programs, medications such as trental, angioplasty, endovascular stenting, or bypass. Diabetes, rest pain, ischemic ulceration, and gangrene are all associated with the risk of limb loss and need an aggressive approach.

Carotid Arteries

Carotid disease can be detected among asymptomatic patients by searching for carotid bruits during the physical examination which is present in about 10% in elderly patients. Noninvasive testing such as ultrasound can detect occlusive disease. Carotid disease reflects systemic atherosclerotic vascular disease. If there is a blocked artery in the neck, it correlates well with blocked arteries in the heart and lower extremities. The symptomatic carotid disease can be characterized as stroke-like symptoms that can lead to retinal strokes and visual loss. If the artery narrowing is more than 70%, then that is when intervention is required, otherwise, prevention should be a priority by monitoring diabetes, smoking, cholesterol, metabolic syndrome, and high blood pressure. If mild or moderate plaque is present, then the LDL goal is less than 70 mg per d/L and statins should be considered.

Aortic Aneurysms:

Thoracic Aortic Aneurysms are commonly caused by atherosclerosis and Marfan syndrome, giant cell arteritis syphilis, traumatic aneurysm, and pseudoaneurysms. Treatments for this condition include invasive surgical repair and even with no associated condition, surgical mortality is high. Abdominal aneurysms can be diagnosed with ultrasound or CT scan and endovascular luminal graft is indicated if not occupying the renal artery space if the aneurysm is more than 4.5 cm in diameter. At times open surgery may be needed. One must be cautious if someone with an abdominal aortic aneurysm qualifies for an ELG. Many of these patients have symptoms of back pain, weight loss but are usually asymptomatic. Other contributors include Burger's disease, popliteal entrapment syndrome, thoracic outlet syndrome, and heparin-induced thrombocytopenia.

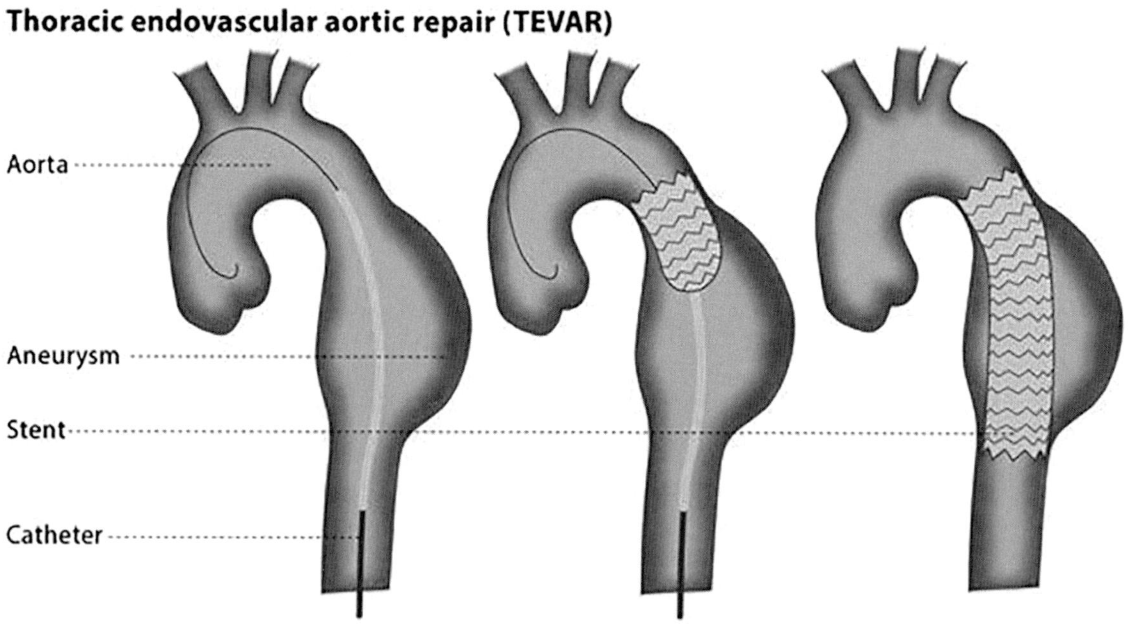

Fig. 25

Abdominal Aortic Aneurysm Graft

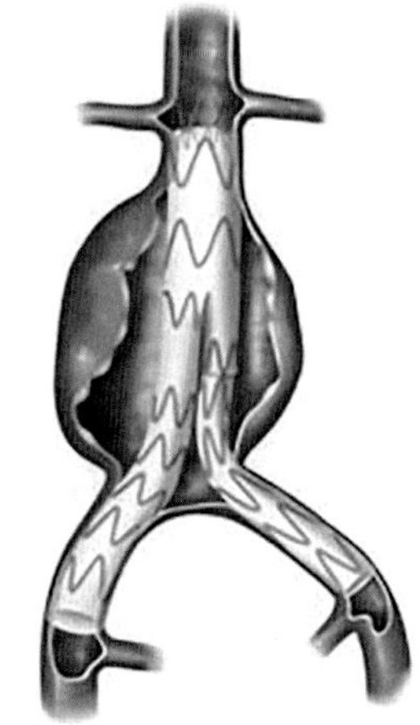

Lower Extremity Venous Disease

Cause of venous disease is usually secondary to deep vein thrombosis, and reasons for these clots can be secondary to lack of exercise, prolonged travel, underlying hypercoagulation state. Other cancers in the body and increase clotting factors can lead to clotting in the lower extremities. Connective tissue disease, inflammatory tissue disease, lymphoma, leukemia, medications such oral contraceptives, coagulation disorders such as antithrombin 3 deficiency protein C or S deficiency, factor 5 Leiden are all other causes that lead to increased clotting tendencies. Coagulation disorders can be managed in an acute hospital setting with anticoagulation such as heparin or enoxaparin or in the outpatient setting with warfarin or other newer anticoagulation agents. Fig. 26

Lower Extremity Ulcers

Lower extremity ulcers are commonly seen among patients with diabetes or lower extremity arterial deficiency which can lead to arterial and venous ulcers. Sometimes neurotrophic ulcers are secondary to central nervous system disorders as well.

Lymphedema

This is another condition that is rare and usually affects women more than men and is prevalent among people under 40 years old. It can happen after the first pregnancy, usually bilaterally more than unilaterally in more than one-half of the patients and one needs to rule out other obstructive lesions such as cancer in the pelvis, ovaries, or prostate which can lead to lymphedema and obstruction in the venous return from the lower extremities going right up to the right atrium. Sometimes a tumor in the inferior vena cava can also lead to lymphoedema. Infection, inflammation, or radiation can affect venous return which increases lymphedema. Treatment strategy includes compression stockings, leg elevation, elastic support, and sequential compression device. Some patients may require surgical decompression if they have recurrent cellulitis from compartment syndrome.

CHAPTER 25

Pregnancy and The Heart Peripartum Cardiomyopathy

"Let us rise up, and be thankful, for if we didn't learn a lot today, at least we learned a little, and if we didn't learn a little, at least we didn't get sick, and if we got sick, at least we didn't die; so let us all be thankful."

– **Buddha**

WATCH NOW

Patient Story

VC is 34 years of age and had fluid retention, shortness of breath, fatigue, and lower extremity swelling who had just given birth to her 4th child. An echocardiogram showed low heart function and an ejection fraction of about 25%. Upon asking her about previous pregnancies, she did mention that she had swelling in her legs and fatigue after her 2nd and 3rd pregnancies but did not follow up with a cardiologist. Her symptoms did eventually dissipate after a few months. However, after her 4th child, her symptoms did return and did not go away. It was explained to her that this was a heart condition that occurs within the final months of her pregnancy and lasts for about 5 months after delivery and sometimes patients recover.

However, others need pharmacologic therapy to support their weak heart. V.C was placed on beta-blockers and ACE inhibitors which improved her symptoms with cardiac rehab and her ejection fraction improved within 3 months. After 6 months, her ejection fraction was 60%. She did not follow up for a long time as she felt good. And one day after a couple of years, she showed up at the clinic. Now she was pregnant with her 5th child and she was in her 3rd trimester. V.C. reported that before her 3rd trimester, she was significantly short of breath and had swelling in her legs and she clearly had all the symptoms of recurrence of her cardiomyopathy and heart failure. Now her ejection fraction had dropped to 38%. V.C was 2 years older now and with heart failure, she was deemed high risk for termination of her pregnancy as she was a little late into her pregnancy. She followed up with her gynecologist frequently and we had optimized her medications and kept a close eye on her.

Finally, she did give birth to a healthy child, and luckily for her, she did not decompensate. "All is well that ends well" is what we kept talking about. What did we learn from this experience? We learned that it is too risky to have a baby/get pregnant when there has been a history of a life-threatening situation in the past and placing your heart at risk is not worth it. Termination of pregnancy at this late in the game is also too high a risk for the mother and she can decompensate. She made a choice of continuing with the pregnancy but under close observation. After delivery, she was placed on medications which improved her ejection fraction and energy levels. V.C was so apologetic for not accepting provider advice on contraceptive medications and the lessons she learned were important. The lessons we learned were to engage our patients on a regular basis with face to face meetings, provide consistent education and increase the patient's trust towards our recommendations as we advise against subsequent pregnancies despite having a healthy heart.

Pathophysiology in Pregnancy

During pregnancy, there is a 20-30% increase in red blood cell mass, a 30-50% increase in plasma volume. Heart rate increases by approximately 10 beats a minute, blood pressure does not change significantly, cardiac output increases by 30-50% all of which are normally tolerated in pregnant women. During delivery, there is between 300-500 cc of blood loss during a cesarean, and there is about a liter of blood loss as well in the postpartum state. During delivery, the venous return is increased due to the relief of renal compression by the inferior vena cava. Hence spontaneous diuresis will occur for the first 48 hours. The cardiac output will increase with alteration and stabilization of hemodynamics about 4 weeks after delivery. Cardiac diseases in pregnancy become difficult to manage due to the changes in systematic, anatomical, hemodynamical alterations.

Vaginal delivery is still the gold standard of delivery, but some patients may not tolerate this delivery due to pulmonary hypertension or valve disease and may need cesarean. Anticoagulation may also cause complications as well. Congenital heart disease during pregnancy can complicate everything. The incidence of these conditions in the general population is about 1% and the offspring of women with congenital heart disease have 5-6% incidence of congenital heart disease. Marfan syndrome can also be present in children as there is a recurrence of the same in the family. Cardiac contraindications to pregnancy include pulmonary hypertension, Eisenmenger syndrome, cardiomyopathy, valvular heart disease, coarctation of the aorta, hypertrophic obstructive cardiomyopathy, peripartum cardiomyopathy if ejection fraction has been low. Pharmacological management has also been complicated in pregnancy as many of the antiarrhythmic medications cannot be used safely.

Digoxin and verapamil are thought to be safe in pregnancy. Beta-blockers can be used for supraventricular tachycardia in pregnancy and continued among patients with congestive heart failure. Diuretics can be a problem with thrombocytopenia and should be used judiciously. Angiotensin-converting enzyme inhibitors are contraindicated during pregnancy. Anticoagulation management is complicated and needs to be personalized based on the condition. Endocarditis prophylaxis is not recommended during deliveries. If one needs endocarditis prophylaxis for specific reasons, then they should be used 30-60 minutes before delivery and 8 hours after. Low dose aspirin can be prescribed safely during pregnancy.

CHAPTER 26

Infections of The Heart

Common infections of the heart include native valve disorders and endocarditis and it is estimated that 15-20 thousand cases of infective endocarditis are present in the United States. It is common among children with congenital heart disease and after repairs of these conditions. Catheter induced infections, complex congenital heart disease, ventricular septal defect, previous pre-existent valve disease, chronic rheumatic valve disease, dialysis, shunt placement, pacemaker wire endocarditis, hypertrophic cardiomyopathy gradient between aorta and ventricle are at risk for endocarditis. Many times, the complications of endocarditis can involve the central nervous system with stroke-like symptoms, abscess, aneurysms, infection, splenic infections, pulmonary infections, skin infections, eye infections, kidney complications.

Most of the time the presentation for this condition is fever, chills, shortness of breath, heart failure, weight loss, vomiting, spitting of blood. The intravenous drug users have a different kind of endocarditis with staphylococcus being the primary reason for infections. IV drug abusers usually get tricuspid valve endocarditis. People with cancer can develop endocarditis as well. There are rare fungal endocarditis infections that typically occur in intravenous drug users or uncontrolled diabetes.

Prosthetic valve endocarditis can also occur in patients with mechanical or bioprosthetic valves and will need prophylaxis for any kind of dental or gastrointestinal procedures and before any kind of invasive procedures. Treatments for endocarditis involve therapy with antibiotics or surgical intervention if the organism proliferates to form sepsis or other complications.

How does one pay another back for a new life?

In the hands of cardiologist Kris Vijay – and others – I owe a second birthday – December 26th, to that new life. It was afforded to me through the diagnosis, treatment, and follow-up of a lingering cardiovascular disease – with Dr. Vijay – more than seven years ago.

But my introduction to a person who has mastered the art of medicine, began more than 28 years ago as a pharmaceutical representative. I was intrigued by his curiosity and unbridled drive in research to find better clinical outcomes.

He was, at the outset of my career, helping to craft better outcomes in diabetes with a managed care company, as a director of treatment protocols, locally. Vijay subsequently completed a fellowship at Good Samaritan Medical Center with the University of Arizona, in cardiology, and worked to achieve high prominence in the field with his research, collaboration, and active work as a practitioner. He is tremendously knowledgeable about the diabetes and cardiovascular diseases. To that point, he is a leader in the field about public education, treatment, and research on those topics. He is a very humble, however. He created a nonprofit, Twin Epidemic, harnessing better treatments for those two diseases – and extending the care to those who have cardiovascular and diabetes who can least afford their therapies. That work extends to India and other impoverished countries around the world with his connection to Project CURE.

This book affords one an opportunity to peer into the man, and those twin maladies – for hope toward better outcomes – sooner. I benefited from that passion toward action: I am thankful, as well.

Brian Mosley, MBA, ACS, ALB
Chief Marketing Officer, Chic Fillet
President, Toastmaster International
Member, Arizona Community Foundation
Member, Fundraising committee, Act One

CHAPTER 27

Prosthetic Heart Valves

WATCH NOW

There are multiple kinds of Prosthetic Heart Valves which consist of bioprosthetic, porcine, pericardial, homograft. Multiple different companies have come up with bioprosthesis for mitral and aortic valves. At present, we do not have any tricuspid valve prosthesis available, but a pulmonic valve is still available. A mechanical prosthesis is also produced by multiple different companies such as Bay Valves, caged valve, ball valve, tilting disc, and bileaflets. There are now new valves available for transcatheter replacement of the aortic valve called TAVR.

In terms of the prosthetic valve itself, the complications include calcification of the bioprosthetic valve or clotting of the mechanical valve. Thromboembolism is common among mechanical valves; hence, they may need anticoagulation long term. Prosthetic endocarditis also can happen on the ring or the cusp of bioprosthesis and mechanical valves usually have vegetation on the sewing ring. Valve ring abscess is a common complication of prosthetic valve endocarditis. Many of these are diagnosed with an echocardiogram and usually, transesophageal echo is needed specifically because of the artifacts that one visualizes with a routine echocardiogram.

Evolution of different types of Valves: see figure below.

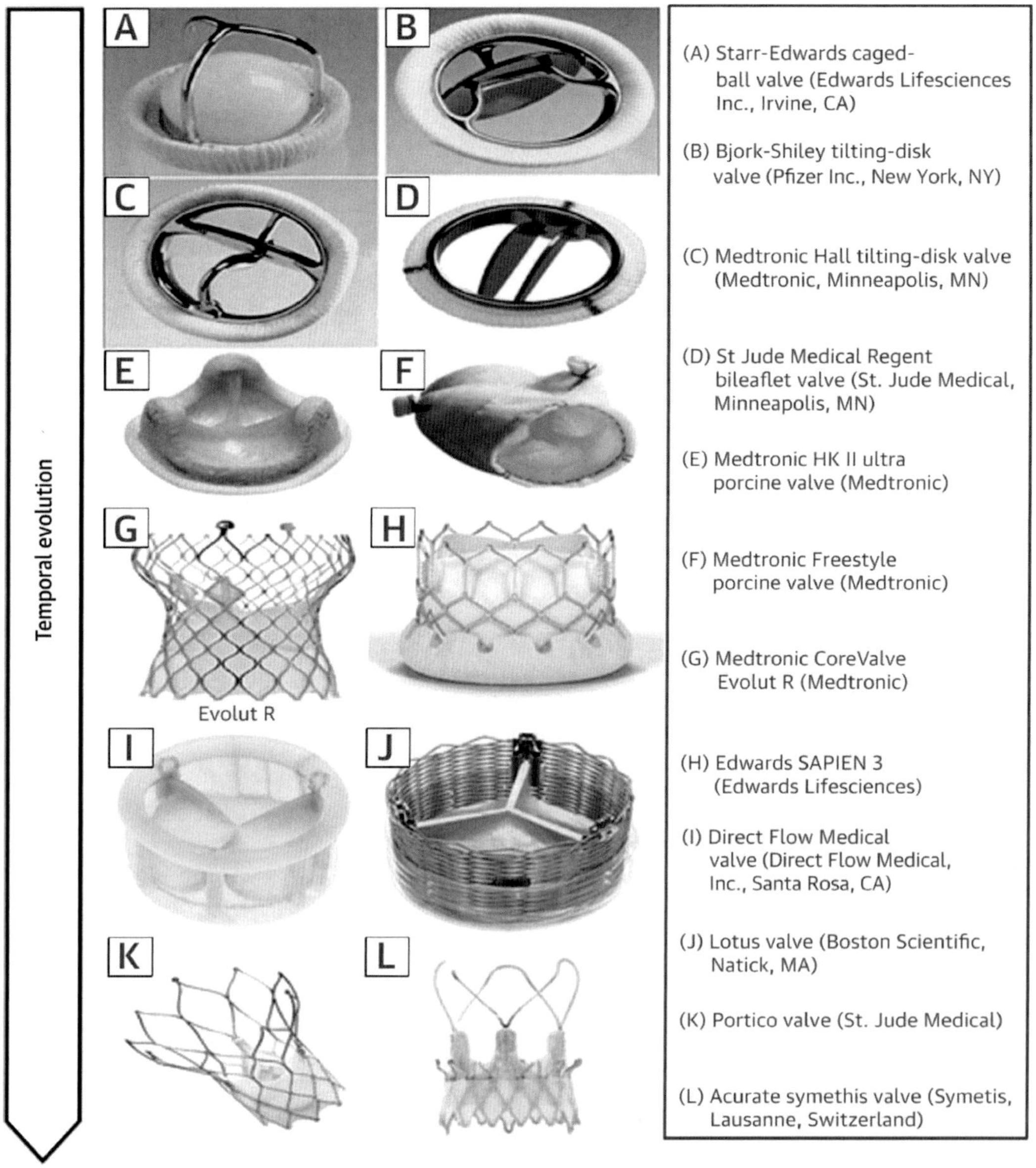

Fig. 27

CHAPTER 28

Systemic Diseases and The Heart

WATCH NOW

Multiple different systemic diseases affect the heart negatively. From a neurological standpoint, Fredrich's ataxia is associated with hypertrophic and dilated cardiomyopathy and is an autosomal recessive neurological disorder with thickening of the left ventricle and has a poor prognosis. Duchenne muscular dystrophy is an X-linked recessive disorder that affects skeletal muscle and cardiac muscle to cause arrhythmias such as atrial flutter, ventricular tachycardia, and significant skeletal muscle involvement with weakness. Myotonic dystrophy is an autosomal genetic muscle disorder that can affect the heart with conduction disorders and heart failure.

Guillain barre disorder is a non-hereditary demyelinating neuropathy associated with autonomic dysfunction sometimes associated with cardiac arrhythmias. Endocrine diseases such as acromegaly are associated with myocardial fibrosis and atherosclerotic disease. Rheumatic diseases are some of the conditions that affect vasculature and granuloma formation with inflammation of the valves, leading to amyloid deposition, pericarditis, pericardial effusion, and constrictive pericarditis. Complete heart blocks can also occur with autoimmune diseases as well.

Hematology/oncology diseases such as anemia can lead to left ventricular dilatation and hypertrophy. Thalassemia is associated with iron overload and myocardial iron deposition from multiple blood transfusions. Complications include recurrent pericarditis, pericardial effusion, pericardial tamponade, and heart blocks. Sickle cell diseases are also associated with anemia, heart attack and pulmonary embolism, papillary muscle dysfunction, and iron overload. Hemochromatosis is a genetic condition that increases iron absorption which increases serum levels of iron and ferritin which gets deposited in the heart muscle leading to heart failure.

SECTION IV

Diagnostics in Heart Failure

CHAPTER 29

History and Physical Exam

WATCH NOW

History is one of the most important ways that a health care provider can assess the patient and influence the diagnosis. History may reveal specific causes for worsening symptoms of heart failure that include shortness of breath, fatigue, weight gain, abdominal distention, and leg swelling.

The history that is important to obtain includes high blood pressure, diabetes, cholesterol, cancer, cardiomyopathy, recent viral infections, or bacteria pneumonia to guide diagnosis and therapy. Many times, these symptoms will be subtle starting with mild shortness of breath on minimal exertion and one would want to brush it off as deconditioned state due to some weight gain.

Weight gain itself could be from fluid retention and one may mistake it as something benign. Some patients have wheezing and may believe it is from their lungs acting up due to asthma or allergy. At times, patients present with coughing episodes, blood in mucus, coldness, pale, dizziness, fatigue, or lightheadedness. Some patients experience a weight gain of approximately 3 to 4 pounds or more over a 48-hour period. Increased leg swelling and abdominal distention may be manifestations of right-sided heart failure. Many others may have sleep apnea like symptoms but are usually misdiagnosed with other sleep disorders.

It is important to recognize sleep issues related to breathing as opposed to other factors. Some patients may have palpitations which indicate atrial fibrillation and can be a contributor to heart failure. Some patients may have chest pain or pressure associated with shortness of breath and may have blocked arteries. NYHA classification is a good determinant of mortality in CHF.

From a physical exam perspective, it is important for the healthcare provider to ascertain whether there is fluid retention and low cardiac output and if they are stable or decompensating acutely. These are the two major focuses of physical examination. Low cardiac output manifests as low blood pressure, cold clammy extremities, dizziness/lightheadedness, obtunded mental status, increase in BUN or creatinine suggesting acute kidney injury due to low perfusion.

To identify congestion, the healthcare provider will watch for elevated venous pressure in the neck or extra heartbeat called third heart sound. One may have leg swelling or abdominal distention which would indicate ascites, reduced air entry into the lungs because of fluid overload with or without pleural effusion. Heart murmurs can indicate valvular heart disease. Systolic murmurs in the apical area can indicate leaky mitral or aortic valve disease when the heart murmur is predominant in the second intercostal space towards the left sternal border. Identifying valvular heart disease and congestive heart failure is extremely important because most patients are asymptomatic in the first few stages of the disease.

This is a wonderful book that encapsulates the best of the art and science of medicine for patients with heart failure. This common illness impacts so many adult lives and the journey taken by the patient, family, and physicians is one of hope, endurance, discomfort, and sometimes despair. Vijay captures the essence of the issue for both the infirm and the bluestocking. Sit back, enjoy, and savor this masterpiece.

Peter A. McCullough, MD, MPH
Professor of Medicine, Vice Chair of Internal Medicine,
Consultant Cardiologist,
Baylor University Medical Center, Dallas TX

CHAPTER 30

Imaging

WATCH NOW

Patient Story

Mr. SW is a 47-year-old gentleman who sought attention for progressive shortness of breath with minimal exertion. All kinds of testing with echocardiogram and stress test were performed and it was found that his ejection fraction was 40% and a coronary angiogram was within normal limits.

He was placed on a beta-blocker and ACE inhibitor and advised that he may have nonischemic cardiomyopathy as his left ventricle was not severely dilated. It was unclear what the underlying reasoning was. From an imaging perspective, he had all the imaging that we would do to evaluate underlying symptom etiology with the use of EKG's, echocardiograms, angiograms, left and right cardiac catheterizations.

However, in this case, what was challenging was that the patient's symptoms were not improving despite optimizing his medications and he felt that he was deconditioned and unable to perform well. A cardiac MRI was done which showed left ventricular noncompaction cardiomyopathy. We changed some of the mediations and initiated cardiac rehab which improved his condition. What is interesting is that he presented very atypically, and his echocardiogram was not very definitive in diagnosing left ventricular noncompaction cardiomyopathy (LVNC).

Hence, it was an eye-opener to detect this genetic condition that may develop before birth but by the time one presents with symptoms, is usually in their adult life affecting men more than women and is a mutated or altered gene that can be inherited. He did later mention that he had a first-degree family member that had heart failure which was attributed to smoking or arterial occlusion but may have been secondary to LVNC. Non-compaction is about the left ventricle having new gaps and channels in the trabeculations. The left ventricle has a characteristic spongy look in the MRI which sometimes affects the right ventricle. Normally, it is well compacted to form a good contractile reserve for the heart muscle to function and perform.

In this case with noncompaction abnormality, it caused him to lose their breath, become fatigued or gain fluid retention. Patients are usually placed on a blood thinner because the risks of a blood clot forming in these trabeculations are high and can lead to stroke. The patient did have transient atrial fibrillation which resolved spontaneously but we had to keep him on warfarin which seemed to improve the flow of the blood inside the heart and with the use of the medications as mentioned above, he felt better. His ejection fraction did drop to 30% and he required a defibrillator, implantable pacemaker, cardiac rehab, and medical therapy.

He started to improve symptomatically, and his EF went up to 50%. The lessons that we can learn here include the diagnosis of noncompaction which can be hidden upon traditional imaging and one needs to start rethinking whether there is a need for more advanced imaging such as MRI. So, we do have an appreciation for this patient who made us address his persistent symptoms with a new thinking process.

Lab Testing and Imaging for Diagnosis

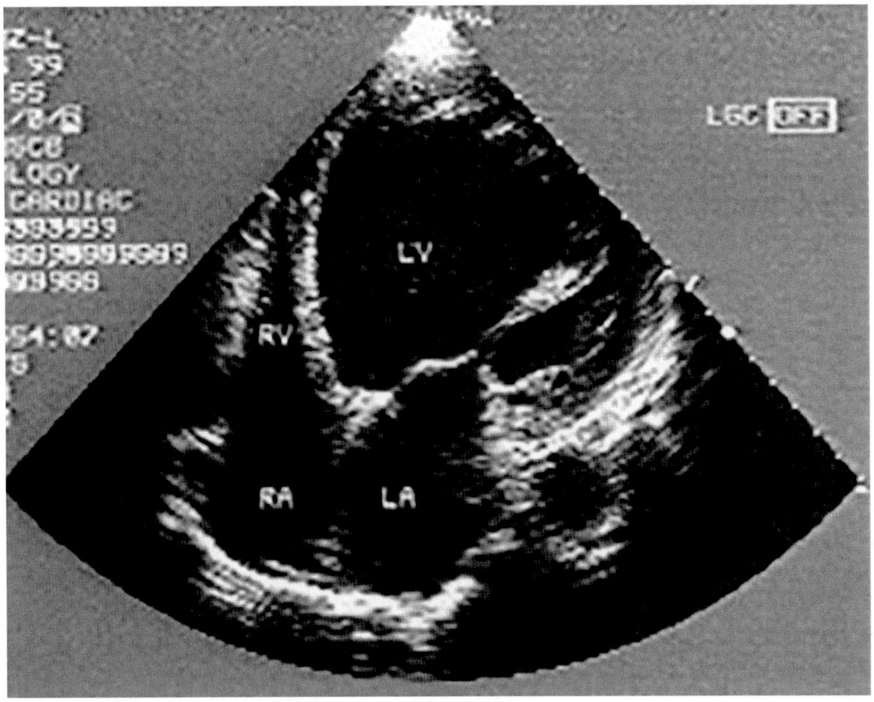

Fig. 28

Enlarged Left Ventricle (LV) shown by ECHO

Lab Testing for Diagnosis is used often for diagnosis; red blood count is used to assess for anemia, white blood count is used to assessing for infection, the low platelet count can also indicate heart failure. Sometimes mean corpuscular volume (MCV) can be used for a signal for liver disease, hypothyroidism, alcoholic liver disease, anemia.

Hemoglobin may be normal but MCV is low which could signal thalassemia or sickle cell anemia. A comprehensive metabolic panel (CMP) involves liver tests, kidney tests, electrolytes, and calcium. This can be a great tool to determine if congestive heart failure has affected kidneys, liver, or caused any electrolyte imbalance. Blood pressure can be exceedingly high, and potassium low which triggers suspicion for primary hyperaldosteronism or a tumor in the adrenal gland.

In addition, if anemia is present due to perceived iron deficiency in conjunction with liver disease, it could signify hemochromatosis especially if they have diabetes and bronze-like skin discoloration. HIV and autoimmune/rheumatic disease can be assessed with HIV testing and an antinuclear antibody (ANA) test, respectively. ESR will tell us if there is an active ongoing inflammatory process.

If one has fluid retention there is a test called a b-type natriuretic peptide (BNP) which assesses if there is increased ventricular volume and pressure overload as well as an NT-Pro-BNP which are cleaved products of this molecule, which will also increase in heart failure. Amyloidosis assessment is also important if there is preserved ejection fraction and there is infiltrative cardiomyopathy. Additionally, there are other blood tests called ST2 and galectin 3 which are some of the newer biomarkers in the cardiorenal space. Management of chronic heart failure diagnosis and therapeutic treatment strategies can be targeted based on the test results.

There are other biomarkers especially with the assessment of cardiorenal syndrome such as urine albumin/creatinine ratio and Nephrocheck and NGAL tests which can detect early kidney injury and treatments geared towards these can prevent nephrotoxicity. Cardiac troponins can also be assessed if suspicious of heart failure. If troponin level is high in conjunction with high BNP but there are no coronary occlusions, then the prognosis can be assessed. If the troponin is elevated, then it is important to determine if there are any blocked arteries through invasive cardiovascular testing.

Electrocardiogram

Electrocardiograms are important cardiac tests that can detect the underlying risk factors for heart failure such as left ventricular hypertrophy, atrial fibrillation, atrial abnormalities, conduction defects, evidence of old heart attacks, lack of blood flow in coronary arteries. Sometimes in patients who may have left ventricular hypertrophy as confirmed by echocardiogram, they may have a low QRS amplitude on the EKG which could trigger a thinking process that would suspect amyloidosis as the etiology.

Echocardiography

Echocardiography is a term encompassing all cardiac ultrasound techniques. We can do a transthoracic, 3rd-dimensional echocardiogram, tissue dopplers, strain rate imaging echocardiogram, and transesophageal echocardiogram.

There are so many ways to use these tests based on symptoms and signs and underlying reasons behind heart failure. An echocardiogram is a powerful tool that can reveal possible heart failure as assessed by measuring chamber dimensions, pressures inside the different chambers of the heart, and ejection fraction. If the ejection fraction of the left ventricle is less than 40%, then the patient has HFrEF and at risk for decompensation.

In patients with reduced ejection fraction, multiple different therapies can be utilized to increase the quality of life and functional capacity. In midrange heart failure, there are limited therapies, but in HFpEF, specific pharmacological therapies are lacking. But there are many things one can do to make patients feel better. The other assessment is that of the right ventricular size or function and the pressure in the pulmonary artery.

Clearly the assessment of the tricuspid valve on the echocardiogram and tissue doppler imaging, as well as right ventricular fractional area change, and pulmonary artery pressure assessment give us guidance to use different types of therapies. Echocardiography is an immensely powerful diagnostic modality and an important imaging test that will continue to be used for determining underlying etiology. Also, a serial echocardiogram over time will guide us in the direction of improving outcomes in ejection fraction, functional capacity, and survival.

Another kind of echocardiogram which includes the 3rd-dimensional echocardiogram determines if there is a hole in the heart, especially atrial septal defect or ventricular septal defect, and also can determine if there is a clot in the left ventricle following a heart attack involving the apex of the heart. It also can view the valves to rule out narrowing or leakiness and rule out any valvular abnormalities. The tissue Doppler imaging gives us information about the relaxation phase of the heart. Also, the strain rate imaging uses more information regarding specific abnormalities inside the heart muscle both with systolic and diastolic heart function. It also gives us information if there is a possibility of amyloidosis. The transesophageal echocardiogram (TEE) is mainly reserved for patients who are suspected of specific abnormalities such as congenital heart disease, valve disease, atrial septal defect, patent foramen ovale, and to evaluate for a clot in the left atrial appendage to assess the safety of cardioversion to convert atrial fibrillation to sinus rhythm. TEE is also helpful to gauge proximal aorta for aneurysm/thrombus/plaque and dissection. At times, if there is confusion about a clot in the left ventricular apex, utilizing a contrast agent in conjunction with the endoscope will give us a better picture of the specific abnormality in question.

Another type of echocardiogram called a stress echocardiogram is utilized by making patients run on a treadmill and at peak exercise, perform imaging to detect if there is any lack of blood flow suspicious for a blocked artery. If there is a suspicion for occluded coronary artery, it will reveal abnormal dynamics of wall motion in the left ventricle. Stress echocardiograms can also be used to detect exercise-induced diastolic dysfunction in patients with preserved ejection fraction with inconclusive diagnostic tests at rest.

Other radiological non-invasive imaging includes a treadmill stress test that uses a treadmill to rule out exercise-induced ischemia. Nuclear stress test to assess for ischemia with imaging increases specificity and sensitivity to detect any kind of blocked arteries up to 90%. Invasive imaging includes coronary angiography which will determine if there are specific blockages in any of the coronary arteries.

Other noninvasive testing includes a CT scan of the heart which sometimes determines structural abnormalities in the heart. A CT scan with dye is called CT angiography which may determine the narrowing of the arteries. If the condition is suspected to be borderline, then one has the option to pursue CT angiography rather than invasive angiography with a catheter. In addition, CT scans of the heart may detect pericardial effusions, pleural effusions, pulmonary fibrosis, pneumonia, lung tumor, and pulmonary embolism. A CT scan of the pulmonary artery itself may determine if it is dilated.

Cardiac magnetic resonance images (MRI) are used to evaluate diastolic dysfunction, left atrial size, left ventricular hypertrophy, non-compaction cardiomyopathy, the viability of the myocardium, congenital heart diseases, after complex cardiac surgery for anatomical deformities, and to screen for TTR amyloidosis. This test is usually more accurate than echocardiograms. Many times, the pulmonary vein assessment, left ventricular time and volume relationship, left ventricular myocardial tagging along with flow propagation velocity to assess for myocardial fibrosis and extracellular volume measurement are all important variables that MRI's may be able to evaluate. Magnetic resonance elastography can be used as a biomarker for patients with preserved ejection fraction as it uses mechanical shell waves to quantify the stiffness of the tissues. Cardiac MR may have an increasing role in measuring abnormalities in congestive heart failure. Time will tell in terms of the availability, sensitivity, and specificity in detecting disease as well as accuracy and cost.

Cardiopulmonary stress tests are used in heart transplant centers which will determine if the VO2 max is higher than the number 14; if higher than 14 then one may not qualify for a heart transplant. If 10-14, then one may be considered for the same, if less than 10, the patient may be significantly at risk for worsening heart failure and death. Hence, a heart transplant may be the last option if all other treatments have failed. This test also determines other variables that can detect if someone with shortness of breath has lung or heart disease or deconditioned state. To differentiate between the three and tease specific abnormalities, a cardiopulmonary stress test may be beneficial.

Other non-invasive imaging that is available includes impedance cardiography which measures intracardiac pressure noninvasively. There are multiple different devices available that detect lung water to thoracic fluid content and intracardiac pressures. Also, other non-invasive techniques include arrhythmia monitoring from a distance for 24 hours to a week to 3 years or even longer if implanted into a patient. This long-term arrhythmia monitor is called an implantable loop recorder which is used for patients with suspicion of paroxysmal atrial fibrillation that cannot be caught with a short duration event monitor.

Invasive imaging includes right and left heart catheterization, which are tests that are performed at the hospital. Right heart catheterization gives us plenty of information about pressures on the right side of the heart, as well as the inferior vena cava, pulmonary artery, and superior vena cava. It also gives us information about the left side of the heart which is called pulmonary capillary wedge pressure detection.

All of these give physicians more information to treat acutely in the hospital setting. Some patients with pulmonary hypertension may need right heart catheterization to determine if they have secondary pulmonary hypertension because of something else that is increasing the pulmonary artery pressure or have primary pulmonary hypertension which has a poor prognosis. Left heart catheterization involves the insertion of a catheter to the heart through the radial or femoral artery which is essentially performed to rule out any occlusion of coronary arteries.

SECTION V

Management of Heart Failure

CHAPTER 31:

Lifestyle modifications and Cardiac Rehab

A study called ACTION-HF was about exercise training among patients with heart failure performed by NHLBI and it showed the patients had improved their exercise duration and had improved their cardiovascular outcomes favorably.

WATCH NOW

Patient Story

Mr. WN was a man in his late 70's who had bypass surgery about 6 months prior and was enrolled in cardiac rehab programs. After his initiation in the cardiac rehab program, he started to feel better overall but a year after his bypass, he started to feel worse. His ejection fraction had dropped to 22% and not performing well, and we optimized his medications which made him feel better and re-enrolled him for cardiac rehab.

Hence, cardiac rehab has been approved since then for patients to go through an exercise program in heart failure. After WN was introduced to cardiac rehab again, he started performing better in cardiac rehab and his ejection fraction had improved to 45%. He had significant improvement in other objective measures. He decided to continue going to cardiac rehab regularly.

We had started a program for patients to spend $15 a week for them to continue cardiac rehab. WN continued for more than 5 years until he was in his mid-80's but had other issues. And he started to slow down. However, WN showed us was that a continuum of exercise programs, supervised or unsupervised in patients with heart disease including heart failure makes a big impact on their own performance in life, the ability to do more, and sustain independence. WN taught us that there is clear benefit in continuing cardiac rehab or getting to a gym even long after an event has occurred. All of this is beneficial for subjects with heart failure.

Lifestyle Modification

There are risks and costs to a program of action.
But they are far less than the long-range risks and
costs of comfortable inaction.

— JFK

- Modifying risk factors are extremely important in the management of heart failure.
- Smoking cessation is extremely important as smoking can erode the inner lining of blood vessels leading to plaque genesis and blocking of the arteries which can lead to heart failure.

DO or Do NOT. There is No "TRY."

— Yoda from STAR WARS

- If overweight, then the person is at a higher risk for these conditions and should aim for a BMI range of 23-27%.

- If they are heavy drinkers, then reducing the amount of overall alcohol consumption would be beneficial. However, 1-2 glasses of wine a day should not be a major issue as long as they do not have other conditions that could get worse with alcohol consumption.
- If the patient has high blood pressure, diabetes, coronary artery disease, then these conditions should be treated individually. For hypertensives, diet, exercise, weight reduction and adherence with low salt diet and medication are extremely important to prevent the onset of heart failure
- High cholesterol should be addressed, and LDL should be brought to goal. Triglycerides are important players in CAD and HF thereof. Hence should be addressed with diet and medications as needed to protect from the risk of cardiovascular events.
- Newer therapies used for diabetes control are now indicated for heart failure. Healthcare providers are still learning about these therapies and it would be a good idea to initiate a conversation with one's PCP, endocrinologist, and/or cardiologist.
- Other lifestyle modifications include monitoring weight regularly. There are so many published studies available that suggest weight monitoring and sodium management are extremely important in reducing the risk of this condition.
- Daily weight checks may prevent heart failure exacerbation by allowing prophylactic use of diuretic therapy or water pills. Sometimes water pills may not remove water and IV diuretics would be more effective in this case. Patients can weigh themselves on a regular basis and contact their clinician for further management instructions. If one has a weight gain of over 4 pounds over a 48-hour period, then there is a possibility that increased salt intake and water retention is contributing to this weight gain. If this is the case, then they need to be seeking attention from a health care professional. Also, they need to be empowering themselves and utilize water pill medications as instructed by their physicians. Some patients can also utilize a sliding scale of diuretics to maintain their weight as well.
- Support from nurses, physician assistants, and respiratory therapists are additional important resources to utilize if one runs into any trouble with increasing shortness of breath.
- Plant-based diet seems to be extremely beneficial in controlling heart failure. In subjects with HFpEF, diet modification, exercise, and weight loss program are the initial therapeutic strategies that may immediately impact with benefit from symptom mitigation and increased quality of life.
- Exercise programs including cardiac rehab are highly researched and evidence points in favor of cardiovascular exercise being beneficial. Sarcopenia or loss of muscle bulk and function is a phenomenon in heart failure, diabetes, and aging. Muscle-strengthening exercises in a dedicated supervised setting are helpful in improvement in functional capacity. Sarcopenia centers are sprouting in the country to address this problem.

- In patients with advanced heart failure, sometimes sodium levels need to be monitored as increased sodium levels can be related to an increase in water retention. Sometimes low sodium levels, also called hyponatremia, can be attributed to a syndrome called inappropriate antidiuretic hormone (SIADH) which can be secondary to lung disease or other pathologies affecting the pulmonary system. In addition, brain disorders or tumors can also be an underlying cause and should be addressed by their clinician.
- Many of these recommendations are based on expert opinion as many of the resources are based on heterogeneous populations. The data can be conflicting and is some studies, a restriction of sodium to 2g a day is recommended in some people and 1g a day in those with advanced heart failure. It is clearly reasonable to restrict fluid intake to about 40-50 ounces a day while restricting sodium intake. Some patients may get too dry with restriction and may need fluid optimization than restriction.
- Beyond lifestyle modifications, medications like beta-blockers and angiotensin-converting enzyme inhibitors or Angiotensin Receptor Blockers or Sacubitril/valsartan combination medications and agents like spironolactone are lifesaving therapies that may be beneficial when considering one's individual situation with other co-morbid conditions.
- Pacemakers, Bi-ventricular pacemakers (also called Cardiac Resynchronization Therapy or CRT) with or without implantable defibrillators are devices that may be beneficial in some patients based on EKG abnormality as well as ejection fraction
- A structured cardiac rehabilitation program provides supervised exercise and support and assists with lifestyle modifications and improving functional capacity. However, few studies prove that these treatments to be extremely effective in mortality reduction. In a large multicenter randomized clinical trial beyond usual care, exercise care was shown to be well-tolerated and safe and as assessed through a 6-minute walk test and peak oxygen capacity.
- They seem to have a major improvement in health outcomes from a functional and quality of life perspective. After heart surgery or among those with low ejection fraction, cardiac rehabilitation therapy has shown to be beneficial. Patients with heart failure with preserved ejection fraction may find this beneficial, however, it is not clear in terms of clinical trial or data. Patients with peripheral vascular disease seem to benefit from cardiac rehab program significantly. Weight reduction, improvement in diabetes, and exercise capacity are all beneficial in patients with preserved ejection fraction.

This book gives an incredible insight into the heart and the miracle it is. It's a real education on the complexity of the heart. It goes into detail about many of the issues the heart can experience and some solutions to help. Few people take time to ponder about their heart unless something goes wrong. A compassionate, caring cardiologist is a true gift to those people who have life-and-death issues with their heart.

This book goes into research that has happened and continues to happen on this incredibly important organ. This book delivers hope with a plethora of solutions to many heart failure issues, new diagnostic equipment, amazing drugs, implantable electronics, exercise, and diet all are all possible solutions to a better quality of life.

Patient stories are featured in this book. The patient is not looked at as 'sick' but as a real and vital person. This critical distinction allows Dr. Vijay his team of cardiologists to go past merely treating the heart failure problem that is in front of them instead to look for the root cause. Caring and learning more about their patients gives them the insight to get to the root reason for the heart failure, which allows for real and lasting healing.

The inspiration I got of this book is the caring and compassion that Dr. Vijay and his team of Doctors and nurses have for those who fell into heart failure issues. Their compassion for the individual allows them to learn daily to help others, which is the true highest calling.

Finally, Dr. Vijay shows us with proper care; there is the hope of a brighter tomorrow. A healthy lifestyle with proper diet and exercise will prevent many issues. Every day is a gift; proper maintenance and care of the heart will make every day worth living.

Marcus Newton – Entrepreneur and Community Leader
CEO Printing Specialists
Chairman of the Tempe Diplomats
Executive Committee Member Project C.U.R.E
Western States Printing Alliance (WSPA) Chairman and now past chair
Thrive AZ – Advisory Board
Military Affairs Committee – Emeritus Member

CHAPTER 32

Controversies in Cardiovascular Nutrition

Many trending foods and supplements are not clearly understood, and scientific inquiry continues to evolve. Several controversial dietary patterns in food and nutrients have caused significant media attention. There is a lot of hype about many nutritional products such as milk, vitamins, shakes, berries, and tea.

WATCH NOW

In this section, we will discuss the main evidence and key conclusions in the utilization of these products.

Dairy products are the leading source of saturated fat in the US and they are loaded with cholesterol and sodium which leads to consequences in chronic disease. However, data is sparse and fragmented; the association with increased cardiovascular risk is evident in observational design studies and meta-analysis, but no major randomized control trials have been performed.

Dairy products have been analyzed in three large cohort studies and one large meta-analysis of 20 randomized controlled trials involving more than 1,600 subjects over 26-week period. The key conclusion in these studies revealed that a high percentage of dietary fat intake with polyunsaturated fat or vegetable fat was associated with 24% and 10% lower risk of cardiovascular disease, respectively. Also, high, and low-fat dairy products cause modest weight gain and a nonsignificant increase in LDL. Hence, the key conclusion for the use of dairy products includes a consensus that food fats of dairy products are a significant source of saturated fat and sodium and should be limited. However, dairy products do contain essential vitamins and protein.

Metabolic abnormalities in cardiovascular risk have had a resurgence with the use of excessive **added sugars** in recent years. There have been scientific reviews funded by sugar industries in the 1960s that claimed that there was insufficient evidence to suggest that there is a correlation between high sugar intake and health consequences. However, more data is coming out that suggests added sugars may contribute to coronary artery disease. The evidence is mainly from a large study called the National Health and Nutrition Evaluation Survey where a total of 11,733 subjects were followed over a period of 14.6 years. Added sugars such as sucrose and high fructose are linked to an increase in cardiometabolic risk and atherosclerotic cardiovascular disease (ASCVD). The key conclusion from this study is that the cardiovascular death ratio was 1.3-fold higher if 10-25% of caloric energy were from added sugars.

People who consume more than 20% of energy from added sugars were at even high risk with a hazard ratio of 2.75 which means more than double the risk. They concluded that consuming added sugars at 10% or less of total daily calories will have a positive effect on heart disease and heart failure. The cardiac metabolic and atherosclerotic cardiovascular risk from added sugars is very real, hence, the conclusion is that clinicians should recommend a diet low in added sugars. Patients should also be taught how to read nutritional food labels to assess for added sugars.

Legumes: High Legume consumption is associated with a reduction in all-cause mortality which includes beans, peas, lentils, and other seeds that are low in fat but rich in protein, saponins, phenols, and complex carbohydrates. There are 4 large studies utilizing legumes.

A meta-analysis of prospective studies showed an inverse relation with all-cause mortality and high legume consumption. Another meta-analysis of prospective randomized studies on the Mediterranean diet revealed a significant reduction of cardiovascular disease.

Systematic analysis, meta-analysis, and randomized controlled trials are showing a significant reduction in body weight, stroke risk, and cardiovascular risk. The conclusion for legumes is that consumption is associated with a reduction in cardiovascular risk, blood glucose levels, and body weight. The Western population consumption of pulses and derived products is exceptionally low; hence, it should be a part of any diet to uphold cardiometabolic health and among patients with heart disease.

Coffee is one of the most commonly consumed beverages in the US and contains polyphenols that are responsible for its taste and is an alkaloid with stimulant properties. It may affect the adenosine receptors and release dopamine in the brain causing a pleasurable sensation. A large meta-analysis showed no positive long-term effects of coffee in cardiovascular patients. The United Kingdom National Health Service (NHS) in Britain showed no association between coffee consumption and high blood pressure. The polyphenolic antioxidant in coffee may improve glucose levels and insulin sensitivity in large studies.

A meta-analysis of 36 prospective cohort studies showed an inverse relationship between coffee consumption and cardiovascular risk. In another large prospective study of 186,000 subjects, who drank 4 cups of coffee a day, an 18% lower risk of premature death was noted compared to nondrinkers. Even 1 cup of coffee a day reduced mortality by 12% compared to nondrinkers. In a large prospective study of 521,000 subjects in Europe, coffee drinkers had a 7-12% lower risk of premature death as opposed to nondrinkers. Conclusion on coffee is that it is correlated with high dose-response protective benefit on all-cause mortality but is not associated with an increase in blood pressure. However, one must be cautious with coffee because many of them are loaded with added sugars and fats that will reduce health benefits.

Tea is another popular drink that is more common in Europe than in the US. However, green tea is also being consumed in the US more commonly over the last decade. A study following 66 patients with proven heart disease randomized to black tea consumption, revealed an improvement in the dilatation of the brachial artery with improvement in endothelial function. A large study in China that included 200,000 men and 300,000 women found daily consumption of tea had an 8% reduction in heart disease and a 10% reduction in major heart attack and strokes. Green tea may be associated with improved cardiovascular disease, perhaps from the EGCG component. In conclusion, plain teas have positive health benefits without added milk, sweeteners, sugars, and cream.

Alcohol consumption and cardiovascular outcomes relationships are extraordinarily complex and are based on age, ethnicity, and genetic factors. A low to moderate intake of less than one ounce has been shown to have benefits with reduced cardiovascular mortality. Other benefits include improvements in insulin sensitivity, and HDL, prevention of thrombosis, stomach inflammation, and diabetes. However, increased and binge drinking is associated with atrial fibrillation, ventricular arrhythmia, cardiac death, cardiomyopathy, high triglycerides, and diabetes.

Most of the studies have been done on men and sparsely among women. In 2017, in 330,000 subjects, the analysis showed that mild to moderate alcohol consumption is associated with reduced all-cause mortality by 29%. The phenolic components in wine such as flavonoids and nonflavonoids include resveratrol and quercetin have been shown to have antioxidant, vasodilatory, and anti-inflammatory properties. The bottom line in alcohol consumption is as follows: low to moderate consumption of alcohol is associated with benefit, however, risk of falls, certain cancers, liver disease are associated with high amounts of alcohol. Also, adding sodas, creme, or added sugars to alcohol has neutralized the benefits as well.

Energy drinks among adolescents in the US are quite common with more than 30% of 12-24 year-old individuals consuming energy drinks regularly. Consumption of energy drinks has been associated with multiple negative side effects. Many of them contains multiple vitamins, 2 to 4 times the caffeine dose, and other potentially harmful supplements. Hence, high consumption of energy drinks can result in high blood pressure, seizures, agitation, strokes, cardiomyopathy, and arrhythmias. Even Takotsubo cardiomyopathy has been described with their use. In one large study, following Energy drink consumption, there is evidence that blood platelets get aggregated and endothelial function gets affected negatively. The International Society of Sports Nutrition recommends that children and adolescents do not consume energy drinks without parental permission. The American Academy of Pediatrics is very conservative in advertising energy drinks. Europe has restricted marketing this to minors. Hence, the conclusion on energy drinks is that it should be avoided due to its negative health effects.

Mushrooms seem to have cardiac protective benefits through multiple mechanisms and many studies have revealed that mushrooms may have anti-inflammatory and antioxidant benefits and are vitamin D producers. Ergothioneine, ergosterol, and beta-glucans are responsible for these beneficial effects. They may prevent atherosclerotic disease, decrease cholesterol, immunomodulatory effects, metabolic syndrome, and type two diabetes. All mushrooms contain ergosterol and get converted to vitamin D2 when exposed to ultraviolet light. In 3 ounces of white mushrooms, one can get 100% of vitamin D.

The evidence in clinical trials with the use of mushrooms is as follows: a cross-sectional study of 720 subjects with type two diabetes revealed overall lower usage of diabetes medications and a better lifestyle. In another clinical study, that compared the bioavailability of vitamin D2, it was clear that mushroom consumption was associated with a lower postprandial triglyceride response. In a randomized controlled trial of 73 patients who were obese, substituting mushrooms for red meat revealed that there was an improvement in inflammatory markers in people who consumed mushrooms. They also experienced lower calorie intake, and weight reduction. Hence, substituting mushrooms for red meat is a recommended strategy in reducing cardiovascular disease.

Fermented foods such as kimchi, sauerkraut, yogurt, and kombucha have the potential to suppress inflammation and some of these agents have cholesterol-lowering properties. Kimchi, which is fermented cabbage, has been known for its medicinal properties which are rich in dietary fiber, vitamin c, beta-sitosterol, and other minerals. In a 2-week study in 22 overweight patients who consumed 3 servings of kimchi, the analysis showed a significant decrease in weight and improvement in fasting blood glucose and blood pressure. Although sodium intake was significantly high (more than 5g a day), the onset of high blood pressure was still low. Fermented milk and yogurt products contain lactobacillus acidophilus which showed an increase in HDL when compared to baseline. Some of the seaweed such as algae and spirulina have bioactive properties that exhibit lowering of blood pressure and improvement in insulin sensitivity. Recent clinical trials have found that there is no high-quality evidence of cardiovascular outcomes benefits with fermented foods and seaweed, but observational data have found that natural probiotics and fermented foods may help with lowering cholesterol and weight. However, there is not enough evidence to recommend these routinely.

Fish and Marine Omega 3 Fatty Acids

EPA is obtained mainly from fish and DHA is present in some fish, meat, and egg products. Intake of fish reduces triglyceride levels, has modest effects on blood pressure, improves insulin signaling, and reduces inflammatory and atherogenic markers. Large meta-analysis using all types of omega 3 fish oil compounds have not shown a benefit on cardiovascular events. Many of these compounds have been commercially made and questions were raised about the impurities in these supplements. These included polychlorinated biphenyls, lead, methyl mercury, and other potentially harmful molecules.

It was not clear if the dose of omega 3 was correct and there have been doubts about the study design and whether one component of the omega 3 was better than the other. Hence EPA only study was performed recently which revealed a significant benefit in reducing cardiovascular disease. The outcome benefit was attributed to the proprietary way it was purified to get EPA only from multiple fish sources. In addition, large doses at 2 gm twice a day was used to increase the EPA levels in the blood. This may have translated to a significant benefit due to its anti-inflammatory, antiplatelet, antioxidant, and anti-coagulant properties. FDA has approved this agent for reducing CV risk in subjects with established cardiovascular disease and a TG level > 150 mg/dL. More data is coming out of the REDUCE-IT trial and we will learn more with time.

Vegetable Acquired Omega 3 Fatty Acids

Most common types of Omega 3 are EPA, DHA, and ALA. EPA is found in fish, DHA is found in meat, and ALA is found in green leafy vegetables, walnuts, canola oil, soybean oil, and flax oil. ALA is rapidly oxidized after intake and has a low conversion to EPA and DHA (about 10% to EPA and 1% to DHA). The two large randomized controlled trials in heart attack survivors have tested the effects of ALA in the Lyon Diet Heart Study and the Alpha Omega Trial. These revealed a trend in the reduction of cardiovascular outcomes with 2g of ALA over 40 months compared to the control group. Mediterranean diets also have increased amounts of ALA and 50-70% lower risk of recurrent heart disease as measured by 3 different combinations of outcome measures. Hence, at present, the current guideline of ALA with plant-based omega 3 is positive and favorable because it favorably affects cardiovascular disease.

In non-fish consumers and vegetarians, there is a clear benefit with vegetable omega 3. Folic acid and vitamin B supplements lower homocysteine levels, however, a large study using folic acid to reduce homocysteine in hyperhomocysteinemia patients did not reveal any cardiovascular benefit. The use of vitamin B12 which contains cobalamin, an essential micronutrient in patients who have a deficiency, clearly benefits in preventing hematological and neurological complications. From a cardiovascular standpoint, data is sparse. It has been touted to have wide-ranging health effects such as improved energy, memory, and movement.

In a study called Western Norway B Vitamin Intervention Trial (WENBIT), 3096 patients underwent coronary angiography along with a supplement of vitamin B12 and folic acid with and without vitamin B6 for one year. Homocysteine levels reduced by 30% but they did not reduce mortality or cardiovascular events. The Norwegian Vitamin Trial also showed no reduction in stroke, heart attack, and sudden death. The data so far in multiple clinical trials with vitamin B12 is sparse. It is possible that too much vitamin B12 or folic acid may have worsening effects such as lung cancer in men which were noted in some studies. Hence, the final word on vitamin B12 and folic acid is that they are recommended to prevent hematologic or neurologic disease but not found to be effective in cardiovascular disease.

In summary, the global population is depending on healthier dietary lifestyle patterns; however, what is unclear is whether there is substantial health benefit with the use of many of these nutraceuticals, functional foods, and nutritional supplements. As a health care provider, it is important to stay abreast of all scientific evidence that provides meaning and reasonable guidance for patients with heart disease and heart failure. Consumers and patients may be gullible and vulnerable to be brainwashed by unethical business practices and upbeat marketing even with a lack of scientific evidence.

Current evidence supports cardiovascular benefits in plant-based proteins and plant-based omega 3's, with some concern about marine sources. Not enough data is available with vitamin B12, although it is helpful in both neurological and hematological consequences. It is safe to recommend the use of legumes, caffeine, tea, low amount of alcohol, mushrooms, fermented foods, and seaweed, The evidence to date, suggests that adverse cardiovascular outcomes with intake of red meat, added sugars and excessive energy drinks are real and should be avoided. It is still not clear if use of dairy products increases the risk of cardiovascular disease.

Dr. Vijay gives us an evidence-based approach to CHF that is credible, easily comprehended and presents" the whole patient" approach. A quote attributed to Mark Twain says, "It's not what you don't know that gets you in trouble, it's what you think you know that is just plain wrong." Dr. Vijay has successfully given us the tools so that we don't engage in practices that are "just plain wrong"

Dr. Vijay is an innovative, highly educated, competent, and the most compassionate physician I have encountered. I am forever grateful for the privilege of making his acquaintance. I am humbled to share his friendship. Spanning the last two decades, we have collaborated on both a professional, as well as a personal level. Kris has excelled in leadership roles within multiple organizations. His goal continues to expand our understanding of congestive heart failure and its therapies. Dr. Vijay remains a staunch advocate of including patients in their healing process. He sets the standard to include the heart failure team including nurses, in whatever accolades and accomplishments come his way.

Dr. Vijay's book explores often ignored and seldom reported aspects of congestive heart failure that go well beyond traditional medicine. Dr. Vijay documents actual patient experiences to present their perspective. Drawing from his own extensive experience, he exposes the physician thought process as well as the significant contributions that nurses add to the healing process.

Finally, in what is an often-unexplored territory, the spiritual side of the healing process is fully described. He expertly includes the science of what we understand to be the best therapy for congestive heart failure in all of its varieties. Dr. Vijay gratefully acknowledges the pivotal role that nurses play in the success of heart failure clinics. Defining his "whole patient" approach, Dr. Vijay includes emphasis from the patients' perspective. He considers the patients' psyche, including their thoughts, fears, questions and their expectations of the physicians and heart failure team.

The book is an excellent example of the team approach to therapy for congestive heart failure. Establishing the" best approach to heart failure" he re-iterates the age-old concept that "there is no me in team". Contributions made by physicians, nurses as well as the patients themselves ultimately lead to success. The volume documents the history of the congestive heart failure and what we have learned to make us successful. Dr Vijay adds to our knowledge base providing us with new insights, that when incorporated, will favorably influence our success.

Thomas Haffey, D.O., F.A.C.C., F.A.C.O.I., F.N.L.A., F.A.H.A., F.A.S.P.C.
Professor of Medicine College of Osteopathic Medicine of the Pacific
Past President: Colorado Chapter of the American College of Cardiology
Past President: Southwest Chapter National Lipid Association Member:
Chair, Political Action Committee – American College of Cardiology
Chair: Political Action Committee – National Lipid Association

CHAPTER 33

Pharmacological Treatment

> *"To conquer oneself is a greater victory than to conquer thousands in a battle."*
>
> **— Dalai Lama**

WATCH NOW

Patient Story

Mr. RC is a 58-year-old male who was told that he had 6 months to live and went to multiple centers of excellence where he was told that he needed a left ventricular assist device and followed up with a heart transplant. He did not want to pursue any of that, and it was not clear why his heart had failed. Possibly he has been taking human growth hormones for bodybuilding and energizing himself. It appears that this may have taken a toll on his ejection fraction with nonischemic cardiomyopathy.

> He clearly has come around and the message to learn from him is to never give up or believe that there is no other treatment strategy other than open-heart surgery. He taught us that, being turbocharged, one can transcend oneself with monumental recovery and have the drive for control, energy for congruence, and compassion towards oneself and others.

He has been highly vested in his own healing and resorted to our recommendations with medical therapy and cardiovascular exercise rather than weightlifting. Slowly, but steadily with optimized medical therapy, pacemaker, and ICD, he has turned around with an ejection fraction that went up to 40% from 7%. He was very thrilled about his success and talked about it with his friends and family, as well as multiple people in his community.

Pharmacological Therapies

In patients who have significant worsening heart failure with fluid retention, low blood pressure reflects low cardiac output and may require hospitalization. In acute decompensated heart failure, one may need IV diuretic therapy, IV infusion therapy on a continuum with furosemide or bumex. Continuous IV administration of inotropic agents such as dobutamine or milrinone can increase cardiac output and decrease afterload in patients with severe decompensated heart failure who are not responding well to standard oral medications. Organ damage can happen with low blood pressure, low perfusion pressure, and a high level of fluid retention. This organ damage can be attributed to low perfusion of either liver or kidney. Patients can also go into cardiogenic shock, requiring continuous IV inotropic support. Some may suffer from hypoxia (low oxygenation) which usually requires intubation from a mechanical ventilator. Others may have blocked arteries and need surgical intervention or stents in the cath lab. IV inotropic support is usually used in the hospital for a few days in the ICU and mechanical ventricular assist device may need to be utilized to stabilize the patient. In selected patients with end-stage heart failure who are not eligible for mechanical assist device, a heart transplant may be needed.

Some may not qualify for a heart transplant and if medical and device therapies have not made an impact in improving their status and patient continues to deteriorate, then palliative care and hospice may be appropriate. Sometimes this care may require IV inotropic support for 6 months to a year and attempts should be made for improvement in the quality of life and comfort care. While the patient is acutely decompensated, priority should be to stabilize blood pressure and heart rate. Fluid volume should be stabilized as well, so they do not experience volume overload or volume depletion. Once this condition is achieved, then utilizing lifesaving medications can be beneficial but can be difficult to manage at the same time. Most cardiologists have adapted to the management of heart failure, but sometimes a heart failure subspecialist may be required to provide the best treatment possible with improved functional capacity and longevity.

Beta-blockers are usually one of the first-line therapies indicated for patients regardless of how good their functional capacity is. Many patient have NYHA class I (no symptoms), class II (mild symptoms), class III (moderate symptoms) class IV (severe symptoms). Hence, functional capacity is an important outcome measure to be assessed. Beta-blockers have been shown to have benefit in every stage of heart failure but patients with a lower stage of heart failure have experienced a long-term benefit, including those with reduced ejection fraction. Normal ejection fraction is somewhere between 50% to 80%, however, those with an ejection fraction of 40-50% may not have any symptoms but may still benefit from beta-blockers. Many of the randomized controlled trials that have included a variety of heart failure medications have shown significant reductions in hospitalizations, cardiac arrests, and mortality. Range of mortality reduction is 23-65% on beta-blockers and the specific ones that have shown evidence in clinical trials among patients with low ejection fraction include long-acting metoprolol, carvedilol, and bisoprolol. The agent nebivolol has been approved in Europe but not in the United States but has shown positive effects in heart failure.

One of the studies in heart failure using increasing doses of carvedilol showed an improvement in Ejection fraction over time. This is one of the goals of many heart failure clinics around the country where we enable the use of this agent at higher and higher doses using baby steps while we optimize and adjust other medications that may drop the blood pressure and not allow for up-titration of carvedilol. Dr. Michael Bristow from Colorado had explored the basis of this principle through what is called the beta receptor signal transduction pathway as depicted in the figure below.

Beta Receptor Adenyl Cyclase Interaction Signaling Pathway

A 3-step model that leads to an increase in contractility of the heart muscle may explain this simplistically.

> Step 1: The Beta-Adrenergic Receptor (BAR in red) couples with Adenyl Cyclase (AC in blue).
>
> Step 2: This coupling (like anything in nature, triggers a new life, new energy) stimulates the dual-direction conversion of cyclic AMP and ATP (green and purple). Simultaneously, calcium and potassium are getting into the cell, sodium is going out of the cell, and calcium is embedding into the sarcoplasmic reticulum forming SERCA 2A molecule

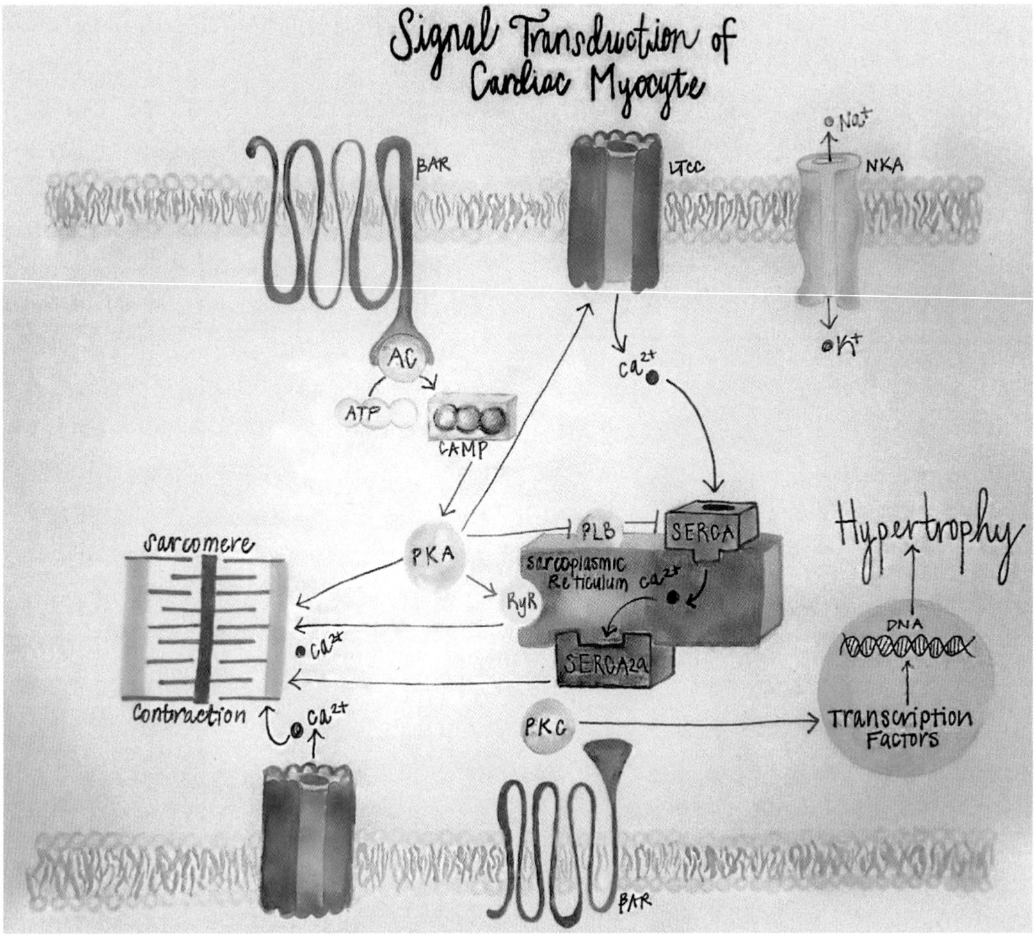

Fig. 29

Step 3: SERCA 2A and Protein kinase A are now stimulating the sarcomere to increase contractility of the heart muscle. Also, protein Kinase C is fueling the transcription factors in DNA stimulating the thickening and function of the heart muscle.

Step 1 is activated by beta-blockers such as carvedilol. Adenyl Cyclase is generated by exercises such as cardiac rehab or EECP.

Step 2 can be activated by medications such as milrinone, sildenafil, and others acting on the phosphodiesterase enzyme.

Step 3 is influenced by other pathways called MAPK, PIPk which work in the neurohormonal milieu interacting with ACEi/ARB/Sacubitril/spironolactone and others.

SERCA 2A, phospholamban, Ryanodine receptors are all molecules, some genetically mediated, some biochemically generated, that coalesce to increase contractility of the heart muscle. Hence it is important to combine medications and exercise as a therapy to improve EF in the long run.

ACE inhibitors have shown significant benefit in treating left ventricular systolic dysfunction. Complications of these medications include angioedema, high potassium, and cough. These medications may not be the ideal ones if patients get side effects. ACE inhibitors that have been studied in research include enalapril, lisinopril, and ramipril. Another one called captopril is not used often anymore because it must be used more than once a day and patient compliance has been an issue. ACE inhibitors are vasodilators; hence, they unload the pressure inside the heart and improve symptoms. They have been linked to fewer hospitalizations and mortality reduction by 30%.

One must be actively watching renal function and potassium levels which can go up with the use of these medications. ARBs have also been used for heart failure and have potential side effects of high potassium and renal dysfunction. Randomized control trials have shown a 35-45% reduction in mortality and improvement in functional capacity. Some trials have tried simultaneous intake of ACE inhibitors and ARBs but have shown worsening blood pressure and kidney function, hence, they are not used in combination. Irbesartan was studied in patients with kidney disease, losartan, and Olmesartan in those with high blood pressure. Valsartan has been studied extensively with positive results. One must follow evidence-based guidelines when using these medications.

Patients with moderate to severe heart failure, such as class NYHA II to class IV who have tolerated ACE inhibitors or ARBs were studied in a large clinical trial called PARADIGM. This study incorporated over 8442 patients and randomly compared enalapril to ARNI which is a combination of sacubitril and valsartan. Studies showed that there was a significant reduction of 20% in heart failure hospitalizations and mortality in patients on sacubitril/valsartan compared to enalapril. However, this medication can also cause a lowering of blood pressure, kidney injury, and high potassium level; hence, one needs to be aware of this and monitor vitals and potassium and kidney function closely. One should not use this combination in conjunction with ACE inhibitors or ARBs as blood pressure can dramatically drop. The cost of these medications is starting to come down which would make them more accessible. Insurance companies are also helping a lot of patients and increasing coverage for these medications.

Patients who are intolerant of ACE inhibitors were studied in a clinical trial called A-HeFT that compared hydralazine and isosorbide vs placebo in African Americans with class III or IV heart failure. Patients had up to 43% mortality reduction and hospitalizations with this medication. Patients who can tolerate ACE inhibitors, ARBs, or Sacubitril/valsartan may not have a need for hydralazine and nitrates but can be used if the other medications prove to be ineffective.

Agents like spironolactone have shown to be beneficial in the RALES study, which showed improvement in advanced heart failure patients when compared to a placebo. This agent has antifibrotic and anti-inflammatory effects on the heart and may be considered as a supplemental medication to other blood pressure medications. Spironolactone has been studied exhaustively but can cause gynecomastia (breast enlargement in men). Hence, one needs to monitor closely. In addition, it has a potassium retaining property which can lead to complications and needs to be monitored closely.

One of the problems we encounter is the co-morbidity of kidney disease in heart failure patients. When this happens, most health care providers will stop ACE inhibitors/ARBs/Sacubitril valsartan combo due to fear of worsening their kidney function and potassium levels. This deprives many heart failure patients of life-saving medications.

Eplerenone is a selective aldosterone antagonist that does not have much gynecomastia effects and a reduction in mortality has been shown in patients with heart failure who have experienced a heart attack. This was observed in a study called EMPHASIS-HF where there was a 37% reduction in risk of death or hospitalization. One needs to watch potassium and BUN/creatinine levels with this medication as well. If potassium is low despite these medications, then one needs to take oral supplements. All of this should be discussed with the health care provider and instruction should be followed.

To prevent high potassium levels from occurring, 2 new therapies are now available and approved by FDA; one is called Patiromer which is a potassium binder and will reduce potassium levels in patients with high potassium and kidney disease. Another agent called Zirconium Silicate is also approved by the FDA with a similar mode of action. We are pleased about the advent of these agents as we can now safely use some of the life-saving medications without the fear of hyperkalemia (high potassium)

Ivabradine is a new agent that slows the heart rate by inhibiting the funny current in the sinus node. It reduced the combined endpoint of hospitalization and death in patients with early-stage heart failure studied in SHIFT clinical trial. Patients with heart rates of over 70 and sinus rhythm with low ejection fraction < 35% may qualify for this medication. One needs to consider this as an add on to other medications.

There are multiple diuretic medications used in heart failure. Thiazides work on the proximal convoluted tubules, loop diuretics which work on the loop of Henle, spironolactone which works on the distal convoluted tubules and collecting duct. Diuretics are the only medications that reduce short term issues such as shortness of breath, lung water (pleural space and interstitial space) edema, reducing the pressure of the heart, and abdominal distention. However, they have not been shown to provide long term benefits in terms of mortality reduction. In recent studies, when diuretics are used in acutely decompensated heart failure patients, IV diuretics have reduced mortality. In patients with acute decompensated heart failure, there are no differences in bolus vs continuous infusion. However, those with right-sided heart failure may benefit from slow continuous infusion with fluid removal in a gingerly fashion instead of sudden high doses to prevent vitals from fluctuating too much and putting them in renal failure.

Commonly used thiazide diuretics include hydrochlorothiazide, indapamide, chlorthalidone, and metolazone. Metolazone is a strong potent diuretic and using only 1-2 times per week may be more than adequate. When using thiazide diuretics, one must closely watch potassium, magnesium, uric acid, blood sugar levels, and monitored closely. Indapamide has shown significant benefit in patients with high blood pressure and reducing strokes. It has not been extensively studied in heart failure yet. Loop diuretics are extremely beneficial in patients with advanced heart failure. Bumex and torsemide are agents stronger than furosemide and need to be used accordingly depending on the severity of fluid retention and the patient's condition.

Usually, diuretics are not used to prevent disease progression and are usually used in conjunction with other medications for patients with heart failure. Many times, patients may require IV diuretics if oral medications are not available and can sometimes be done at outpatient heart failure clinics. Patients receiving diuretics need to have blood pressure and electrolytes checked frequently and replaced. Kidney function needs to be monitored regularly as well. Digoxin has been utilized for heart failure but recently used mainly to control heart rate.

Clinical studies show that these medications have shown to reduce hospitalizations but not mortality. Digoxin used with beta-blockers can be effective in lowering heart rates in patients with advanced heart failure and atrial fibrillation. Low potassium and low magnesium are common with diuretics and should be replaced to avoid toxicity with digoxin which can worsen these conditions. It is important to utilize digoxin cautiously as levels can be increased by certain medications such as amiodarone, verapamil, azithromycin, Clonidine, and cyclosporine. Digoxin dose needs to be decreased in patients with kidney disease.

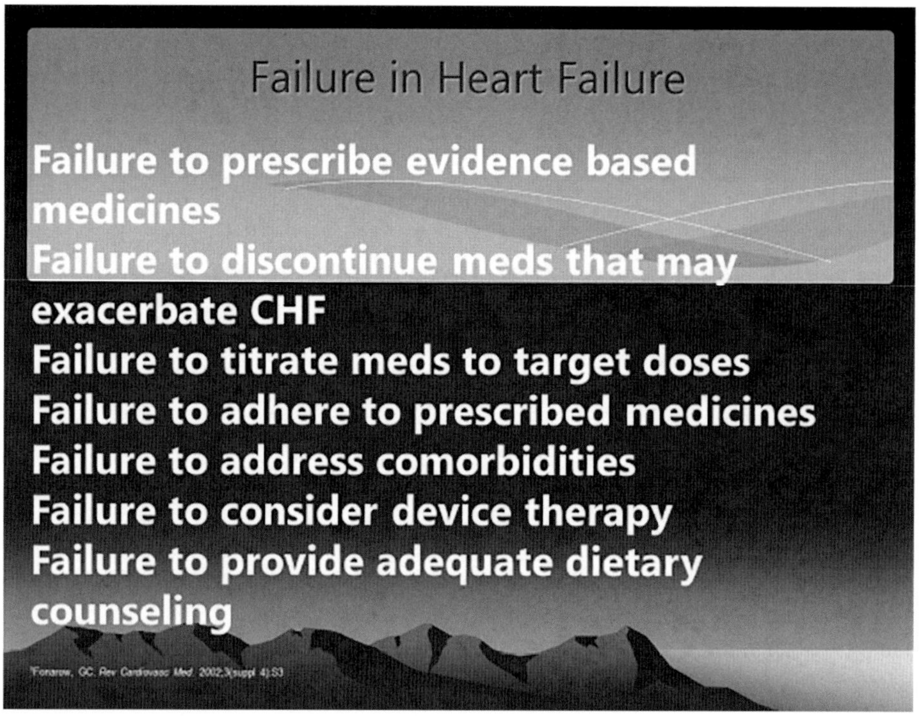
Failure in Heart Failure
Failure to prescribe evidence based medicines
Failure to discontinue meds that may exacerbate CHF
Failure to titrate meds to target doses
Failure to adhere to prescribed medicines
Failure to address comorbidities
Failure to consider device therapy
Failure to provide adequate dietary counseling
Fonarow, GC. Rev Cardiovasc Med. 2002;3(suppl 4):S3

Fig. 30

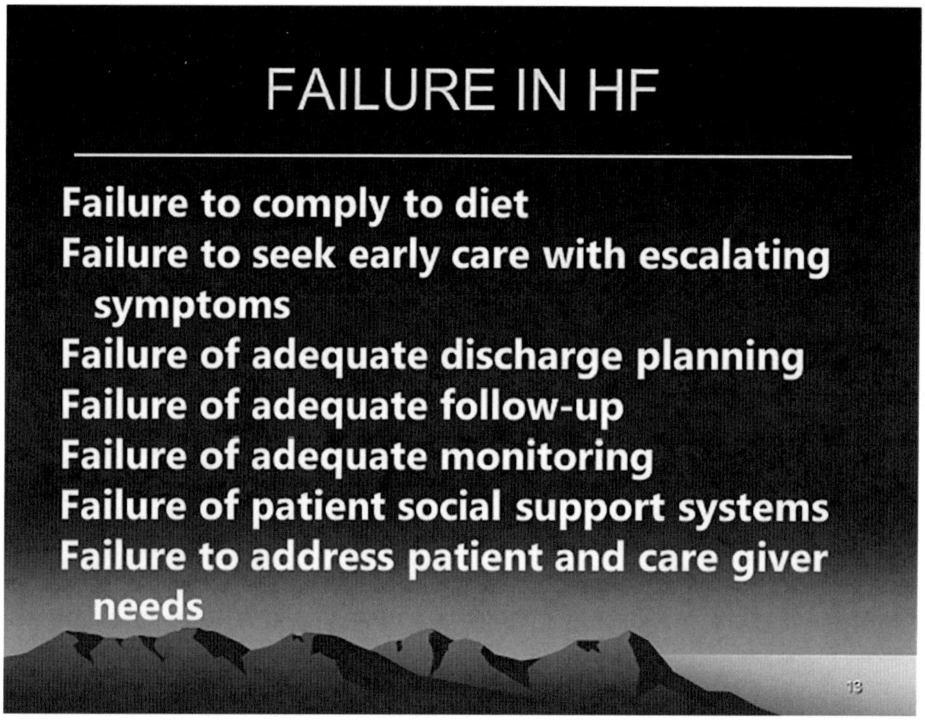
FAILURE IN HF
Failure to comply to diet
Failure to seek early care with escalating symptoms
Failure of adequate discharge planning
Failure of adequate follow-up
Failure of adequate monitoring
Failure of patient social support systems
Failure to address patient and care giver needs
13

Fig. 31

Goals in heart failure management include improvement of symptoms, utilizing lifesaving medications, to make them live longer, improve quality of life and functional capacity, and prevent initial hospitalization and recurrent hospital admissions. Hence, risk factors should be controlled adequately such as hypertension, angina, atrial fibrillation, diabetes, and high cholesterol. Smoking cessation is advised, and resources to help them quit is particularly important. Aspirin is an especially important agent in heart failure patients, specifically in those with coronary artery disease or cerebral ischemia/stroke.

Most of the time, one to 2 baby aspirin from 81-160mg should be more than enough as higher doses may inhibit the good prostacyclin and may have a rebound clotting effect. Clopidogrel is now used for post-stent placement individuals for 2-3 years after surgery and can be used for vascular disease. Ticagrelor is a new antiplatelet agent that has been shown to be slightly more effective than clopidogrel, however, the bleeding complication is a little higher. If one has failed clopidogrel and had recurrent stent restenosis, then ticagrelor may be a good alternative.

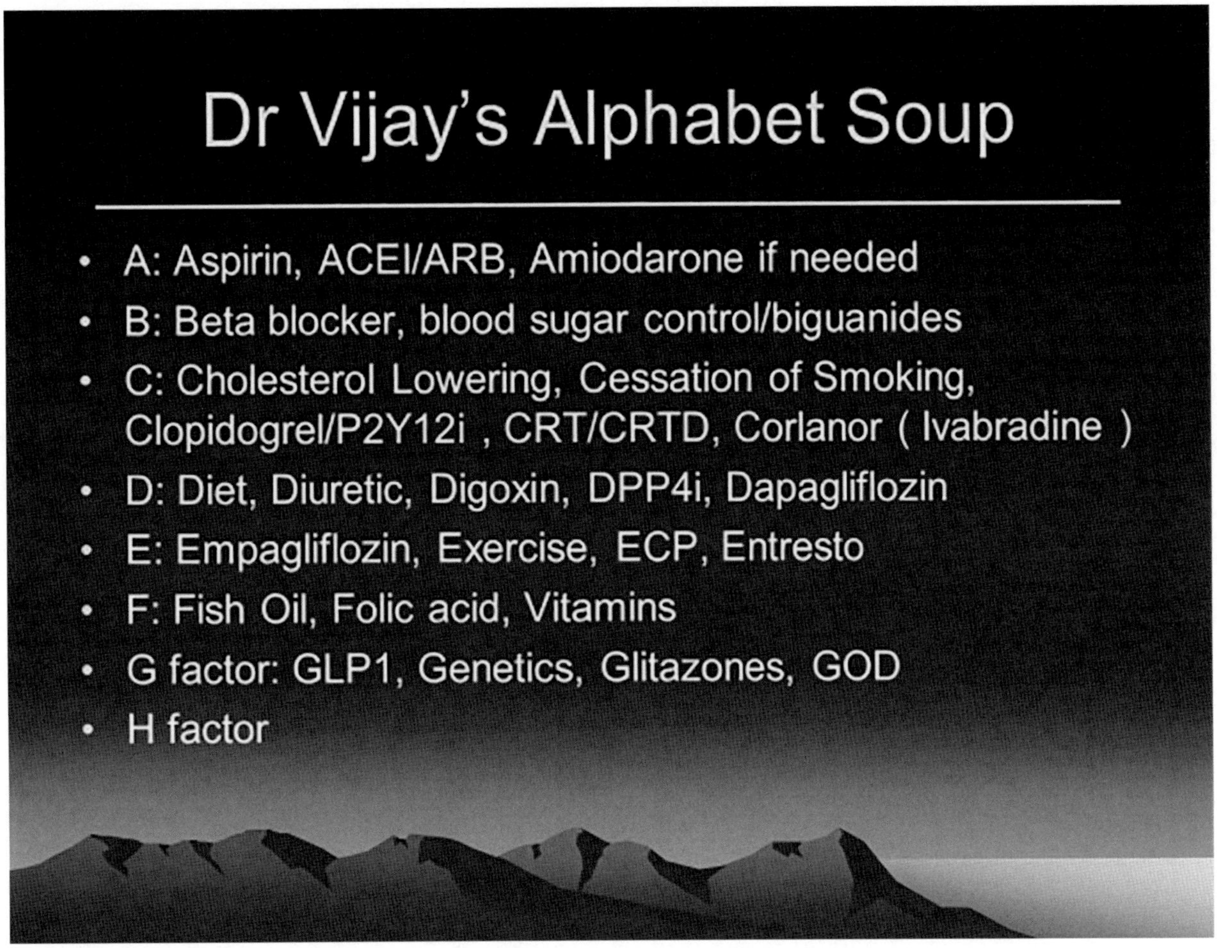

Fig. 32

Warfarin is the most cost-efficient and commonly used anticoagulation, but, is not indicated for patients with heart failure who do not have another indication for blood thinners. However, conditions that may need anticoagulation include atrial fibrillation or a clot inside one of the chambers of the heart. In addition, anticoagulants are needed after a surgically replaced metallic prosthesis of the aortic or mitral valve. Patients on warfarin should monitor their blood-thinning parameter called INR and keep it in therapeutic range with the help of nurses at a coumadin clinic. Warfarin's side effects include bleeding.

Issues with these drugs include drug interactions, efficacy monitoring, diet restriction as greens can reduce the INR due to vitamin k present in them. Side effects of these medications include intracranial hemorrhage, gastrointestinal bleeding, nose bleeds, easy bruising, hence, one needs to weigh the benefits and risks of these medications. Newer anticoagulants include Rivaroxaban, apixaban, and dabigatran. These newer anticoagulants work in different pathways and do not have drug-drug interactions as much as warfarin. Also, there is no need to worry about consumption of green leafy vegetables and there is no need to monitor their blood for INR

Management of a Diabetes Subject:

> Now with new data, management of a patient with diabetes should begin with asking the question: Does this patient need to be prevented from the risk of having heart failure/heart attack/stroke/cardiovascular death and progressing kidney disease: the bigger larger picture of the ocean of cardiovascular disease. The message from Antoine de Saint Exupery epitomizes this concept.

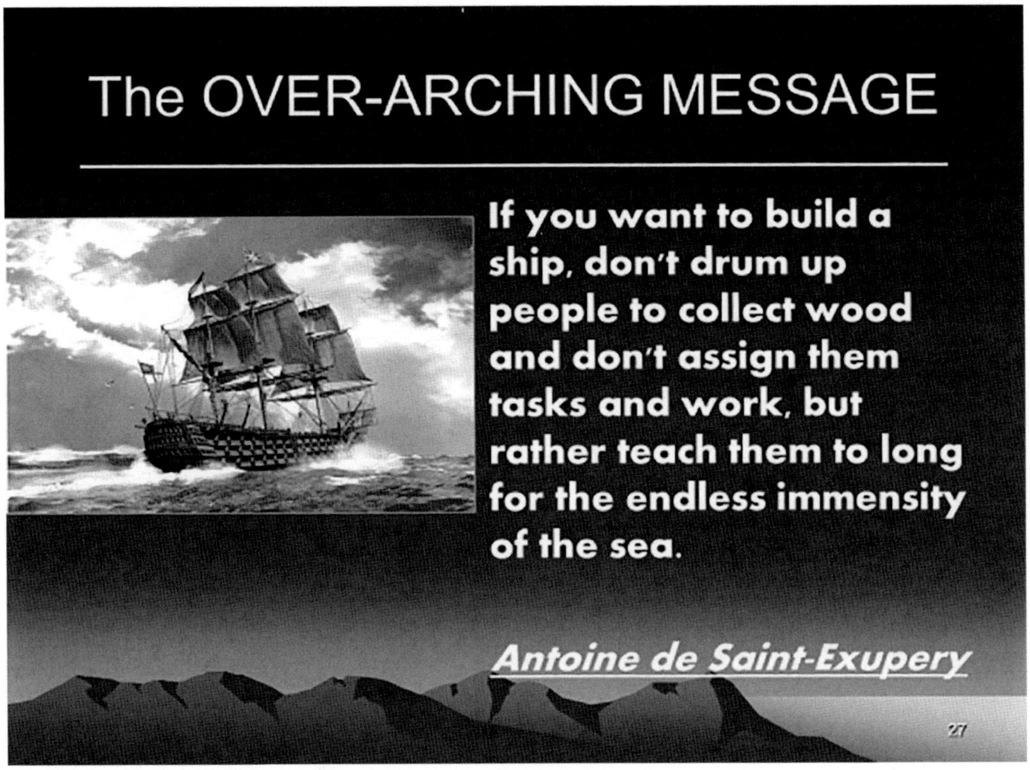

Fig. 33

Treatment strategies based on comorbid conditions

condition	Rx to be considered
Prediabetes	Metformin, RAASi, Statins if needed , LSM, Omega 3, Fenofibrate if high TG > 500
T2DM with no complications	Metformin, statin, RAASi, consider SGLT21i / GLP1/DPP4i/Pio
T2Dm with severe post prandial Glucose excursions	GLP1/Acarbose/Amylin/meglitinide
T2DM with microvascular disease	Metformin plus SGLT2i/GLP1/DPP4i/Pio Asa, RAASi, Statin
AGE > 40 yrs	Consider adding statins
Women	ASA only if T2Dm and 2 other risk factors as risk > benefit
T2DM and CAD	Met , SGLT2i/GLP1/ asa, statin, BB, if stents, then P2Y12 i

28

Fig. 34

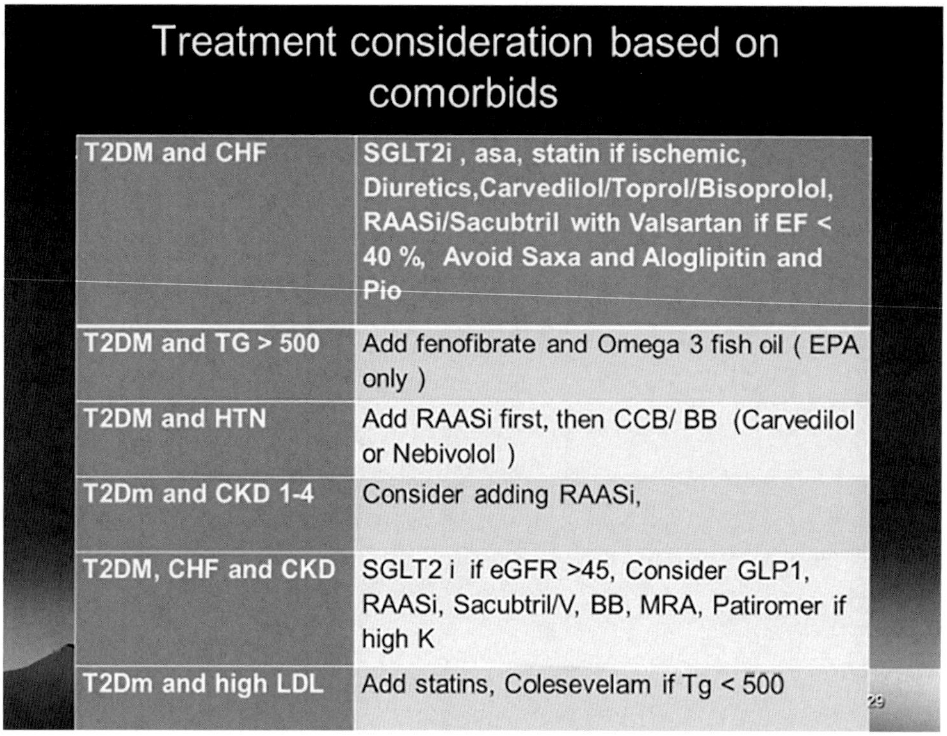

Treatment consideration based on comorbids

T2DM and CHF	SGLT2i , asa, statin if ischemic, Diuretics,Carvedilol/Toprol/Bisoprolol, RAASi/Sacubtril with Valsartan if EF < 40 %, Avoid Saxa and Aloglipitin and Pio
T2DM and TG > 500	Add fenofibrate and Omega 3 fish oil (EPA only)
T2DM and HTN	Add RAASi first, then CCB/ BB (Carvedilol or Nebivolol)
T2Dm and CKD 1-4	Consider adding RAASi,
T2DM, CHF and CKD	SGLT2 i if eGFR >45, Consider GLP1, RAASi, Sacubtril/V, BB, MRA, Patiromer if high K
T2Dm and high LDL	Add statins, Colesevelam if Tg < 500

29

Fig. 35

Treatment Algorithm based on risk for cardiovascular disease (CVD)

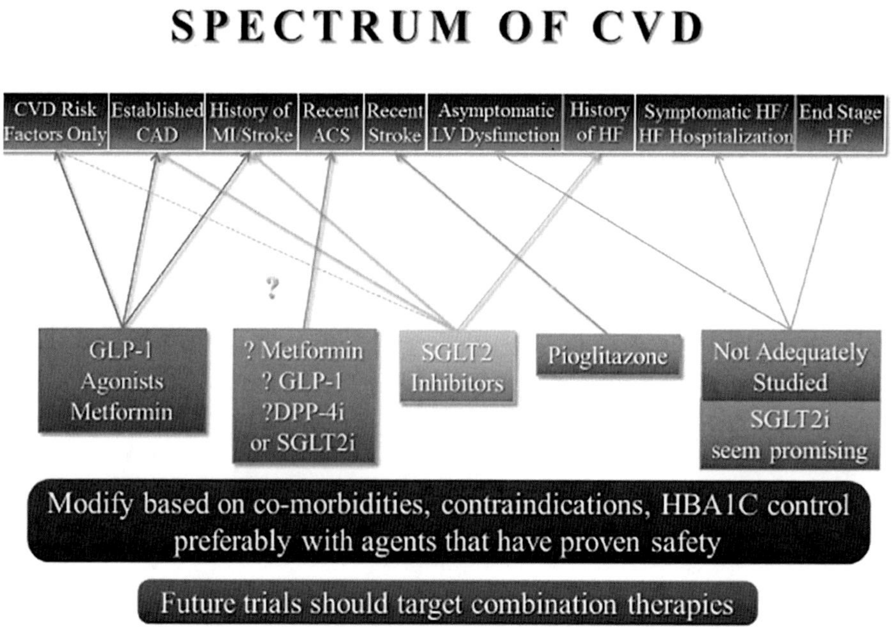

Fig. 36

I have had the honor to know Dr. Kris on many different levels, personally and professionally. A man of great intellect and I feel most importantly great integrity.

Passionate caring approach to patients is evident not only here in the USA but to international medical missions I witnessed with him firsthand in India. Rich or poor made no difference. The love and compassion was evident as he listened to his patients and they listened intently to what he told them.

We have spent many days together in London, New Delhi, Ladakh, India and here in Phoenix. Talking with high level doctors and administration in several countries, it was clear they showed a high level of respect, trust and admiration for Dr. Vijay. His unique whole vision and approach to cardiac medicine and treatment is well received and valued by colleagues and especially patients. This book is a culmination of vast knowledge and experience that will undoubtedly save lives and relieve much suffering.

As an Executive Director of Project C.U.R.E. Phoenix and as an international assessor of hospitals worldwide, I have worked closely with Dr. Vijay certifying him as an assessor of hospital needs for Project C.U.R.E. What a humanitarian asset to our worldwide community. Congrats on this magnificent new book!

Charles G. Irion, MBA, Global Philanthropist and Humanitarian,
Award Winning Author, Publisher, Entrepreneur, Artist, Actor and Executive Producer.
Active Volunteer with a myriad of charities, including Executive Board Member and International Assessor for Project C.U.R.E.
www.charlesirion.com

CHAPTER 34

Role of Device Therapy in Heart Failure: Cardiomems

A bird doesn't sing because it has an answer,
it sings because it has a song.

—Maya Angelou

WATCH NOW

Patient Story

JO was a wonderful Irish gentleman in his 80's who had an amazing sense of humor and every time he was seen at the heart failure center, there would be a sense of joy with a lot of jokes being passed around. JO would have significant fluid retention now and then and struggled with intravascular volume depletion with kidney failure vs truly having worsening heart failure with increased venous pressure making him short of breath.

Because of the confusion of the two states, he did undergo CARDIOMEMS implantation. This device measures pulmonary artery pressure noninvasively after implantation. It is implanted in one of the branches of the pulmonary artery in a short a period of time. Using a wand from outside or even from a distance while laying on a pillow with the hardware inside the pillow, we can detect all of the intracardiac pressures. A study called CHAMPION trial clearly demonstrated a reduction in 30-day readmissions if we monitored their pressures and took actions by preventing fluid retention with the use of diuretics.

The study has clearly shown significant benefits that led the FDA to approve the diagnostic device in patients who are struggling with heart failure readmission. Patients who also have right-sided heart failure, renal dysfunction, or high pulmonary pressures seem to benefit from this procedure as well. Cardiomems device can differentiate fluid retention from fluid depletion and thus allows us to intervene with the right combinations of medications. JO significantly improved with monitoring and treatment from this device which has allowed him to stay out of the hospital for a time.

> What we learned from JO is that it is important to respect the lightness of being, allow yourself to be kind-hearted, and have a wonderful sense of humor and camaraderie which will and transform many of us to balance the aspects of the physical and the spiritual.

He was energized with the use of this device and had a wonderful personality that allowed him to heal. He continued with us for a couple more years before passing away from worsening kidney failure. He was placed in hospice towards the end of life.

Cardiomems Device

Cardiomems is a device that gets placed in a branch within the pulmonary artery. It has a sensor that sends an external signal that can be detected and translated to digitally acquired numerical variables such as pulmonary artery pressures. These numbers can help the clinician adjust medications and improve outcomes. A study called CHAMPION showed significant data that suggests an improvement in 30-day hospital readmissions, mortality, functional capacity, and quality of life.

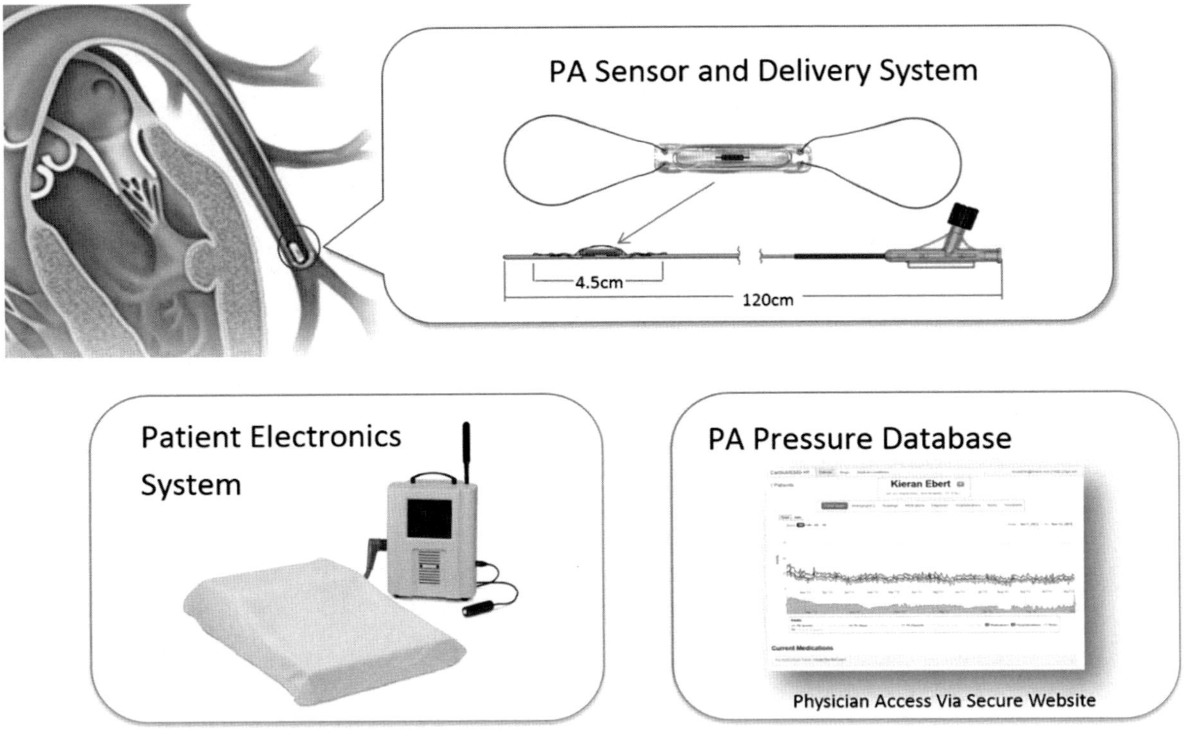

Fig. 37

Lifevest Variables

Lifevest saves lives. It has saved many lives of my patients who went on to receive an implantable defibrillator and are still alive because of that. CPR saves lives. Automated External Defibrillator saves lives. Researchers have studied these concepts intensively over the years and we, as the general public are, indeed, reaping the harvest of hard work that has gone on behind the scenes. We are all indeed extremely grateful for that to the scientists and the industry, regulators, firefighters, and all the workers in the background who make it all happen.

Let me tell you a very touching moving story.

> It was an experience that truly made me start thinking about the limited time that we have on this earth. It brought me a perspective on life and death and realize that life is about storytelling and I have told the real-life stories multiple times about 9/11 events and what happened over the next 4 days of my life.

I was right across for WTC on that morning at Brooklyn Marriott at a research investigator's meeting. The study was called the PAD (Public Access Defibrillation) Trial sponsored by NIH. Many investigators and coordinators had come from all over North America to have this meeting on Flag Day. PAD trial was comparing CPR versus CPR plus AED in out of hospital cardiac arrest after a 911 call.

We had to prove that AED had incremental value. The study was positive for CPR plus AED and hence nowadays you see first responders using both CPR and AED to save lives after a cardiac arrest. Since it was about firefighters as first responders, many of our coordinators were EMT personnel. Since one has to call 911 to dispatch, it was apt that this trial was scheduled on September 11th! Soon after the crash into the WTC occurred the second time around, we were told to evacuate immediately.

There was chaos, pandemonium, and stampede all over the place. When went to the front of the hotel and told the cops we were doctors and firefighters, they quickly got us inside a van and took us to Ground Zero. We were about 10 of us and immediately took steps to initiate an emergency room like setting, blood drive, and helping people running away from the disaster zone. Many had injuries, trauma to multiple portions of the body, smoke inhalation, diabetic coma, hypoglycemic coma, etc. We were there for 4 days. Our families had no access to us due to cell phone outage. Finally, made it home after reaching Baltimore by train and the first flight out four days later.

> It was indeed a traumatic experience from a mental, and psychological perspective, and spirit was shattered. We took solace in the fact that we were able to help so many who were needy. At a time of crisis, we found an opportunity to go towards the crisis and help save lives!!

For the next few years, I was showing a lot of pictures from New York City at that time. Also, rather than focusing on the destruction, it gave us a sense of hope for those people who had escaped. We have many of those stories told by our own PAD trial team. Many team members' relatives and friends had died during the attack. Many escaped from the World Trade Center that day. Hence, when we heard the stories a year later from the PAD trial team members, it was heart-wrenching.

The stories that they were telling were seemingly emerging out of their own pockets of memory. There were vivid images as if it were drawn from their lifetime of pictures that were embedded inside their brain. We discussed how we should be celebrating our lives and what it truly means to be so blessed to be alive and not have a physical trauma and come out untouched. So many have had severe psychological trauma after 911 that we were also addressing in our patient populations at the time. It made us believe in embedded values such as individuality and teamwork. Love and kindness, respect for oneself, and each other. It taught me the meaning, value, purpose, and context of my own existence. Perhaps, throughout our lifetime, while we deal with suffering, we also have to incorporate the aspects of humility, contemplation, clarity of mind, mindfulness, and compassion.

The current guidelines for **Cardiac Resynchronization Therapy** with a Defibrillator (CRT-D) for primary prevention include those with a high risk of cardiac arrest, an ejection fraction of 35% or less, mild to moderate symptoms and a prolonged QRS duration on EKG of more than 120 ms. Patients with ischemic cardiomyopathy qualify after 40 days of an event, but non-ischemic or dilated cardiomyopathy subjects must wait for 90 days after initial diagnosis. Until then a Lifevest is used to protect them from death due to cardiac arrest. Left bundle branch block that occurs with abnormal electrical conduction with an increased QRS duration of over 130 ms may qualify them for a third lead on the left side of the heart if LVEF is < 35%.

Pacemaker wires are usually placed on the right atrium and right ventricle and a third lead along the left side of the heart. CRT's can reverse some of the dyssynchronies and are usually not indicated for asymptomatic patients or those with a narrow QRS on the electrocardiogram. Biventricular pacing may be beneficial for converting the heart to a synchronized contraction. If the lateral walls and septum do not contact together, then there may be decreased cardiac output to the rest of the body. If there is an issue with synchrony, then the lateral walls and septum move side to side, rather than push together and force blood out the aorta. CRT has been shown to improve ejection fraction and CRT-D improves survival.

Implantable Defibrillator

Every day think as you wake up, today I am fortunate to be alive.
I have a precious human life; I am not going to waste it.
I am going to use all my energies to develop myself, to expand my heart out to others; to achieve enlightenment for the benefit of all beings.
I am going to have kind thoughts towards others.
I am not going to get angry or think badly about others.
I am going to benefit others as much as I can.

—Dalai Lama

Patient Story

TE was an embodiment of many of Dalai Lama's philosophical paradigms. He was about 58 years old when I met him and was being taken care of at the VA hospital for many years and was in heart failure. He knew that his ejection fraction had dropped to about 30% and within a few months he was close to 15% and did not qualify for a heart transplant at the time. He was not interested in being seen at the VA as he was not responding adequately. He was a risk-taker and wanted to seek attention outside of the VA.

He knew that the VA was grounded in their own framework of taking care of heart failure with the resources that they had. However, they were reluctant to send patients outside the system. Hence, when he sought attention somewhere else, they refused to pay for his services. So, he took some loans to seek care somewhere else. At that time, enough data was coming out for BiV ICD and he was one of the first ones who received this device after which he started to turn around and felt better. He also increased his exercise and initiated cardiac rehab which raised his ejection fraction.

He was willing to take risks because he believed that the cost of proactive action was far less than the risk of comfortable inaction. Hence, when he ventured outside the system and started to feel better, he suddenly had new hope. Over the years, he became a good friend as we engaged in cutting edge technology and medical therapy with newer medications that had received approval. He also participated in new clinical research trials and believed in the advancement of science. He started feeling better and lived for another 15 years. He told me many times that he wanted to help my nonprofit in helping the underserved community with heart disease and diabetes. He had also introduced me to a few of his connections who would possibly fund a stem cell clinical trial but unfortunately, he passed away. He had a good quality of life for more than 15 years after he was told that he had 6 months to live and he is thankful to all of us as a team as he followed with us in our heart failure clinic.

I believe that the lessons I learned from TE were immensely powerful and our friendship assisted me in recalling our conversations over the years in terms of helping the underserved community that struggled from a socioeconomic and financial disadvantage. Second, our friendship encouraged me towards a conscious recommitment to the meaning and purpose of what we were doing from a heart failure perspective and reinforced our better natures. Third, the relationship with reconnecting regularly, truly helped me embrace a positive approach towards believing in the hope and dream that newer therapies and technology brought forth to us to take care of our heart failure patients.

Enhanced External Pulsation Therapy (EECP

Patient Story

WB is a 64-year-old female who had mildly reduced ejection fraction around 40% with coronary artery disease, stent placement, diabetes with intermittent diastolic heart failure. She improved with fluid management, salt reduction, controlling blood pressure, however, she was still symptomatic and had done an angiogram with no more vessels that needed stenting, so she was a candidate for EECP. After educating her on this therapy, she was willing to consider this. She was explained that it involves inflatable cuffs that were applied on her lower legs, upper legs, lower abdomen, gluteal area, and alternatively inflate and deflate in a synchronized fashion with the heartbeat.

When the heart would squeeze, the cuffs deflate and when the heart is relaxing, the cuffs would inflate. This would happen for about an hour a day, 5 days a week, and would also take about 35 sessions or so. The patient was willing to consider this and was recommended to go through one of the centers that had the device. She also explained that following the 35 sessions, what we have learned in clinical trials is that there would be a new natural development of small blood vessels that would supply the heart muscle, improve blood flow to the heart, create angiogenesis and hopefully improve her quality of life.

The experience that WB had was amazing and not only improved how she felt, but also improved her functional capacity and ability to walk on a treadmill with no limitations and fewer symptoms. Her experience parallels that of many who have undergone EECP and have a 95% satisfaction rate. Most people start to feel better within about 15-20 sessions. After they complete the 35 sessions, there seems to be an overall improvement in bioenergetics and the capacity to do more. The benefits of EECP have been explained through a lot of biometric assessments. It seems to have a lot of benefits in improving many of the biomarkers such as VEGF, and nitric oxide, suppressing endothelin, and inflammatory markers, improving cardiometabolic markers and blood flow to multiple parts of the body. There is some weight loss that occurs with this therapy as well which improves blood flow to the kidneys and the brain through increased carotid blood flow. It is not clear whether these subtle benefits can be extrapolated to patients with Parkinson's disease or other diseases such as erectile dysfunction, peripheral neuropathy, peripheral vascular disease.

All of these studies need to be performed objectively in the longer term, but in the short term, we are seeing benefits like Ms. WB experienced which has been life-changing for many patients. The first step to embrace the concept of what EECP can do has to come from within. The patient has to be empowered, open-minded, and have a belief in healing. EECP is like exercise training for the heart. It connects the science of physical and shear stress principles with neuro associative conditioning that can translate to a vibrant endorphin release and improvement in feeling happier, healthier.

EECP seems to benefit most patients who are not candidates for any more open-heart surgery or intervention of coronary arteries or those who have diminished functional capacity because of heart failure with reduced ejection fraction. There is a recent study among those who have preserved ejection fraction, where the use of EECP seems to improve their functional capacity and reduce hospital readmissions in 30 days. We have seen in so many patients whose EF was stuck at 20% or so, their heart from being plastic, now has transformed to being elastic, moving and shaking, improving their Ejection Fraction!! What we have learned with EECP therapy is that it can transform patients' lives as they improve their QOL and Ejection fraction with more energy and vigor.

EECP

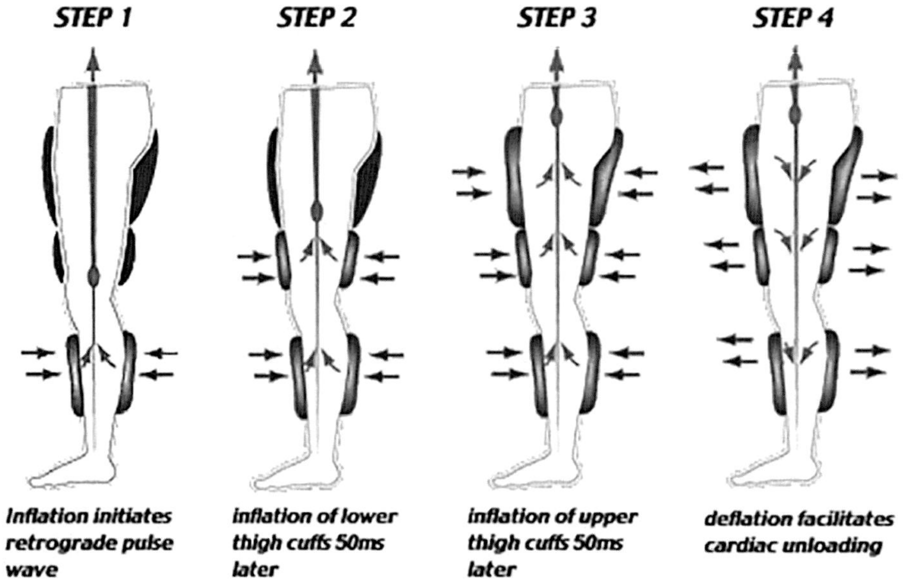

Fig. 38

Enhanced External Counterpulsation (EECP) is a mechanical form of therapy used to treat intractable forms of angina in patients who have the coronary disease but are not eligible for more angioplasty or stenting. It is a mechanical procedure where cuffs are placed around one's legs, thigh, and abdomen, and the cuffs are squeezed synchronously with each heartbeat. As we know, the coronary arteries fill during the relaxation phase of the heart. When the heart squeezes in systole, the cuffs delate and when the heart is relaxing in diastole, the cuffs inflate. During this time when the cuffs are inflated, it allows blood flow into the coronaries with more strength. This might create new blood vessels and increase collateral circulation across the whole heart. Angiogenesis or new blood vessels are formed and there is release nitric oxide, along with other growth factors. It might act as a form of exercise therapy for the heart.

It is done 1 hour per day, 5 days a week for 7 weeks for a total of 35 sessions. Ischemic cardiomyopathy is another indication if they have low ejection fraction with associated angina. Some patient's manifest shortness of breath as their anginal equivalent and may benefit from this therapy. The benefit beyond blood flow during diastole also can be from the suctioning effect during deflation of the cuff that acts as a vacuum and reduces the work from the heart muscle. This may improve the condition of the endothelium and oxygen demand of the heart muscle. It has been recommended by many approved organizations and insurance companies. Many cardiology groups have chosen to ignore this form of therapy even though there are clear data and evidence of heart failure symptoms improvement.

Aquapheresis is a therapy that is used to remove fluid overload which is caused by heart failure, liver congestion, kidney failure. Many times, with the use of diuretics, it may be hard to remove excess water without worsening kidney function and losing electrolytes. If there is not adequate fluid removal despite diuretic therapy, then Aquapheresis can be a technique to remove fluid in the body without losing major electrolytes. Blood contains excessive water and sodium that is withdrawn using central venous catheter. It is a form of ultrafiltration that may require anticoagulation during therapy to prevent blood from clotting.

Up to a pint of excessive fluid can be removed in an hour, but usually, the average rate is about 250-500cc per hour and can be controlled unlike inability to control volume of fluid removal with diuretics. The fluid is also isotonic to blood therefore electrolyte balance is maintained. Aquapheresis therapy kit consists of a console (a machine that pumps), a blood filter circuit, and a venous catheter. The benefit has been significant to the extent that insurance companies and FDA have approved these therapies in patients who are getting complications to diuretic therapy.

TAVR

So many patients who have had severe aortic valve stenosis have also experienced heart failure. I have had multiple patient experiences who have undergone TAVR and have had a successful outcome. Before TAVR, many patients feel symptomatic with shortness of breath, chest pain, syncope, fatigue, and death. They experience significant limitations and are more vulnerable to risk for hospitalizations. They seek further help and those who have heart failure are not able to have open heart surgery due to high risk.

The TAVR team has a challenge in their hands. There is significant apprehension among patients who need to undergo surgery or new procedures involving their heart. Hence, the TAVR team might have to instill a sense of hope and confidence and invoke trustworthiness before enrolling them in a TAVR program. The outcome of the TAVR procedure is truly grounded in their knowledge base and their own hope of recovery and positive quality of life.

Most patients seem to have benefited from this procedure and undergo cardiac rehab and many of these patients' lives have changed for the better. We have had patients in their 60's to their 90's who have struggled with aortic stenosis and heart failure. They have not only been helped with a new percutaneously placed Aortic valve but there has also been an improvement in heart failure.

TAVR research started with high-risk populations and moved down to the low-risk populations now and been extraordinarily successful in its outcome. TAVR has taught us multiple lessons with the most important one being the aspect of giving patients a sense of hope in alleviating their anxiety and fear. The patient has to trust the TAVR team in terms of their competence, credibility, compassion, kindness. When both physical and spiritual outcomes improve, and when they compare their life struggle before TAVR with improvement post-TAVR, they are extremely grateful for the availability of technology, accessibility to the TAVR team, affordability of it all and the outcome benefit they can enjoy. They will become a believer in the technology that has made a positive impact on their lives.

TAVR Procedure

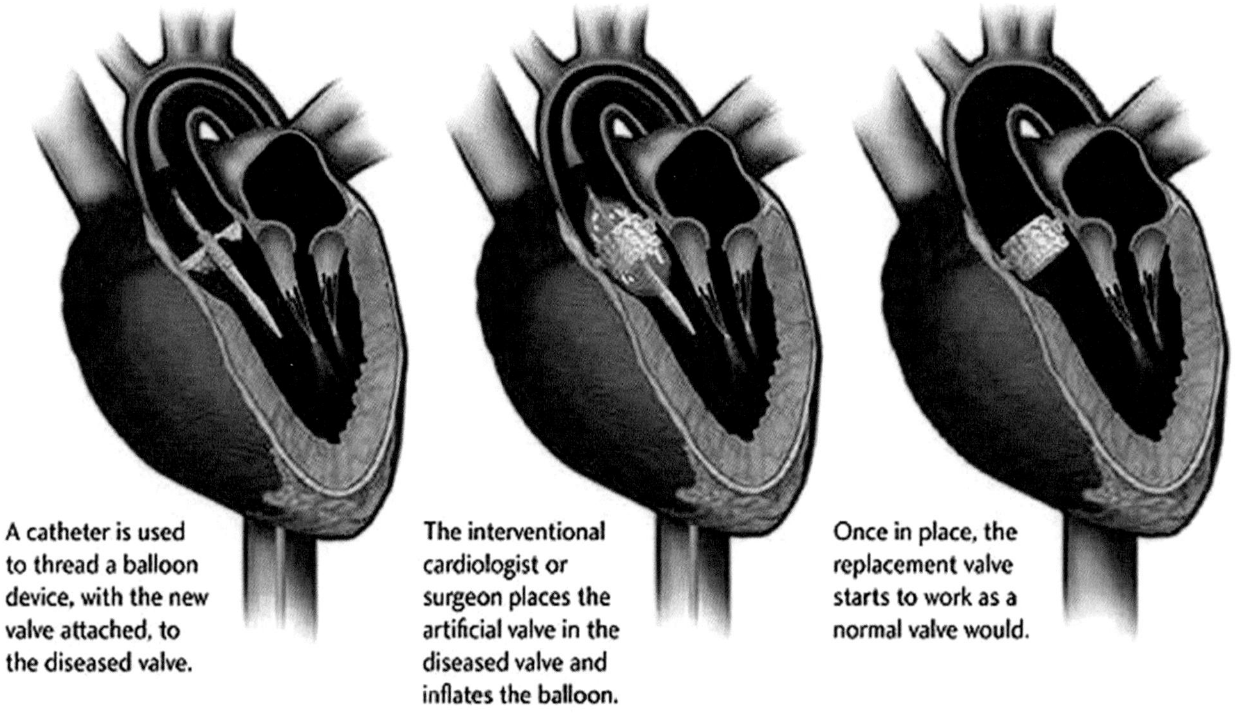

Fig. 39

TAVR is a transcatheter aortic valve replacement that is minimally invasive that is used to open a tight aortic valve that has stenosed. This is a good option for patients who are at moderate to high risk for open-heart surgery. The decision to perform a TAVR is made by the interventional cardiologist or heart surgeon who work together to weigh the benefit and risks.

This procedure may improve aortic valve stenosis symptoms such as shortness of breath, or fatigue. It benefits patients with a high risk of heart surgery, persistent symptoms, or kidney failure. The risk of this procedure includes bleeding, strokes, heart rhythm issues, and other disorders with the blood vessels but is still significantly lower than open-heart surgery.

Mitraclip placements are a less invasive alternative to mitral valve repairs and are usually performed among patients with comorbid conditions who are too high risk for open-heart surgeries. It begins with an incision in the leg through the vein to reach the heart and the device clips a portion of the mitral valve leaflet to reduce the backflow of the blood from the left ventricle to the left atrium which would allow blood to be pumped more efficiently into the aorta and all parts of the body. The indications and optimal candidates are those with significant leakiness and degeneration of the mitral valve and are symptomatic and at high risk for open-heart surgery. Usually, this procedure is done in the hospital and recovery takes between 1-4 days. Most of the patients who get discharged do not need special assistance as recovery is generally easier but strenuous movements are not recommended.

LVAD

Patient Story

Mr. MA was 72 years old and I met him a couple of years ago when he was hospitalized. However, he was traveling between Canada and Arizona as he lived out here. He had done some amazing things in his life starting as a car dealer salesperson and built a large dealership in Canada. He gained tremendous respect from his community and was kindhearted with a high level of dignity and a demeanor of warmth.

He had devastating complications of his heart failure which was slowly getting worse with extensive fluid retention and a low ejection fraction of 10% when he was hospitalized. At the time, we had to keep him on multiple different drips to prevent cardiac arrest and multiple medications to improve his heart pump. He was on a continuous drip with blood thinners as well as he had a small clot in his ventricle. Given all of this, it appeared that he was not going to make it. His wife who is a few years younger than him was quite attached to him and wanted him to live.

He needed an LVAD and in the US, they had refused a heart transplant because of his age and he requested to go back to Canada. However, with all of these drips going, it was an exceedingly high risk to transfer him by plane to Canada. After multiple phone calls, one of the hospitals accepted him as they recognized his name. Both the patient and his wife had the financial resources to travel and offered that I come with them which I was very humbled to be of service to him. We flew on an Air medic jet plane and reached Edmonton in a short time.

As soon as we reached the hospital, the air ambulance people called the ICU and the team came straight to the entrance of the hospital, and soon he was in ICU to get him stabilized. I was in contact with the team of surgeons and cardiologists at the hospital over the next few days who quickly implanted an LVAD within 72 hours which made him feel better. We had the honor to visit him over a year and a half later to spend a couple of days when he gave us a beautiful tour of the vineyards around British Columbia. Unfortunately, MA passed away 6 months after that, but we had great memories of MA and his family. The stories about Mr. MA are not unique but clearly, his life was precious, and he had given back to the community in unimaginable ways. To have met a wonderful person and family itself taught me many lessons over the years.

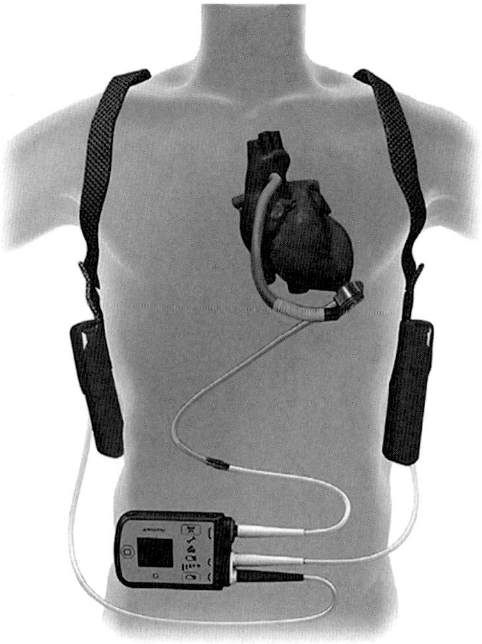

Fig. 40

Left ventricular assist devices (LVAD) is a mechanical pump that is implanted in someone's chest to help a weakened heart pump. Unlike an artificial heart pump, the LVAD does not replace the heart but simply helps the heart do its job. It can be a destination treatment or bridge to transplant and works by attaching one of the ends to the left ventricle and the other end is attached to the aorta. The blood then flows from the heart into the aorta via the pump where the sensors assist in moderating the flow.

The device is connected to an external driveline, which connects the pump and the external control power source. The pump and these connections are implanted during open-heart surgery. The benefits of LVADs include the improvement of the weakened heart and multiple heart failure symptoms. Sometimes the heart can make a full recovery and work better than before. However, if this is not the case, then one may require a heart transplant. Older LVADs usually require individuals to carry a battery with them but most of the smaller, newer LVADs do not require battery packs.

I can't think of a better person that Dr. Kris Vijay to educate the general public on the topic of congestive heart failure given his innate ability to translate technical information into concepts that are simple to understand. With an extensive wealth of knowledge and unsurpassable clinical experience Dr. Kris Vijay succinctly and comprehensively lays out in his book what everybody should know about congestive heart failure. I would not doubt Dr. Vijay's congestive heart failure book would become a frequent source of information, not only for patients but also for physicians. Dr. Kris Vijay has touched the life of many in his numerous roles including mentor, professor, healer, humanist, researcher, philanthropist, author, and spiritual advisor. With this book, Dr. Vijay will be able to reach as many patients as the publisher prints.

Michael Castro MD FACP
Associate Program Director
Abrazo Health Network Internal Medicine Residency Program.
Former Chief of Staff
Abrazo Arrowhead Campus
Abrazo Arizona Heart Hospital

I am very pleased to recommend Dr. Kris Vijay's new book, "Invoking Your Inner Therapist in Heart Failure, Untold Patient Experiences From Prevention to End Stage."

I have enjoyed his presentations and friendship for nearly 30 years and have high regard for his dedication and skills in patient care, research, and teaching.

Dr. Vijay has in this new book distilled four decades of experience in patient care and research, providing patients' stories to explain and illustrate the wide variety of causes of heart failure, outlining the appropriate evaluations to reach the correct diagnoses, optimizing evidence based treatments including new technologies, and showing the positive outcomes in his patient's lives resulting from improving their physical, emotional, and spiritual health.

It is a remarkable story of providing excellent clinical care, lifting up lives, changing detrimental habits and mindsets, and showing that patients suffering with heart failure can be stabilized and can recover heart function leading to improved quality of life.

I highly recommend this book.

John F. Rausch, Jr., MD, MS, FACP, FNKF, FCRS
Board Certified Internal Medicine
Past Board Member of the National Kidney Foundation of Arizona, 2010 – 2016
Past Chairman of the Board of the National Kidney Foundation of Arizona, 2014 – 2016

CHAPTER 35

Heart Transplant

WATCH NOW

Patient Story

Mr. TA was a big guy over 400 pounds who had extensive heart failure, primarily because of a viral infection and his arteries were all clean and yet he was struggling with walking issues and ejection fraction was 10%. At the time he was first hospitalized we tried to make him feel better with medications but was unable to tolerate medications and blood pressure was low. He kept getting readmitted to the hospital since he was generous in weight, it was thought that he was not a candidate for a heart transplant.

> He made himself in charge of losing weight and lost between 60-70 pounds and yet his heart pump was still weak. This is the time that we had to quickly call our resources at Mayo and transfer him, because of his own actions that showed us how empowered he was in fighting for his life. His child was less than 2 years old at the time. He did get a new heart transplanted and his pure determination made him feel better and live longer.

However, because the patient was in his 50's, he was determined to get a new heart if he had to.

With heart transplant and many new medications to prevent rejection of his heart, he was closely followed up regularly.

He did remarkably well and had an ejection fraction of 55-60% with weight loss. It was at this time that he wanted his daughter to grow up in the middle east in Lebanon where his wife's family and his family hailed from. I reached out to one of my cardiology friends who was practicing in Lebanon and he was excited to take care of Mr. TA. I have not heard from him recently but hope that he is doing very well. This is another story of a power that one had within oneself to become emboldened. While he still confessed about his flaws in dietary indiscretion, he still had the courage that rekindled his urge to live and be robust and available for his family. We learned many of these values from this patient.

Heart Transplant

A heart transplant is an invasive surgery that is performed when the heart is failing and replaced with a healthier donor heart. This procedure is usually reserved for people with worsening heart function who have attempted medical therapy and device treatments. It is performed when there is severe cardiomyopathy secondary to atherosclerosis, valvular heart disease, or congenital heart defects. Many times, abnormal heart rhythms such as atrial fibrillation or ventricular tachycardia that are unable to be fixed with ablations or cardioversions may require a heart transplant. However, sometimes the heart and kidneys may fail together, and some centers have heart and kidney transplants performed at the same time which are known as multi-organ transplants.

Sometimes heart-lung transplant may be needed in some patients who have respiratory failure as well. Patients who may not be candidates for heart transplants include advanced age, cancer, kidney disease, smoking, or infections. Problems with heart transplants include

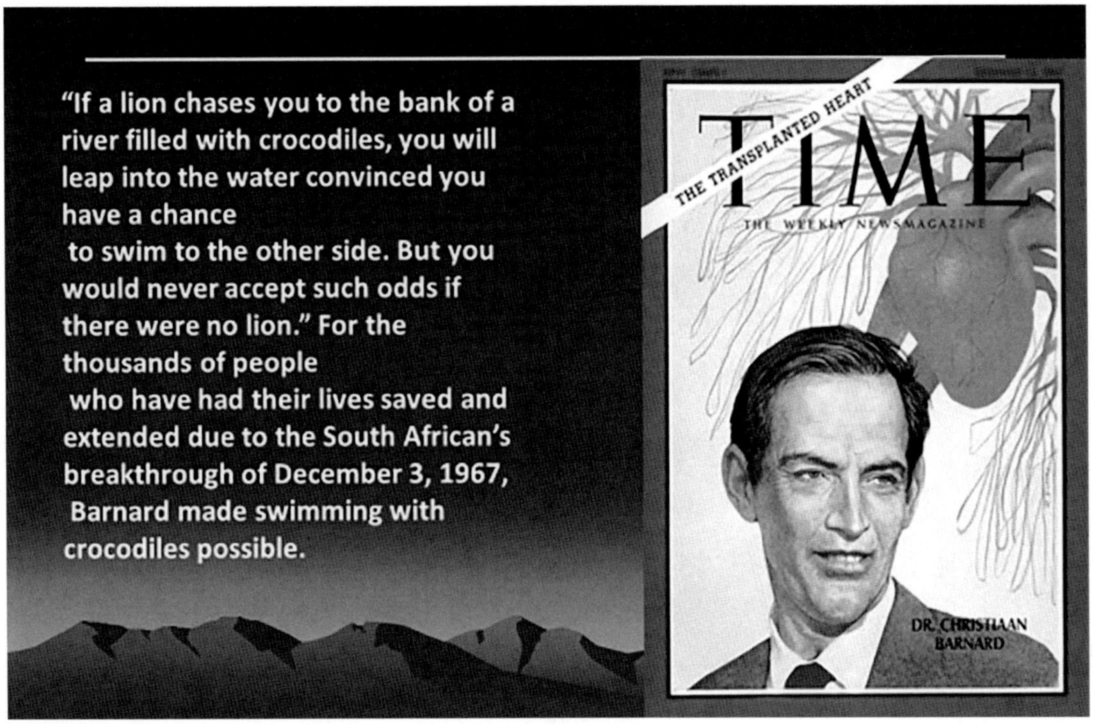

Fig. 41

rejections of the donor's heart, cardiac allograft vasculopathy, need for immunosuppressants, and infections arising from an immune-compromised state. To prepare for this surgery, the physician has to assess them at an inpatient or outpatient setting and send them to a heart transplant center. Many of the scientific registries of recipients are available in the database at each respected site.

SECTION VI

Miscellaneous Topics in Heart Failure

CHAPTER 36

Nutraceuticals in Heart Failure

Faith is a function of the heart. It must be enforced by reason. The two are not antagonistic as some think. The more intense one's faith is, the more it whets one's reason. When faith becomes blind it dies.

— Mahatma Gandhi

Nutraceuticals are used to describe medical or nutritionally functional food, also known as medical foods, designer foods, phytochemicals, functional foods, and nutritional supplements. They include products such as yogurts, fortified cereals, vitamins, and herbal remedies. In even genetically modified foods and supplements. Many countries have different terms for these foods; hence, it can result in confusion. A market research report in 2018 projected that the worldwide market would account for about $100 million in 2020.

Nutraceuticals are classified as dietary supplements or functional foods. They are derived from food sources that are utilized to provide health benefits. In addition to the basic nutritional value found in foods, they may be marketed as preventing certain chronic diseases, improving health, supporting a function in the body, or delaying mortality.

A dietary supplement in the US is a product that contains a dietary ingredient, such as vitamins, minerals, herbs, amino acids, enzymes, or botanicals. Dietary supplements can also be extracts or concentrate found in such forms as tablets, capsules, soft gel caps, liquids, or powders. They do not have to be approved by the FDA before marketing, however, manufacturing companies must register their facilities, conform to FDA standards, and follow good manufacturing practices (GMP). Functional foods are fortified or enriched during processing and marketed as providing specific benefits to certain portions of the body. Some additional complementary nutrients are added to fortify existing products such as Vitamin D to milk. Each country has a different definition of functional foods. For example, In Japan, all functional foods must meet three established requirements which include: Presence in naturally occurring form, consumed in the diet daily, and regulate biological processes in controlling certain diseases.

> These supplements have also been marketed with a lot of hype than actual clinical testing.

History of nutraceutical comes from the founder or chairman of the Foundation for Innovation in Medicine, Stephen DeFelice. Criticism has been high for nutraceuticals because they are not regulated.

> However, there may be significant benefits when pharmaceutical, organ transplants, and devices therapies fail.

It is not clear whether there are significant benefits when using these supplements. Scientists dispute the belief that they are truly effective in the prevention of chronic diseases. The concept of multivitamin supplements was sold to the US by an eager nutraceutical company to generate profit without any scientific data for supporting their usage.

While there is sparse data from many of these compounds, one must have faith in believing that there may be benefits in prevention of non-communicable disease states with utilization of some of these products. Absence of evidence does not necessarily equate to evidence of absence!!

The following nutraceuticals will be discussed specifically in terms of its risks and benefits in cardiovascular disease.

Role of Nutraceuticals in Statin Intolerant Patients

The following should be considered before considering nutraceuticals in patients who are not tolerating statin therapy. They are at a high risk of cardiovascular outcomes if they have partial or complete intolerance to statins, and their low-density lipoproteins are not controlled and not at target levels. Statin intolerance may be secondary to muscle symptoms and have significant side effects such as body aches and pains. Some of them may have pain from neuropathy. Some may have liver or kidney disease and are tolerating medications at small doses. Some of the nutraceuticals may be utilized in statin-intolerant subjects beyond the use of ezetimibe or PCSK-9 inhibitors.

Artichoke has a mechanism where the interaction of luteolin and chlorogenic acid inhibits HMG-CoA-reductase enzyme (similar mechanism to statins) thereby decreasing cholesterol production. A study was performed in close to 900 patients which showed a reduction in LDL from 11-22%. It seems to be tolerated and the safety has been documented long term.

Berberine is a compound that has benefits in reducing LDL cholesterol anywhere from 24-25%. Mechanism of action is through PCSK-9 inhibition and from a decrease in intestinal absorption of cholesterol, increase fecal excretion, and promoting hepatic cholesterol turnover. Side effects of berberine are mild to moderate gastrointestinal discomfort, but no major adverse events have been noted in the liver or kidneys.

Bergamot has been shown to reduce LDL cholesterol by 61mg per deciliter in a study of 107 subjects with metabolic syndrome. There is a reduction in small dense LDL as well and the mechanism of action is through HMG-CoA-reductase enzyme and ASAT inhibition of formation of cholesterol esters. Naringin is a byproduct of bergamot that inhibits oxidation of LDL and initiates AMP-activated protein kinase that has some scavenger activity. There is increased fecal excretion of cholesterol and bile acids, as well as the increased turnover of cholesterol and reduced intestinal absorption. All this has been shown to improve LDL. Bergamot seems to have a good safety profile with no major side effects. However, the vascular side effects have not been demonstrated.

Nutraceutical Fibers

Fibers such as Metamucil and Citrucel have been shown to be well tolerated long term with no complications. There have been some suggestions of a reduction in cardiovascular risk. The reduction of LDL cholesterol has been anywhere from 8-20mg% with an LDL reduction of 10-15%. The mechanism of action is through its prolonged gastric emptying time and increase in satiety and inhibition of hepatic cholesterol synthesis with increased fecal excretion of cholesterol and bile salts.

Nutraceutical Garlic

Garlic has been commonly used in food products as an additional component of ethnic foods. It seems to have a reduction of LDL cholesterol by roughly 9 mg% in certain studies. It seems to also have a reduction in total cholesterol, triglycerides, platelet aggregation, and blood pressure. The mechanism is through inhibition of HMG CoA reductase, and squalene monooxygenase, which reduces the stability and availability of cholesterol. They do not seem to have any direct vascular effects. Side effects are usually gastrointestinal and well-tolerated.

Green tea seems to reduce LDL cholesterol up to 8 mg% and may have associated low blood pressure and total cholesterol as well. In a large study among 1500 patients with elevated LDL, it seems to have some benefit in diabetic subjects where it seems to reduce pulse wave velocity having some direct vascular effects. The mechanism of action is through inhibition of expression of inducible nitric oxide synthase and activating AMP kinase and inhibiting HMG-CoA-reductase. The epigallocatechin gallate (EGCG) is another chemical found in green tea which seems to have some anecdotal benefit in reducing dementia through its possible anti-amyloidogenic potential. The safety of green tea has been fairly established and its consumption is well tolerated. Some people may experience a rash or transient elevation in blood pressure or gastric disorders. High doses of green tea can cause iron and folic acid deficiency and one needs to be careful about this.

Plant stanols and sterols are commonly used compounds that are available in stores and LDL has been shown to reduce 12-18% and safety profile is shown to be established mid-term. Direct vascular effects have not been demonstrated. There is one large study with over 2000 subjects with high cholesterol that showed a reduction in cholesterol from about 12mg/deciliter. The mechanism is inhibition of secretion of apo B by enterocytes and modulation of cholesterol synthesis and preventing the initiation of the inflammatory cascade.

Red yeast rice is another component that is easily available across the world. They are low potent statin and shown to have an LDL reduction of 36-90mg% and increase flow-mediated vasodilation. More than 6000 patients were studied with 1200 to 4800mg a day for a month which showed a significant reduction in LDL. The mechanism of action is through its reversible inhibitory action on the HMG-CoA-reductase enzyme which is similar to what a statin does. Side effects with red yeast rice are similar to that of statins which consist of muscle aches, myopathy, liver injury, and kidney injury.

Spirulina is another compound commonly available that seems to have hit the headlines in the 21st century. It reduces LDL cholesterol by up to 40-45mg% and increases HDL. A study of 522 overweight, diabetic with dyslipidemia patients, showed a significant reduction of LDL over a 12-week-period with 1-2g per day dosage. The mechanism of action is through activation of athero-protective heme oxygenase 1 enzyme and decreases total cholesterol and triglycerides through increased hepatic glycogen levels and maintains glucose kinase expression in the liver. This seems to be one of the most exciting nutraceuticals with some presumed benefit. Vascular effects have not been demonstrated.

Soy protein is commonly available across the world and seems to have an LDL reduction of somewhere around 5-10mg% at 25-35mg dosage. More than 2600 diabetic patients were studied where this was shown to have statistical significance in total cholesterol reduction.

It works through reducing APO B receptor activity, decreasing the synthesis of cholesterol, and removing cholesterol from the blood. However, caution needs to be expressed with chronic use of high consumption of soy products containing isoflavones as it can interfere with thyroid function or fertility and reduction of vital vitamin absorption. It can increase estrogen activity and has shown some vascular effects, however, there is not enough data on this.

Studies show that a combination of red yeast rice with other substances, including policosanol, berberine, sterols, artichokes, and other antioxidants have shown a reduction in LDL when used together.

Selected Role of Micronutrients in Heart Failure:

Despite the use of medications in patients with heart failure, some patients continue to feel unwell due to ineffective pharmacological or device therapies and the quality of life feels unsatisfactory. They may also have depression or noncompliance issues as well. The increased risk of poor diets is associated with lower quality of life in heart failure. However, many of the heart failure guidelines have not specified any nutritional strategies. Some of the micronutrient deficiencies occur with significant importance in chronic heart failure. Clinical research investigating the effect of micronutrients is still extremely limited, hence, lack of evidence should increase caution with these therapies. The aim is to present the specific role of each of these micronutrients.

CoQ10 is a naturally occurring antioxidant, a component of the electron transport chain and participates in aerobic cellular respiration, which generates energy in the form of ATP. It is synthesized in the mitochondrial membrane of the cell. In healthy subjects, it is present in high concentrations in the heart, and exerts 3 biological roles which include mitochondrial energy production, stabilizing the cell membrane, and powerful antioxidant effect. CoQ10 deficiency is associated with patients who experience statin-induced muscle aches and pains.

In addition, CoQ10 or ubiquinone may be depleted in heart failure patients. In patients with heart failure, low CoQ10 is correlated with reduced functional capacity, increased BNP levels, and reduced ejection fraction. The administration of CoQ10 has been analyzed in small studies where some show benefits or neutral effects. However, in observational studies, CoQ10 seems to be an independent predictor for mortality in patients hospitalized with heart failure which has also been confirmed in large cohort studies. The replacement of CoQ10 to standard therapy has not shown to significantly affect the endpoints that we assess in heart failures such as mortality and functional capacity.

A large study that was done using 420 subjects who were randomized to CoQ10 vs placebo for about 106 weeks with an assessment of hospitalization for worsening heart failure, cardiovascular death, or requiring mechanical assist devices or heart transplant. Over a 2-year-period, data analyzed revealed a 43% risk reduction but no statistical significance. Two other studies showed no benefit. Due to conflicting results, large randomized controlled trials are needed to prove a beneficial improvement in the quality of life and reduction of hospitalization for heart failure.

Vitamin D

In patients with heart failure, intracellular ionized calcium utilization is impaired and heart contraction is negatively affected. Vitamin D plays an important role in bone mineralization and maintenance of serum calcium levels. In animal models, the administration of vitamin D seems to increase the contractility of the heart muscle. However, 3 recent randomized double-blind placebo-controlled studies on the effect of vitamin D on functional capacity as detected by the cardiopulmonary stress test, 6-minute walk test, and isokinetic muscle testing did not show any improvement in physical improvement despite an increase in plasma vitamin D levels. Hence, it is not clear if vitamin D supplementation is a good therapy to decrease fatigue, frailty, and functional decline.

Iron is a key element in hemoglobin metabolism. It acts as an enzyme in oxygen transport and storage. It is involved in oxygen metabolism in the heart and skeletal muscles. Iron deficiency is one of the most common nutritional deficiency disorders affecting 30% of the general population. Lack of iron may initiate a pro-inflammatory state which can impair intestinal absorption of iron creating a vicious cycle. Usually, it is diagnosed with the measurement of serum iron, total iron-binding capacity, ferritin levels, and transferal saturation levels. Multiple different trials have demonstrated that correction of iron deficiency improves symptoms such as exercise capacity among heart failure patients.

In the most recent study called the CONFIRM HF, the effect of intravenous iron on functional capacity was studied, which revealed a 61% relative risk reduction in heart failure hospitalization in patients with worsening heart failure when receiving IV ferric carboxy maltose or iron infusion. In addition, multiple combinations of trials (meta-analysis) revealed reduced heart failure hospitalizations with an iron infusion or oral replacement while improving quality of life. Hence, the recommendation is if someone who is iron deficient and has heart failure, patients will benefit from replenishment with iron therapy both intravenous and oral therapy.

Thiamine is a coenzyme of oxidation-reduction reactions in the glucose metabolism and citric acid cycle. It is a vitamin B1, which has been shown to be involved in bioenergetics, hemoglobin production, synthesis of the stress response, and neuromodulation. Thiamine deficiency can be associated with alcoholism, poor nutrition, cancer, pregnancy, hemodialysis, chronic diarrhea, and chronic diuretic use. Beriberi is the disease due to thiamine deficiency that can lead to heart failure, and loss of muscle strength. Subclinical thiamine deficiencies are common in heart failure patients who are on long term furosemide or other diuretics. They may have increased basal metabolic rate and at times manifest as malnutrition with advanced age. Only 2 small placebo randomized controlled studies thiamine administration in heart failure improved ejection fraction and quality of life. However, another study showed that it did not improve outcomes in acute heart failure. Two recent systematic reviews and meta-analysis confirmed the benefit. At present, thiamine supplementation has its benefits on heart failure, but larger studies are needed to test this prognostic and therapeutic significance in cardiovascular outcomes.

Creatine is a substance naturally found in skeletal muscle and the heart. It stores and transfers high energy phosphate. It is synthesized from arginine, glycine, and methionine in the kidneys, liver, and pancreas. A dietary supplement in healthy people of about 20g per day for 5 days, increased skeletal muscle bulk and strength. In heart failure, creatine concentration is reduced due to increased sympathetic activity. Creatine supplementation study in chronic heart failure was performed a few years ago, however, it did not correlate with improvement in ejection fraction. But it increased skeletal muscle energy which phosphates and increase in performance, increased strength, and endurance. Few studies have shown the role of supplementing creatine in heart failure. Hence, not enough data is present regarding prognostic significance. In terms of safety, one needs to watch kidney function closely.

3 main amino acids are beneficial for cardiovascular health which includes **taurine, l-carnitine, and arginine**. Amino acids are protein monomers that are fundamental to a large number of complex processes found in vitamins and nutritional supplements. Amino acid availability is reduced in heart failure where it causes a hypercatabolic state and induces fatigue due to cachexia. Amino acid deficiency transitions red fibers in the heart muscle to white fibers. Red fibers are more efficient than white fibers. A combination of amino acid supplementation has demonstrated improvement in red fibers, myocardial performance, and protein synthesis but no large-scale data has shown a reduction in risk of cardiovascular disease.

Taurine is a semi-essential amino acid that results from citric acid decarboxylation and is expressed at a high level in cardiac muscle. It has antioxidant properties and regulates the myocardial key protein in the excitation-contraction coupling mechanism that stimulates the heart muscle. It is also involved in the modulation of enzymes that stimulate the heart muscle such as phospholamban and sarcoplasmic reticular calcium ATPase or SERCA 2A. It is involved in mitochondrial metabolism and modification. Taurine deficiency is associated with impaired metabolism in the heart and altered mitochondrial function. Mitochondrial myopathy and Mitochondrial encephalopathy that result in stroke-like episodes are secondary to taurine deficiency. A few weeks of taurine therapy seems to improve exercise capacity and ejection fraction. In Japan, taurine is an approved supplement for heart failure. However, long term effects or mortality outcomes have not been demonstrated.

L-carnitine is a nonessential amino acid and cofactor in fatty acid transport in the mitochondria and glucose metabolism Many studies have been done in heart failure patients and supplementation seems to improve cardiac metabolic and left ventricular function. HF patients have a 50% depletion of L carnitine. Supplementation with L-carnitine has been studied and revealed positive effects in exercise capacity but did not change any hemodynamics or neurohormones. They improve skeletal muscle metabolism and 2g per day seem to improve survival in a small study. At present L-carnitine seems to have some benefits but has not been touted as a common medication for patients with heart failure. It may improve their functional capacity.

Arginine is a semi-essential amino acid and a substrate of nitric oxide synthase and leads to vasodilation and restores endothelial function. Some studies have tested their supplementation and showed improvement in endothelium-dependent vasodilatation, muscle blood flow, functional capacity, and exercise duration. However, long term data of this amino acid for heart failure has not been demonstrated. Mixed amino acid supplementation has been studied to see if there is an improvement in exercise or oxygen capacity and seems to have mixed results. There are no studies that show improvement in heart failure.

L-carnosine is a dipeptide of beta-alanine and l-histidine which is present in high quantities in the myocardium, skeletal muscle, and brain. It seems to show anti-aging properties as well as antioxidant and immunomodulating features, favoring nitric oxide formation in the endothelial cells. Recent data suggest that carnosine may be effective in preventing type two diabetes in obese patients. It seems to improve exercise quality in stable heart failure patients. Further data is necessary to evaluate ejection fraction improvement and survival in heart failure.

WATCH NOW

I have had the pleasure to know Dr. Kris Vijay for more than 10 years.

"Invoking your Inner Therapist in Heart Failure – Untold Patient Experiences From Prevention to End Stage" is an easy-to-understand guide unlike any other available.

It is gratifying to see that Dr. Vijay's endless optimism and boundless joy shines through in this valuable text for patients and families. His heartfelt stories of individuals experiencing symptoms and what they feel, think, learn and live are vital for all of us.

In a world where personal experiences and clear communication of what to expect from a diagnosis are rare, Dr. Vijay fills the void. I recommend families and patients read this and use the tools provided to yield a calmer way to deal with changes as we age.

Lianna S. Collinge, CAE
CEO
Arizona Chapter of the
American College of Cardiology
www.acc-az.org azacc@acc-az.org
AZ CA CO WA Chapters of the American College of Cardiology

Arizona
CHAPTER

CHAPTER 37

Amyloidosis

WATCH NOW

Patient Story

KM is a patient who we have known less than 6 months and has had kidney disease, uncontrolled diabetes, uncontrolled foot ulcers and is in wound care, with diastolic heart failure. Hence, it was believed that he could have amyloidosis as there were multiple red alerts and we felt as he was not responding to therapy commonly used for heart failure. So, we started thinking outside the box and found that he had ATTR amyloidosis.

He was placed on a medication called tafamidis which recently approved by the FDA to decrease cardiovascular mortality. It is a new medication and was hard to ger, as only a few pharmacies had it in the country and we had to struggle to get it to the patient. It was extremely expensive. The pharmaceutical company, insurance company, case management company, specialty pharmacy, and nurses in the clinic were all supportive and worked hard to get the patient access to this medication. After KM initiated this medication, he felt better, and his wound healed after amputation and needed a prosthesis. The story of amyloidosis is being brought upfront for three reasons: If any suggestion that patients with heart failure are not responding quickly to the standard of therapy or have kidney issues, then one needs to trigger the mind to think amyloid and do a workup with objective measurement to figure out if they truly have TTR amyloidosis.

We learned a few lessons dealing with TTR amyloidosis. First, we have been under the erroneous belief that no medication is available for amyloidosis. Recently two drugs were approved by the FDA. Hence, it gives us more reason for us to be proactive and think outside the box and think about amyloidosis as a possibility in some patients who do not respond with the standard of care and who have red alerts along with diastolic heart failure.

The second lesson that we learned is about a sense of hope and dreams that is vibrant in the health care community and from the patient perspective. The new drug therapy that is truly transformation is now available to the patient and we can make it available at a low cost.

Third, the humility and belief in healing some heart failure patients with HFpEF when no other medications are helping is a testament to our understanding of the disease and its prevalence. It allows us to be recharged in our determination to use empathy, kindness, and compassion to make our patients feel better and live longer.

Amyloidosis

Amyloidosis in general is a group of diseases in which abnormal proteins called amyloid fibrils build up in tissues and are responsible for deposits of protein all over the body. These aggregate of proteins get folded in shapes that cause many copies of proteins to stick together called fibrils. These fibrils get deposited in the brain, liver, eye, and heart. Normally, some bacteria have amyloid protein for hormone and pigment formation. Amyloid was thought to come from starch, then it was felt to be a proteinaceous material like albumin or egg white. There are different kinds of amyloid, but we will focus on cardiac amyloid. Before diagnosing cardiac amyloidosis, we must rule out other types of amyloidosis.

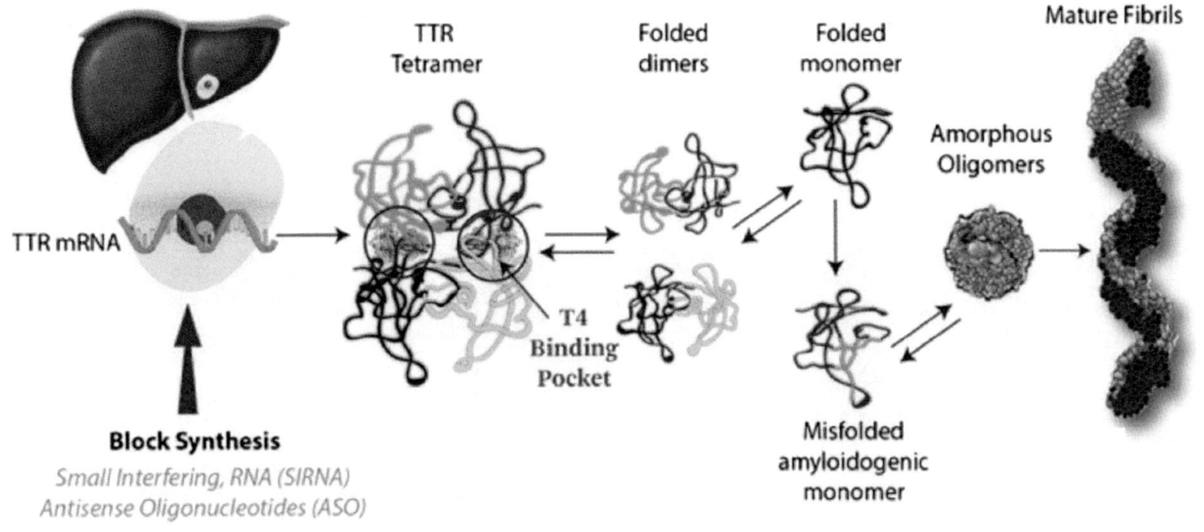

Fig. 42

The beta-amyloid can be deposited as amyloid precursor proteins such as those in Alzheimer's disease. Alpha-synuclein is an amyloid protein that gets deposited in Parkinson's disease. There is a beta-amyloid that can contribute to the condition of Huntington's disease. Even a brain tumor condition called prolactinoma that secretes prolactin hormone is a type of amyloid that gets deposited in the pituitary gland. AL amyloidosis is the second most common which is light chain immunoglobulin which used to be called familial polyneuropathy. There is a type of medullary carcinoma of the thyroid that deposits calcitonin as the amyloid protein. Lattice corneal dystrophy (Finnish) is a type of amyloidosis where gelsolin is deposited in the eye and can lead to vision issues. Among diabetics with kidney disease, there is a beta 2 microglobulin that gets deposited in the kidney which is a type of amyloid as well. There are also functional types of amyloidosis such as pseudomonas, E. coli, malaria, and spider silk.

The most common amyloidosis which is AL amyloidosis is secondary to light chain deposition in various tissues in the body. It is highly prevalent around 200,000 cases in the United States. About 30-40% of AL amyloidosis can also have cardiac involvement and is present in patients with multiple myeloma or Waldenstrom's macroglobulinemia. It causes an enlarged heart, kidney, and liver as well as stroke, adrenal malfunction, bleeding, fatigue, and weight loss. It is usually detected by serum protein electrophoresis and immunofixation as well as serum free light chain tests. Urine protein electrophoresis may show Bence Jones protein. Treatment for this condition has not shown to decrease mortality and patients who do not treat it usually have an extremely poor prognosis. The mean survival is about 13 months but in the last 20 years, has improved to 40 months. Treatments for this condition include autologous bone marrow transplant and stem cell rescue. Some chemotherapeutic agents such as Melphalan or steroids such as dexamethasone have been helpful. Bortezomib and ixazomib seem to help as well.

Cardiac amyloidosis is a kind of amyloidosis where deposition of the protein in the heart muscle can lead to symptoms and worsening prognosis.

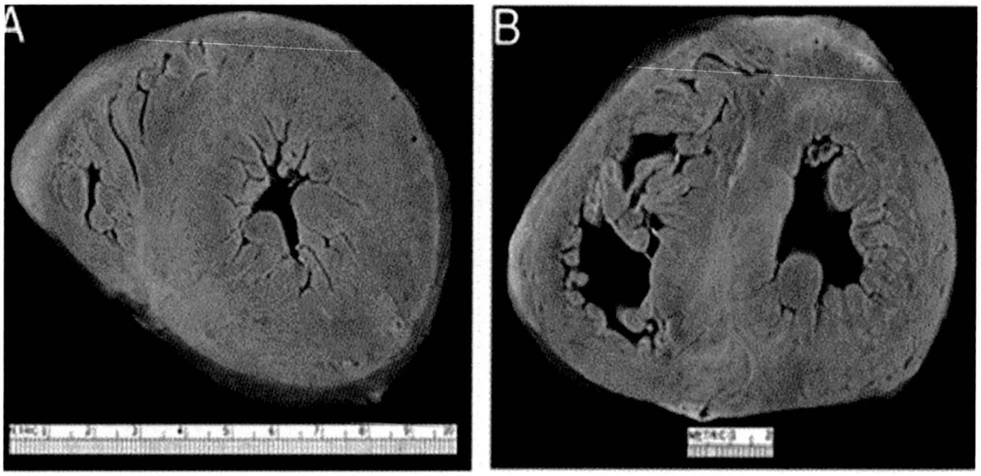

Fig. 43

CARDIAC AMYLOIDOSIS

There are multiple types which can be familial or senile. The familial type includes transthyretin (TTR) cardiac amyloidosis. The reason why we rule out other types of amyloid to ascertain it is TTR is that the treatment is different. Symptoms of amyloidosis include shortness of breath, abdominal distention, clotting formation, neuropathy, hypotension, pericardial effusion, and eye bleeds. Also, this can cause heart conduction system defects as well. The underlying cause of amyloid includes the misfolding of amyloid protein and the deposition of these proteins in the heart.

There is sometimes a genetic factor and hereditary types are endemic in some portions of the world. Andrade discovered hTTR in a town near Porto in Northern Portugal where he found Val30 Met mutation in a family. In Northern Sweden, in a city called Skelleftea 1.5% of the population had a mutated gene associated with hTTR amyloidosis. This is different from senile Amyloid which occurs in the supra-centennials who are 110 years of age or over. About 20-40% of patients may present with polyneuropathy and the TTR gene is present on the 18q12.1 chromosome There is a mutant type variant called V122I and is found in 3.4% of African Americans. Outside the US, V30M is the most frequent pathogenic variant while the phenotype can vary by region. V30M is the most common TTR variant among those with polyneuropathy. In a study from on autopsies, 25% over 80 years old had amyloid deposition.

ATTR types include a mutant type called hTTR or wildtype wTTR. The way to diagnose ATTR amyloidosis is by eliminating AL amyloidosis. Apart from blood tests, CT scans and cardiac MRI's can be used to screen certain forms of amyloidosis as well. An echocardiogram can pick up some red alert signals and to confirm TTR amyloidosis, a PYP scan is needed. It is specific and sensitive to detect the disease. If the PYP scan is positive, then there is a high chance that there is cardiac amyloidosis. If the clinical suspicion is high and the PYP scan is negative, then a biopsy from the right side of the heart with a Congo red stain of the tissue may be needed.

Treatment for ATTR amyloidosis is available with a new therapy called tafamidis meglumine which seems to stabilize the tetramer of the amyloid fibril and prevent the progression of the disease. Studies are showing promise in improving quality of life and survival. Other therapies have either anecdotal evidence or in clinical studies. These include diflunisal, liver transplantation, patisiran, inotersen, and epigallocatechin gallate. Amyloid degradation has also been shown to work with doxycycline. Other treatments for cardiac amyloid include diuretics, ACE inhibitors, ARBs, MRAs, beta-blockers, pacemakers, left ventricular assist devices, and heart transplantations.

CHAPTER 38

COVID-19 and The Heart

"Something to ponder...

Make no mistake... when loved ones are removed from your home by ambulance because the virus has hit them hard, you are not going to be able to follow them there, sit by their hospital bed and hold their hand. You are not going to be able to pop in at 7:00 pm for visiting hours. They are going to have no one other than the exhausted and brave hospital staff to see them through days or weeks of barely breathing through a ventilator until they either die or recover. They are not going to be well enough to text you.

You are not going to be able to phone the ward to check in on them regularly (staff will be too busy for that). During that time, they will be completely alone, while you sit at home waiting to hear whether they have made it through.

Imagine that person is someone you love dearly. Because it's going to be a reality for many in the coming weeks.

And if that person in the hospital happens to be me or you or someone you know, going through that ordeal completely alone, it would be nothing less than terrifying.

Never in my life have I wanted so strongly to say that if anyone is not feeling even a little afraid right now, not only for themselves but for their loved ones and others in general, then there is something wrong with that picture.

While I see end-stage heart failure daily and prepare the family psychologically and spiritually, I am there with family comforting them and they are there with their loved ones at the end of life and there is some kind of a closure.

That is not the case with COVID 19. Those at the end-stage are alone and so are the near and dear ones. What a difficult situation to absorb."

WATCH NOW

COVID-19 can affect the heart just as much as the lungs. In some patients who are critically ill, it is recognized that the cardiac function is severely affected. The virus may affect the heart directly before affecting the lungs. It may affect the kidneys and inner blood vessel lining as well. Hence, one has to be cautious in patients who have pre-existing heart conditions to avoid this virus and protect themselves from the viral infection. Discussions that are currently happening during the pandemic include social distancing, masking, hand washing, wearing PPE near someone who may be at risk.

Patients who are at higher risk include diabetic people, the elderly, cancer, obesity and immunocompromised. Those who are on multiple different medications including immunosuppressants are subjects who need to monitor symptoms closely. Hence, there has to be a bidirectional approach where everybody has to be cautious and believe that the other person could be infected but asymptomatic.

Especially, someone with heart disease gets exposure and get into trouble, they may land up in the emergency room and likely will lead to hospitalization if symptomatic. This will prevent them from seeing anybody and becoming quarantined. Due to this fear, patients do not get tested if they truly are in dire distress from heart issues. Other fears include being anxious about catching COVID-19 in the hospital. Hence, one must not be afraid of seeking attention or going to the hospital or the doctors if they manifest symptoms of cardiac disease

Covid-19 and The Heart

Covid-19 is a coronavirus in 2019 also called SARS-COV-2 as it is similar to the coronavirus of SARS that occurred many years ago. When an infected person expels the virus in droplets, and someone else inhales it, it can start to spread. The Virus has multiple spikes called glycoproteins which try to attach to a receptor on the cell in human tissues. The specific receptor that COVD 19 attempts to attach to is called ACE2 receptor. It is commonly found in the lungs. It is also found in the endothelium, heart, intestines, and kidney. Once SARS COV2 attaches to the ACE 2 receptor, it enters the cell and starts to replicate rapidly. It then gets released into the other tissues and starts to create an inflammatory reaction by upregulating many interleukins and cytokines.

If a cytokine storm ensues, the patient decompensates and needs aggressive management and support. As the virus multiplies, the infected person releases copious amounts of it in the first week or two. They may have minor symptoms such as cough, loss of taste, fever, sore throat, or possibly none at all. If the immune system does not combat this virus, then it can march down to the windpipe and attack the bronchial tree which will develop pneumonia and fill the lungs with a fluid leading to a condition called acute respiratory distress syndrome (ARDS). About 5% of the people have severe disease and this has been leading to significant amounts of comorbidity and mortality around the world.

COVID-2 seems to affect the heart in multiple different ways. It appears as though it may cause arrhythmia with ventricular tachycardia, arterial/venous clots, cytokine storm, and acute myocarditis which can lead to heart failure. At present, there have been diagnoses available with a nasal swab and testing for the virus with reverse transcriptase PCR. There is also antibody testing available which detects IgM antibody present soon after the viral load starts to wean off and an IgG antibody that starts to increase and sustain over a longer time. Many of the questions about immunity, recurrence, neutralizing antibody, length of protection are all unclear. Nasal swabs test for the virus is the most effective at the moment due to its high level of specificity and sensitivity.

In terms of therapy, there are not many therapies that have shown significant benefit in suppressing the disease rapidly. Remdesevir, an antiviral is approved for use for ICU patients to reduce length of stay in the ICU. Dexamethasone is also approved for severely sick patients. No treatment is available yet for mild disease or prophylaxis. No vaccine is available yet. Many clinical trials are ongoing. In terms of prevention, the national strategy includes social distancing, hand washing, quarantining, restrictive access to hospitals, use of hand sanitizer, risk screenings, respiratory masks, PPE, and hospital evaluations in isolated rooms.

Dr. V. MOHAN,
M.D., FRCP (Lond, Edin, Glasg & Ireland), Ph.D., D.Sc.,
D.Sc (Hon. Causa), FNASc, FASc, FNA, FACE, FTWAS, MACP
Chairman, Dr. Mohan's Diabetes Specialities Centre
President, Madras Diabetes Research Foundation
Awarded Padma Shri by President of India &
Dr. B. C. Roy Award by Medical Council of India

Dr. Mohan's DIABETES SPECIALITIES CENTRE
MADRAS DIABETES RESEARCH FOUNDATION

It is a great pleasure for me to write a few lines about the excellent book by my good friend, Dr. Kris Vijay, entitled 'Invoking Your Inner Therapist in Heart Failure - Untold Patient Experiences From Prevention to End Stage.

Heart failure today has become very common. In fact, statistics shows that today heart failure is more common that atherosclerotic cardiovascular disease. Thankfully, as we begin to realize the importance of heart failure, newer therapies and newer approaches to heart failure classifying it in to heart failure with preserved ejection fraction and heart failure without preserved ejection fraction are also coming in. More importantly, newer therapies to tackle heart failure are rapidly being developed. It is in this background that the book by Dr. Kris Vijay becomes extremely important, as it encompasses the new developments in medicines and devices, in the field of heart failure. The book is full of success stories from patients which instills hopes in individuals affected with heart failure. Such books are rare.

Dr. Kris Vijay has written this book in a simple language and style which is suitable even for lay public. He describes heart trenching stories when nothing more could be done, but then, shows how life can surprise us with amazing things that can happen which some of us called miracle, when we combine divinity and spirituality with medical care.

Dr. Kris Vijay has excellent leadership skills. I have known Kris for many years now and the leadership role he plays in the triple epidemic of diabetes, heart disease and kidney failure is unparalleled. His dedication to this field of cardio-renal-metabolic medicine has won him many laurels. He has organized several meetings and conferences on this subject and has also published many guidelines with particular emphasis with relevance of these topics to South Asians. It has been a great pleasure to collaborate with Dr. Kris Vijay in some of his academic pursuits. I am sure this book will be a valuable addition not only for general physicians and specialist, but also for medical students and indeed, even for the lay public and in short, for everyone. There are many books in the world today, but when such a masterpiece is written by an expert like Dr. Kris Vijay, including all his personal experiences, it becomes a gem to be treasured. I wish Kris Vijay all the very best with the publication of this book and beyond.

Dr. V. MOHAN, M.D., FRCP (London, Edinburgh, Glasgow, Ireland), Ph.D., D.Sc., D.Sc (Hon. Causa), FNASc, FASc, FNA, , FACE, FTWAS, MACP, FRSE
Chairman and Chief Diabetologist, Dr.Mohan's Diabetes Specialities Centre,
Director & President, Madras Diabetes Research Foundation,
Awarded Padma Shri by Govt. of India

CHAPTER 39

CardioOncology

WATCH NOW

Cardio-oncology is a new subspecialty that was developed to detect, monitor, and treat cardiovascular disease. It occurs as either a side effect of chemotherapy or radiotherapy. Both cancer treatment morbidities can cause heart dysfunction.

Cancer itself can be associated with heart disease and medications for these heart issues may exacerbate the condition of some of these cancers. Hence, it is important to assess cancer patients with heart disease and vice versa. Using a 3D echocardiogram, it is important to watch left ventricular function to assess myocardial deformation that can occur with chemotherapy. Other biomarkers such as BNP may facilitate early detection of cardiac toxicity.

A major cause of mortality and morbidity in the cancer population is that of heart disease. Hence, it makes sense to periodically monitor cancer patients undergoing treatment and especially those receiving anthracycline or trastuzumab for breast cancer. There are multiple kinds of cancer therapies and many of them have cardiovascular side effects.

Cardiac assessment before starting chemotherapy is essential and should be continued throughout cancer treatment and even years after therapy.

High-risk individuals may receive high detailed management of plan in collaboration with oncology and heart failure teams. If one develops heart failure despite a lack of symptoms, then it is important to address the causative agent and discontinue it as soon as possible. Important questions that need to be answered are: whether and to stop the cardiac medications, if so, when, and when will heart dysfunction reverse itself after cancer treatment? Cardio-Oncology is a field in evolution that will lead to further understanding of the mechanism in the effect of heart disease as we learn more about the toxicity of some cancer therapies.

Following are some of the therapies used in cancer: multitargeted tyrosine kinase, vascular endothelial growth factor inhibitors such as bevacizumab or HER2 targeted therapies such as. trastuzumab, pertuzumab; protease inhibitors such as bortezomib; anthracyclines such as doxorubicin and epirubicin; alkylating agents such as bendamustine; microtubule inhibitors such as paclitaxel, Platinum-based antineoplastic drugs such as cisplatin, antimetabolites drugs such as fluorouracil and radiation therapy. Tyrosine kinase inhibitors can cause cardiac myocyte damage and lead to heart failure, hypertension, ischemia, and vascular effects. Protease inhibitors, anthracyclines, alkylating, and HER2 therapies can contribute to heart failure and myocyte damage. Microtubule inhibitors can cause arrhythmias; Platinum-based antineoplastic drugs, antimetabolites, and radiation therapy can also cause occlusive vascular disease and structural heart disease.

As cardiac subspecialties increase in the 21st century, it is becoming important to have collaboration among different specialties and disciplines to provide optimum care. Early detection and management of cardiovascular disease in cancer patients throughout all stages of treatments have to be prioritized. As newer therapies are approved and the magnitude of long-term cardiovascular mortality is likely to increase with unknown complications, it is important to have a close partnership and open discussions of patient management between patients and the physicians, between cardiologists, oncologists, and the cardio-oncology team.

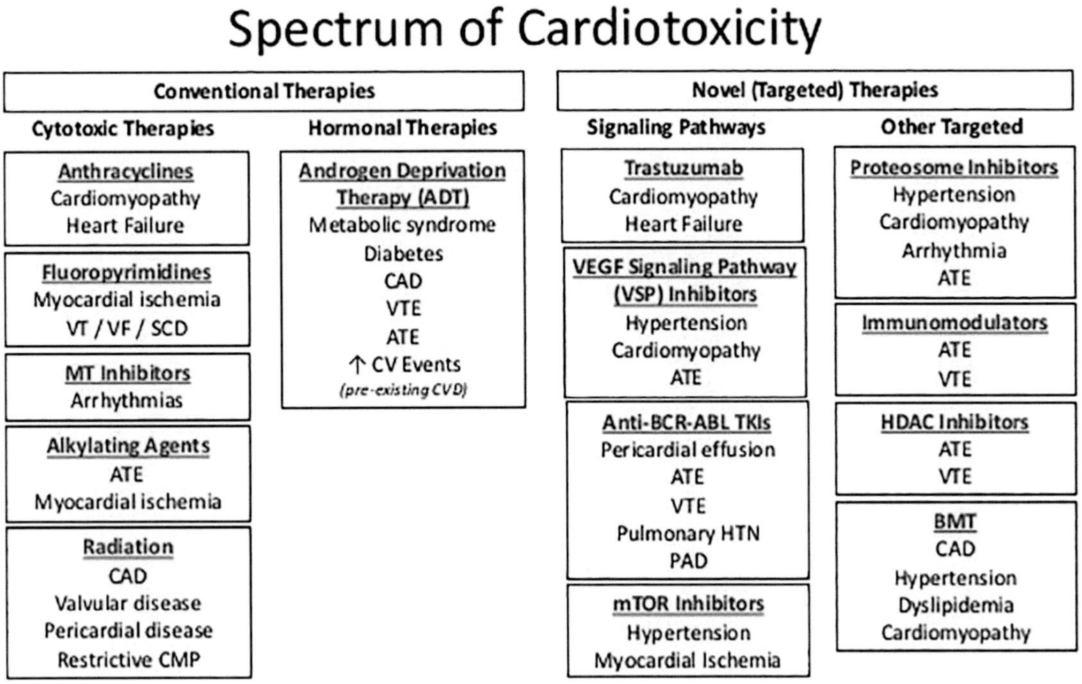
Spectrum of Cardiotoxicity
Conventional Therapies
Cytotoxic Therapies
Anthracyclines
Cardiomyopathy
Heart Failure
Fluoropyrimidines
Myocardial ischemia
VT / VF / SCD
MT Inhibitors
Arrhythmias
Alkylating Agents
ATE
Myocardial ischemia
Radiation
CAD
Valvular disease
Pericardial disease
Restrictive CMP
Hormonal Therapies
Androgen Deprivation Therapy (ADT)
Metabolic syndrome
Diabetes
CAD
VTE
ATE
↑ CV Events
(pre-existing CVD)
Novel (Targeted) Therapies
Signaling Pathways
Trastuzumab
Cardiomyopathy
Heart Failure
VEGF Signaling Pathway (VSP) Inhibitors
Hypertension
Cardiomyopathy
ATE
Anti-BCR-ABL TKIs
Pericardial effusion
ATE
VTE
Pulmonary HTN
PAD
mTOR Inhibitors
Hypertension
Myocardial Ischemia
Other Targeted
Proteosome Inhibitors
Hypertension
Cardiomyopathy
Arrhythmia
ATE
Immunomodulators
ATE
VTE
HDAC Inhibitors
ATE
VTE
BMT
CAD
Hypertension
Dyslipidemia
Cardiomyopathy

Fig. 44

CHAPTER 40

Newer Therapies in Heart Failure

WATCH NOW

Beyond the therapies utilized to make the patient feel better and live longer, multiple other pharmacological agents are recently approved or in clinical trials. We have used diuretics to ascertain that their fluid status is stable and can improve symptoms despite not affecting mortality. Over the past 30 years, we have also studied multiple other agents that have improved survival in patients with heart failure such as ACE inhibitors, ARBs, sacubitril/valsartan, potassium retaining diuretics, anti-aldosterone inhibitors, and beta-blockers. We have had some success with ICD implantation and biventricular pacemaker therapy as well.

We have had heart failure hospitalization reductions with digoxin and many other agents that are still in trials which include molecular targets, immune modulator therapies, free fatty acid inhibitors, Rho-kinase inhibitors, Myosin activators called omecamtiv, calcium sensitizers, phosphodiesterase inhibitors, unloading agents, and SGLT-2 inhibitors. Indications for the same are still pending from the FDA. Antagomir is still being studied for the same.

Two studies, TICLOVER TIMI 58 and DAPA HF reveal that dapagliflozin reduced heart failure, hospitalizations, and cardiovascular death among patients with and without diabetes. Another study called the VICTORIA trial evaluated the efficacy and safety of an agent called Vericiguat which is a guanylate cyclase stimulator that seems to reduce hospitalizations and death and is awaiting FDA approval.

FDA has granted fast track designation for Omecamtiv. This means that the drug, if analysis shows benefit, will get reviewed sooner for approval.

GALACTIC-HF (one of the largest Phase 3 global cardiovascular (CV) outcomes studies in heart failure ever conducted), is designed to evaluate whether treatment with omecamtiv mecarbil, when added to standard of care, reduces the risk of heart failure events (heart failure hospitalization and other urgent treatment for heart failure) and CV death in patients with HFrEF. GALACTIC-HF enrolled 8,256 patients in 35 countries who were either hospitalized at the time of enrollment for a primary reason of heart failure or had a hospitalization or admission to an emergency room for heart failure within one year prior to screening. Dose selection for omecamtiv mecarbil in this study uses a blood test. Top-line results from GALACTIC-HF are expected in Q4 2020.

CHAPTER 41

Nursing care

By

Desiree Little

Desiree Little, MSN, APRN, NP-BC, CHFN
Heart Failure Nurse Practitioner
Abrazo Arizona Heart Hospital: Cardiorenal Center

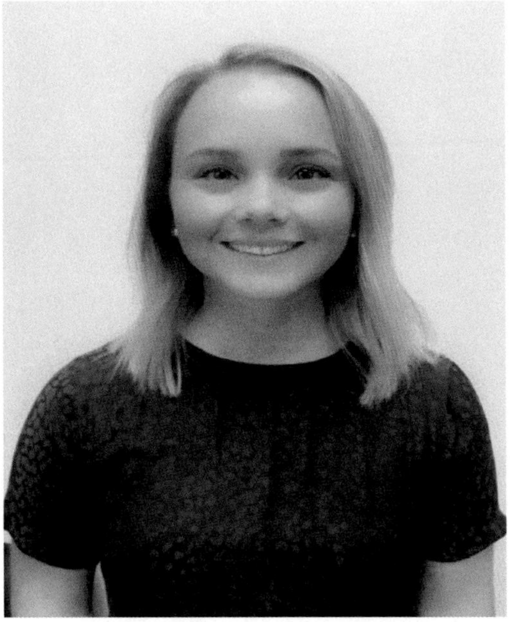

Patient Story

CA is a 58-year-old male who was hospitalized multiple times for recurrent heart failure a few years ago. Since then, we embraced him as a patient who has done well with our recommendations. At one point, his ejection fraction was low at 20% and had recurrent coronary arterial occlusions and kidney failure. He was struggling with medical therapy He did not follow dietary advice and had high salt, sugar, and fatty food regularly.

Once he enrolled in our program, he started to feel that someone cared about him and his recovery. He started to come weekly as we place him on life-saving medications, controlled his fluid balance, ascertained a better diet with low salt and fluid restrictions. We were able to use some lifesaving medications. He was not a candidate for any more revascularization of his coronaries. He used to be hospitalized 2-3 times a month for heart failure and now he realized he was not requiring to be hospitalized anymore.

He required a Biventricular (3 lead) pacemaker and defibrillator. This helped improve his symptoms. When we had the opportunity to change his perspective on life, he started to believe. CA went through multiple therapies including EECP, medication changes, and became emboldened in his calling to heal. Last year he had a mini stroke for which he was hospitalized but other than that, his rehospitalization rate for heart failure has been reduced significantly. He has done well from that perspective and now that he is feeling better and his ejection fraction has improved, he has started doing charity work. He is giving back to the community through his church because he feels that the care and compassion, he has received from nursing staff should now be transferred to other people in his own way.

He has had one big opportunity to live again and he is tremendously grateful for that. CA's generosity reminds me of the movie "Pay It Forward". In this movie, there is a powerful message of the science of neuro associative conditioning that teaches a positive vocabulary to deal with life metaphors. Clearly, he is now attempting to master his own destiny and do charity work for the community. This reflects what he has always believed in and resonates with how a strong internal charge has helped him pursue life with joy and courage.

Nursing Perspectives in Management of Heart Failure

Nurses have been the pillars in the management of heart failure patients; if acute decompensated HF, then at inpatient setting and if chronic HF, then at the outpatient setting. Regardless of the setting, nurses have given their best at every encounter to make the patient comfortable and watching for their best outcomes. They have believed in the success of their patients in a way that many unsung heroes and unknown soldiers have given their all. Reminds me of Mr. Holland in Mr. Holland's opus:

Ms. Gertrude Lang:

Mr. Holland had a profound influence on my life and on a lot of lives I know. But I have a feeling that he considers a great part of his own life misspent. Rumor had it he was always working on this symphony of his. And this was going to make him famous, rich, probably both. But Mr. Holland isn't rich, and he isn't famous, at least not outside of our little town. So, it might be easy for him to think of himself as a failure. But he would be wrong because I think that he's achieved a success far beyond riches and fame.

Look around you. There is not a life in this room that you have not touched, and each of us is a better person because of you. We are your symphony, Mr. Holland. We are the melodies and the notes of your opus. We are the music of your life.

—Mr. Holland's Opus

Heart failure nursing is the provision of holistic care to the specific individual with heart failure diagnosis due to any etiology. This care can take place in an inpatient or outpatient setting and can address the acute or chronic needs of patients and their support systems (AAHFN, 2018). In this chapter, a heart failure nurse's perspective of commonalities amongst the heart failure population is discussed, enhanced with key concepts of the heart failure nurse's role scattered throughout.

Having cared for hundreds of heart failure patients, three commonalities amongst them that standout are:

- They have/are experiencing frustration with their disease process.
- Their appreciation of holistic care by giving them a "medical home"; and
- Their search for what their prognosis is and if they are getting better.

Frustration. Finding that beautiful balance of optimized guideline medical therapy coupled with lifestyle modifications of fluid and sodium restriction can become exasperating for patients. Most heart failure patients limit the amount of fluid and sodium they consume to allow the heart to work efficiently with hopes that the fluid does not back up into the lungs and systemic system. However, inevitably the heart failure patient will have fluid retention during their course of disease resulting in asymptomatic patients. While the patient, provider, and, nurse work together to find the "perfect cocktail" this quote comes to mind, "Life is full of ups and downs. The trick is to enjoy the ups and have courage and perseverance during the downs"-unknown author.

A key role of the heart failure nurse is patient education; this is the foundation of heart failure management.

Nurses help patients make informed decisions and adhere to medical recommendations. The patient should understand why they are asked to restrict fluids, limit sodium intake, exercise, and participate in daily-weight monitoring in order to be successful. Helping a patient to understand why eating a hamburger loaded with 1,200 mg of sodium will make them gain weight resulting in becoming symptomatic can help them to make better choices.

Dietary advice is given. Early symptom recognition of a heart failure exacerbation with an action plan with what to do and whom to call is paramount to keeping them from hospital admission. Educating them on why they are taking their medication and how they are helping their heart can increase compliance. Do you know how many people think they are taking carvedilol or sacubitril/valsartan to control their blood pressure when in reality they are taking it to strengthen their heart! Nelson Mandela once said, "Education is the great engine of personal development. It is through education that the daughter of a peasant can become a doctor, that the son of a mineworker can become the head of the mine, that the child of farmworkers can become the president of a great nation."

> A key role of the heart failure nurse is to provide holistic care to the patient and give them this medical home.

Medical Home. The most loyal person is a heart failure patient that you have helped to get them through their "lows" of their condition. There is an unsettling amount of heart failure patients that "fall through" the cracks and their care consist of multiple trips to the hospital in acute decompensated heart failure. When these patients find a care team to help them to achieve optimize heart failure therapy and begin to feel better, their appreciation and trust in you are endless. A medical home is a place where the heart failure patient can come to get care, somewhere they can call when they become symptomatic, somewhere they feel unjudged so that they can get the care they deserve.

Triaging a phone call from an asymptomatic patient with decision-making if taking an extra water pill can help or if they need to go to the emergency room can make a colossal difference to the heart failure patient's progress. Ensuring that patients have all their medications and if not identifying barriers to why and finding an alternative option, if necessary. Collaboration with other specialists, such as nephrology, electrophysiology, interventional cardiology, pulmonary, and primary care provides holistic care to the comorbid patient. Collection of diagnostics reports, such as electrocardiograms, echocardiograms, angiograms, etc. to ensure the healthcare provider has the most up to date data to create the patient's plan of care. Lastly, just being a voice on the other end of the phone or in-person to the anxious heart failure patient to walk them through their plan of care can assist in adherence and understanding.

Prognosis. Since the invention of Dr. Google, heart failure patients often present with anxiety because of the information they have gathered. While a specific answer on their progress is often complex, an offer of quality improvement strategies can help guide therapy and give the patient data to see if their condition is improving. These strategies consist of periodic surveys and six-minute walk tests.

INSPIRE HF FRAMEWORK

1. Individualize priorities and identify the nature of co-morbidities with patient-centered targeted goals and therapies, and shared decision making.
2. Nutrition intervention instruction through education for cardiometabolic renal comorbidity; sugar, salt, and fluid intake optimization and weight monitoring and reduction programs.
3. Stabilize and assess fluid status utilizing multiple modalities: clinical presentation, biomarkers, evidence-based medical management, and innovative device-based therapies.
4. Psychosocial motivational empowerment through assessment and management of anxiety, depression, socioeconomic assessment and support, coping skills, and motivational interviews with the evocation of positive messages.
5. Initiate guideline-directed medication therapy (GDMT) enabled by pharmacological agents to support hemodynamics in collaboration with other specialties to optimize treatment options.
6. Revisit comorbidities with biomarker assessments and continuously reevaluate interventions, health outcomes, quality of life (QOL), readmissions, worsening renal failure, and mortality; and
7. Education regarding the prevention and slowing of disease progression for diabetes, metabolic derangement, cardiac, renal, and other comorbidities in simplistic terms to invoke self-care and enroll in weight management and exercise programs.

A key role that the heart failure nurse plays in administering these strategies and creating a comparison to the patient's previous efforts. One of the surveys utilized is the Kansas City Cardiomyopathy Questionnaire (KCCQ), which is a well-validated and widely used 23-item instrument that measures patient-reported symptoms, function, and quality of life for patients with heart failure. The other is the Minnesota Living with Heart Failure Questionnaire, which is a 21-item instrument to assess the health-related quality of life of patients with heart failure in adults. The goal is to see improvement in scores; if there is no improvement then a change in the plan of care can be considered. The six-minute walk test consists of the patient walking a given route to see how far they get within six minutes. The goal is to reach a farther distance with each walk. The data from these quality strategies allow the healthcare provider and patient to see their own progression or regression. Due to the multiple comorbidities that are associated with HF, we have developed a framework called INSPIRE HF which is followed on every patient.

Quality or quantity? A question that heart failure patients face during their course of the disease. Heart failure nurses will be there for these patients through both tough decisions and triumphs. The heart failure nurse's role is to provide holistic, passionate care and comprehensive education to every heart failure patient they touch. Florence Nightingale once said, "I think one's feelings waste themselves in words; they ought all to be distilled into actions which bring results.", which is the foundation of how a heart failure nurse practices.

WATCH NOW

CHAPTER 42

Psychosocial Aspects of Heart Failure Psychosocial

WATCH NOW

Patient Story

Mr. PK is an 80-year-old male who has been with us at the heart failure clinic for the past 2-3 years and has done remarkably well in terms of improvement in functional capacity and ejection fraction from 30% to 45%. He is very thankful to the nurses who have been monitoring him closely. The reason that we are thankful to the patient is the gratitude that he instills to the nurses in terms of what they have done for him.

Clearly, the initial nursing assessment in assessing symptoms has been more from a subjective standpoint in assessing the patient but also from objective measures to assessing their cardiac variable, respiration rate, O2 Saturation, rhythm monitoring, blood pressuring monitoring, cardiac output measurement, perfusion measurements, mental status, lab work, psychosocial components. and examining for retention or depletion of fluid status.

> One of the most important aspects of this continuum of care is the psychosocial aspect of Heart Failure. Anxiety and depression are extremely common in this clinical setting The Minnesota Living with HF questionnaires as well as the Kansas City Cardiomyopathy questionnaires are two especially important measures we get to assess objectively.

The key role of the nurse is to rapidly assess and treat in an appropriate environment to improve clinical status. Whether it could be managed in the outpatient or hospital setting is the question that needs to be answered at every point of contact, particularly when a patient is symptomatic. Beyond the objective measurements and observing for improvement, the nurses need to be dealing with discharge planning, referrals to multidisciplinary disease management programs from a nurse navigator perspective with all subspecialty intervention.

Nurses have to draw from their own personal experiences as well as scientific literature in understanding the cognitive psychology of every patient with heart failure. The neuroscience and neuro associative conditioning along with behavioral and communication skills are important in giving them practical steps to change their thinking process to adopt these measures to positively impact the patient's lives.

The human mind operates through a series of multiple feedback loops and through our understanding of what metacognition is and a tool for reflecting on the thinking process of our patients, we may be able to influence their brain response towards healing. Due to our patient's satisfaction and gratitude to the nurses and a better outcome, we feel that there is a value perspective and a value proposition that has allowed us to utilize this psychosocial element as a powerful tool among heart failure patients.

Psychosocial Aspects of Heart Failure

He who has health has hope.
He who has hope has everything.

– **Thomas Carlyle**

Congestive heart failure can be considered as an end-stage disease. Patients generally rely on a battery of pharmacological interventions and device therapies leading to perhaps left ventricle assist devices or heart transplants if they qualify. But short of these treatments, most patients have to rely on medications and devices and adjustment of these therapies. Alongside these aspects of management lies a serious underlying condition that is essentially ignored in the management of heart failure patients. In recent years, the psychological impact of heart failure is being explored which is reflected by the absence of standardized psychological assessment.

Many patients have to deal with depression and/or anxiety and the data shows that 80-90% of patients with heart failure manifest anxiety or depression or both. We also have issues with coping lifestyles and social support. One has to ascertain that psychological issues in heart failure are not neglected.

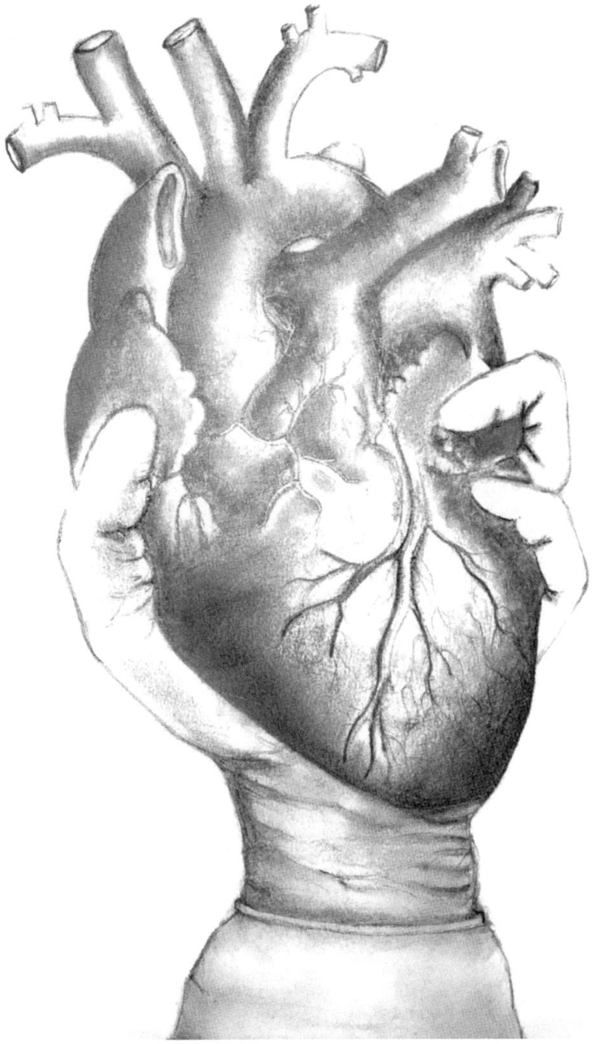

Fig. 45

Prevalence of Anxiety in Heart Failure

A Metanalysis of 36 studies has found that clinically significant depression affects about 21.5% of heart failure patients. One-third of heart failure patients report elevated depression symptoms in depression questionnaires. Also, there are about 19% of patients who meet the criteria for a depressive disorder based on a diagnostic interview. Anxiety is also highly prevalent in about 13-20% of patients with heart failure who were filling a diagnostic requirement questionnaire. The rates range from 70-80% in older adults. In most patients who have had a heart attack, there is almost 90% of patients who go into heart failure and exhibit a significant amount of anxiety and depression. There is a clear link between anxiety, depression, and adverse medical outcomes in heart failure.

In a large study, patients with anxiety and depression had an 18% increased risk of adverse cardiovascular events. In another study of 18,000 veterans without heart disease, the diagnosis of major depression was linked to a 21% increased risk of heart failure which doubled up over a five-year period. Depression is indeed a poor prognostic marker in patients with heart failure. Anxiety and depression have been linked to frequent hospitalizations and increased mortality. Patients with PTSD and developmental heart failure has been shown in clinical trials. A longitudinal study on PTSD conferred a 47% increase in incidents of heart failure over a 7-year period. Although the literature may be lacking between anxiety disorders and health outcomes in patients with heart failure, it is clear that anxiety is associated with poor health, poor quality of life, and poor heart health, and higher rates of mortality in patients with coronary disease. In patients who have had panic attacks and PTSD, there is evidence of an increased rate of hospitalization and mortality.

Mechanisms Linking Depression, Anxiety, and Heart Outcomes

Both physiological mechanisms and behavior may explain the relationship between anxiety, depression, and heart failure. Many patients have poor self-care including non-adherence to a diet in low sodium and physical activity or taking their medication. These patients may have a poor quality of life and higher rates of hospitalization and mortality. It means they are less likely to maintain a healthy diet and exercise regularly compared to non-depressed individuals.

There is a thin line between psychological symptoms and psychiatric symptoms. Inflammation is implicated in the pathogenesis of severe types of heart failure and maybe a driver of ventricular remodeling that is associated with enlargement of the heart, increased fibrosis, and dilatation. inflammatory markers called interleukin 6 is linked to both short-and long-term cardiovascular mortality. It appears that there may be a higher level of inflammation in patients with depression and anxiety and this has been validated in clinical trials that have shown increased levels of CRP and interleukin 1 & 6, TNF alpha, and Monocyte chemoattractant **protein**-1 (MCP1). Also, in certain other studies, there has been an increase in homocysteine level and fibrinogen level and there is a suggestion that platelet aggregation is significantly elevated with patients with anxiety and or depression.

The autonomic nervous system may be implicated in the relationship between anxiety and depression and cardiovascular tone. The parasympathetic and sympathetic systems control the heart rate, blood pressure, vasoconstriction, and vasodilation. In patients with anxiety and depression, there may be a relation between hyperactivity of the sympathetic nervous system and hypoactivity of the parasympathetic nervous system, linked to an imbalance and hence a geometric remodeling of the structural heart components. Endothelial dysfunction may be another factor that is being contributed by anxiety and depression. A study shows a lower level of l-arginine and ADMA ratio indicating reduced nitric oxide availability leading to endothelial dysfunction and cardiac symptoms. Flow Mediated vasodilation also has been abnormal in other studies in patients with anxiety or depression. The endothelial function markers such as soluble intercellular adhesion molecule ICAM, VCAM, and e-selectin are all shown to be abnormal and associated with PTSD and heart failure.

Diagnosis of Anxiety and Depression in Heart Failure

Due to overlapping symptoms shared between heart failure and mental health issues, it is important that the healthcare provider exclude an underlying psychiatric diagnosis. Full diagnostic and statistical management of mental disorders (DSM) has been the primary resource to document depression and anxiety based on specific criteria. To increase recognition among these people, many organizations have developed multiple screening tools. The American Heart Association recommends a 2-step depression screening called 2 item patient healthcare questionnaire (PHQ). In addition, they have a 9-item patient questionnaire called PHQ9 among patients who may have positive PHQ-2. This 2-step procedure is highly specific, although sensitivity maybe around 50%.

A condition called generalized anxiety disorder (GAD) is prospectively associated with poor cardiac outcomes in patients after a heart attack and may be prevalent in patients with hospitalized heart failure patients. There is a GAD 2 & 7 screening tool that has demonstrated adequate specificity and sensitivity as well. Other kinds of screening tools include prime MD, Hamilton Depression Rating Scale (HAM-D), Beck Depression Inventory (BDI), Geriatric Depression Scale (GDS), Hopkins Symptom Checklist (HSCL), Hospital Anxiety and Depression Scale (HADS), Physical Symptom Checklist (PSC-51) and Center for Epidemiologic Studies Depression Scale (CESD-R). Which tools to use may be dependent on specific aspects of the disease and symptoms.

Management of Depression and Anxiety in Heart Failure Patients

Don't ever let somebody tell you, you can't do something, not even me. Alright?
You dream, you gotta protect it.
People can't do something themselves, they wanna tell you, you cannot do it.
If you want something, go get it. Period.

– Will Smith, "The Pursuit of Happyness"

Beyond medical therapy for anxiety or depression, non-pharmacological therapies have also been effective. The most important one includes cognitive behavioral therapy which is the only psychotherapeutic application that has been tested systematically in heart failure patients and has shown benefits. The CBD trial that has shown significant benefit was the Depression and Self Care of Heart Failure Trial which had more than 158 patients diagnosed with major depression and seemed to improve symptoms wise. In studies called SADHART-CHF and MOOD-HF found that sertraline was as effective as a placebo in reducing depressive symptoms, but several factors could have led to a neutral trial.

Possibilities explanations include the overlap between somatic symptoms of heart failure and depression. While we expect antidepressants to improve somatic symptoms, those related to heart failure generally do not improve. Hence, there might be other variables that do not allow pharmacological therapy to cause an impact. Another explanation includes the negative findings of these trials may be biologically distinct from typical depression that is present in the absence of heart failure. There are still recommendations of selective serotonin reuptake inhibitors (SSI) in heart failure, which have had few adverse effects and benefits and the benefit/risk ratio may be higher. One needs to watch the QTC prolongation on the EKG regularly.

The integrated health models in the management of depression and anxiety beyond pharmacological therapies are important and include non-physician care managers supervised by a psychologist or psychiatrist. Collaborative care programs have been effective. Improvement in mental and physical health outcomes including blood pressure, A1C, LDL cholesterol, has been shown to be beneficial in the integrated health model. Patients entering disease management have examined the efficacy of multicomponent collaborative care intervention which seems to find improvement in functional capacity, but the depression scale has not been altered significantly.

A large study called the ARISE-HF was performed to establish a prognostic framework for optimizing health outcomes in patients with heart failure and multi-mortality and specialty statements. They have identified 5 potential key steps that could systematically improve health outcomes. ARISE stands for Acknowledgment of Multi-Morbidity as a syndrome associated with poor outcomes.

- Routinely profile the standardized protocol adapted to local health care systems in our patients hospitalized with heart failure to determine the extent of concurrent multi-morbidity
- Identify individualized priority and person-centered goals based on the extent and nature of multi-morbidity
- Support individualized home-based multi-morbidity and case management to support standardized heart failure management
- Evaluate health outcomes well beyond acute hospitalizations and encompass all causes and person censored perspective in infected individuals.

This multi-morbidity and heart failure study include the following comorbidities: Anemia, atrial and ventricular arrhythmias, cognitive impairment, dementia, depression, anxiety, diabetes, musculoskeletal disorders, and sleep disorders. Thus, identifying the key areas of multimorbidity as well as addressing the psychosocial aspects of the disease process and utilizing ARISE HF as a framework to improve quality of life and health sequelae may be potentially beneficial in overall health outcomes.

Almost every patient who has come through our system over the years with heart failure has struggled with feelings of despair, disappointment, overwhelmed with physical inability, and many things to take care of outside of their cardiac condition to move on with life on a daily basis. Many patients get stretched with no sense of hope with anxiety and depression. They have lost their capacity to think positively and change some of the aspects and

Intangible but Striking Benefits of Positive Feedback in Heart Failure Outcomes

The greatest disease in the West today is not TB or leprosy. it is being unwanted, unloved, and uncared for. We can cure physical diseases with medicine, but the only cure for loneliness, despair, and hopelessness is love. Many in the world are dying for a piece of bread, but there are many more dying for a little love. The poverty in the West is a different kind of poverty – it is not only a poverty of loneliness but also of spirituality. There's a hunger for love, as there is a hunger for God."

— Mother Teresa

become successful in their own physical capacity until they move on. Their emotional destiny is intertwined with their physical relationship in mastering their own life to set a legacy before they die.

From a healthcare provider perspective, we do not want to give them a false sense of hope but there is something to say about positive thinking that truly translates their feeling of being overwhelmed to being turbocharged. It is noticeably clear that there is something about the improvement of physical struggles in heart failure by addressing the psychological, psychosocial, and financial status if we can impact that component. If we increase their knowledge about their lifestyle modifications by helping them quit smoking or improving their dietary patterns with salt restrictions, the trust and psychological impact can follow.

There is no universal code that applies to every patient to put them inside a compartment with a cookbook approach. Certain norms might sustain their overall cardiovascular status and psychosocial status; however, once we illuminate their dilemma and enlighten them about the aspects of cardiovascular disease with education, they may start to trust you with their personal struggles. It is indeed challenging to be grounded with knowledge about everything regarding heart failure.

It is our job as healthcare providers to attempt to educate in ways that bring out courage and a certain level of passion and invoke certain energy from within. We have to attempt to link the nature of suffering from that of the physical, psychosocial, and financial components. If we only focus on the psychological component, then the patient will not heal in a way that we want. Hence, it is important to make them feel better by helping them breathe easier and make their fatigue go away. It is a combination of the education component and treatment of the psychosocial element.

The neuro conditioning with motivational interviews and empowering them by addressing the accessibility of care, affordability of medications, devices, and therapies, will allow them to master their own clinical condition. In a quickly evolving world, the enduring appeal of traditions from a religious, and faith perspective can help to deliver powerful messages of an all-pervading love.

This may be inborn or divinely inspired, and if they believe in the higher power, it is possible that an element of wonder and worship can help stimulate endorphins and good cytokines which in turn can help the heart heal. We educate them with figures and drawings because we believe that a keen visual testimony to the power of acceptance is important. We believe that of by addressing the psychosocial elements such as anxiety, depression, and relationships, we can overcome fear and increase a sense of resilience that makes them capable of fighting against the odds.

HOSPITAL & RESEARCH CENTRE, DAMBUCHAN LEH (194101) LADAKH.

Recipient of Social Reform and Empowerment Award by J&K Government

I have known Dr. Kris Vijay for more than seven years, and I feel well qualified to write this endorsement of his book, and recommend to patients, students in medicine, residence in training, faculty, primary care providers, cardiologists and all those who have believed in the struggles of everyday life. He brings immense credibility in this narrative. As the remarkable title of this book alludes to invoking your inner therapist, he genuinely believes in the education of self, motivating one to understand the concepts and energize oneself with the vocabulary of empowerment.

He has explained the anatomy, physiology and pathology of the heart, and all systems that are associated with it in a unique and simplistic form that it seems incredible that he is able to bring life metaphors to gain excitement and vitality.

The contents of this book are a testament to the comprehensiveness of a topic that is truly complex. It is also alarming if it affects you or your near and dear. Dr. Vijay has beautifully described the risk factors, their transformation to disease, how to understand the tests that one may need to build on a therapeutic model that is so sumptuous to the point of healing as you read through this book. The quotes in every chapter followed by patient stories are inspiring, the illustrations are captivating, the bolded messages give one goose bumps and the neuro associative genre is definitely inimitable and brilliant.

On a personal note, Dr. Kris has positively influenced the health and morale in our community in Leh, Ladakh is some amazing ways. He has been a volunteer to our community at The Ladakh Heart Foundation partly funded by the DALAI LAMA Trust. Over the last seven years, many times, he has brought with him about 25 or so health care providers and volunteers to perform screening, diagnostics, education, and therapies that are not available due to the mountainous terrain at 13,000 feet.

Our whole community is infinitely grateful for the service provided by him and his team. His passion and compassion to serve the underserved is very palpable. His team is building a sustainable model for us in Ladakh. We hope that after the COVID 19 has subsided, they will return her with more vigor and enthusiasm to help the needy.

Dr. Kris has proven again and again that his energy to help others is internally satisfying and I am sure he wishes to impart this message to all readers. His compelling descriptions will embolden you to take actions in your positive beliefs. To one and all, I suggest you read the book in its entirety, and I am sure the knowledge you will gain will make your life more productive and fulfilling.

My absolute best wishes,

Lama Thupstan Chogyal

Director, Ladakh Heart Foundation and Research Center

Leh. Ladakh, Kashmir, India

Ladakh Heart Foundation Hospital And Research Centre, Agling Dambuchan, Leh Ladakh, Pin 194101, Post.Box No.150
Tel: 01982-253291/255888, E-mail: ladakhheartfoundation@yahoo.co.in, www.ladakhheart.com

CHAPTER 43

Technology and Advances in Cardiovascular Space

"His creativity, like that of other great innovators, came from standing at the intersection of humanities and technology. He peeled flesh off the faces of cadavers, drew the muscles that move the lips, and then painted history's most memorable smile on the Mona Lisa. He explored the math of optics, showed how light rays strike the cornea, and produced illusions of changing perspectives in The Last Supper.

Walter Isaacson on "Leonardo Da Vinci"
(describing his ability to combine art and science, his willingness to be imaginative, question existing knowledge, and think differently.)

The following topics will address some of the cardiovascular technologies to watch over the next 10 years. Artificial intelligence (AI) in cardiology is a hard topic and similar to machine learning. Once a science fiction idea, now machine learning is becoming mainstream.

Some of the AI intelligence elements are already in use without the awareness of the healthcare community and are integrated into the cardiology and radiology reporting systems.

> Multiple technologies are trending, and the most recent Consumer Electronics Show revealed a huge area of digital technology mainly pertaining to heart disease. There is a likelihood that technology will play a major part in cardiovascular practice in the future.

AI is helping augment cardiology and their medical imaging; at present ejection fraction calculations found on point of care imaging systems like the GE VSCAN is an example of advancement made in AI.

Premium cardiac ultrasound systems such as Philips also use AI to automatically identify

the anatomy. They also form automatic measurement before the physician even begins to view the pictures. Several vendors are offering calcium score imaging software that detects build up in the coronary arteries. Creating report quantification in seconds with color-coding the calcium in visual segments is some of the benefits of AI. Algorithms are also used to efficiently detect arrhythmias and send alerts through portable technology. They also send alerts to the healthcare provider. Apple watch and Kardia have come together as a viable technology to be used by patients at home to monitor heart rhythm.

The next technology that is already available includes transcatheter valve replacements which are already increasing in research. The TAVR is being used frequently for aortic stenosis. Mitral valve replacement (TMVR) is still being studied in Apollo Intrepid Clinical trial. Tricuspid valve clip is being studied in the TRILUMINATE trial and some of the technology companies will convert these into routine procedures. Everyone carries a smartphone and millions of people are using this to track their health with Apple Watches and Fitbit devices. It is not surprising that technology companies leverage these devices to entice consumers and have them interact with health care professionals to better monitor their health. Health tracking information is now available for patient use 24/7 and uses multiple variables and app algorithms that have been created to detect arrhythmias to alert patients to contact their doctors.

Clearly, variables have a significant role to play moving forward. A large number of healthcare systems are integrating variables into their remote monitoring patient programs. In some situations, professional-grade variables like an inexpensive stick of EKG monitor is now offered by many vendors and are replacing traditional Holter monitors. Many of the hospitals are also using variable consumer-grade devices such as glucose monitoring systems which are continuous glucose monitoring like Freestyling Libre. Wireless machines, such as blood pressure monitors interface with smartphone apps and track cardiac rehab, diabetic care, and heart failure care remotely. Big Data is in demand. To that end, variables can be connected through a smartphone with an internet connection and data collected remotely. Hence, there is a potential benefit of improving the health of patients. However, the accuracy of these devices is not noticeably clear.

Smartwatches currently use photo ethnography to detect irregular rhythm. This is a piece of noninvasive technology that uses a light source and photon detector at the skin surface to measure the variations of blood circulation. This technology is commonly used to monitor heart rate, possible extra beats, ambient temperature, or light. The challenge of finding appropriate patients for variables should not be minimized and underscore the need for robust data on effectiveness in this population. Remote dielectric sensing technology as well as lung fluid measurement with a device called REDS is approved for use in the US.

Technology innovation is outpacing the availability of the clinician in healthcare systems to incorporate infrastructure for use of data. Vulnerability to cyber hacks is a major issue at present. Variable devices can become crucial in clinical trials to monitor data and at present, they are sparsely used in this way. In the heart failure patient population, there are still certain challenges that require industry to ascertain accuracy, reliability, and consistency on data that is gathered frequently. Virtual reality (VR) and augmented reality (AR) in cardiology are being used by many cardiology device vendors. Boston Scientific is using a VR headset with a preloaded live electrophysiology device implanted with cases that offer a 360-degree view in the electrophysiology lab.

Once the physician views these images, they can offer key opinions when proctoring and speed the transfer of how to interpret data and utilize it for therapeutic intervention. Apple uses a VR simulator to train interventional cardiologists on how to perform intravascular optical coherence tomography (OCT) imaging. These are all images that utilize technology to view the coronary arteries better. Philips Healthcare is creating an AR system that can use hand movement or voice commands and call up live procedural ultrasound to their AR visor. This will allow them to review CAT scan images, 3d holograms, CT scans, and help them navigate their procedural ramifications accurately. Telemedicine is gaining significant ground in the COVID 19 era and will probably be here to stay for the long run.

WATCH NOW

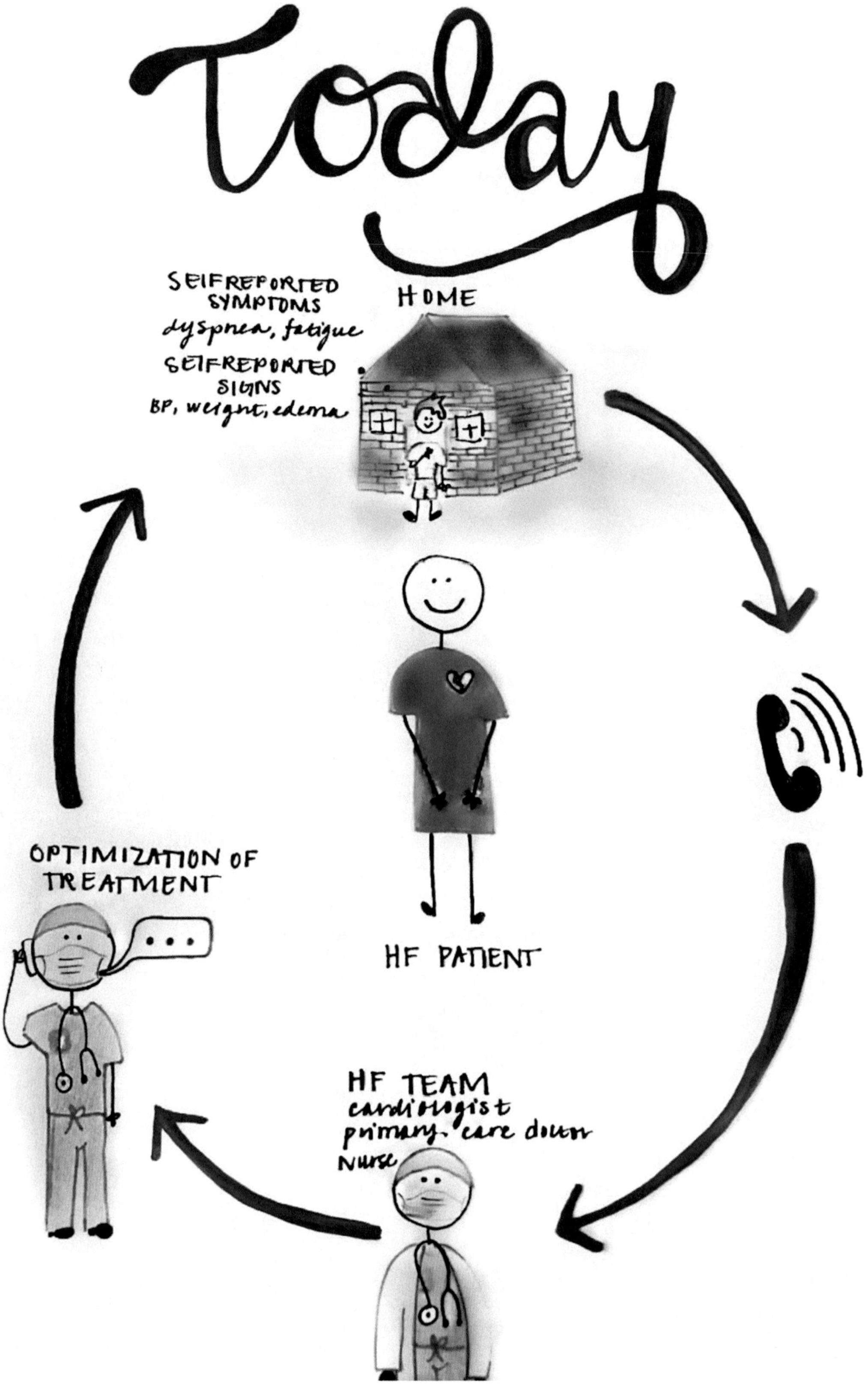
Today
SELFREPORTED SYMPTOMS
dyspnea, fatigue
SELFREPORTED SIGNS
BP, weight, edema
HOME
HF PATIENT
OPTIMIZATION OF TREATMENT
HF TEAM
cardiologist
primary care
Nurse

Fig. 46

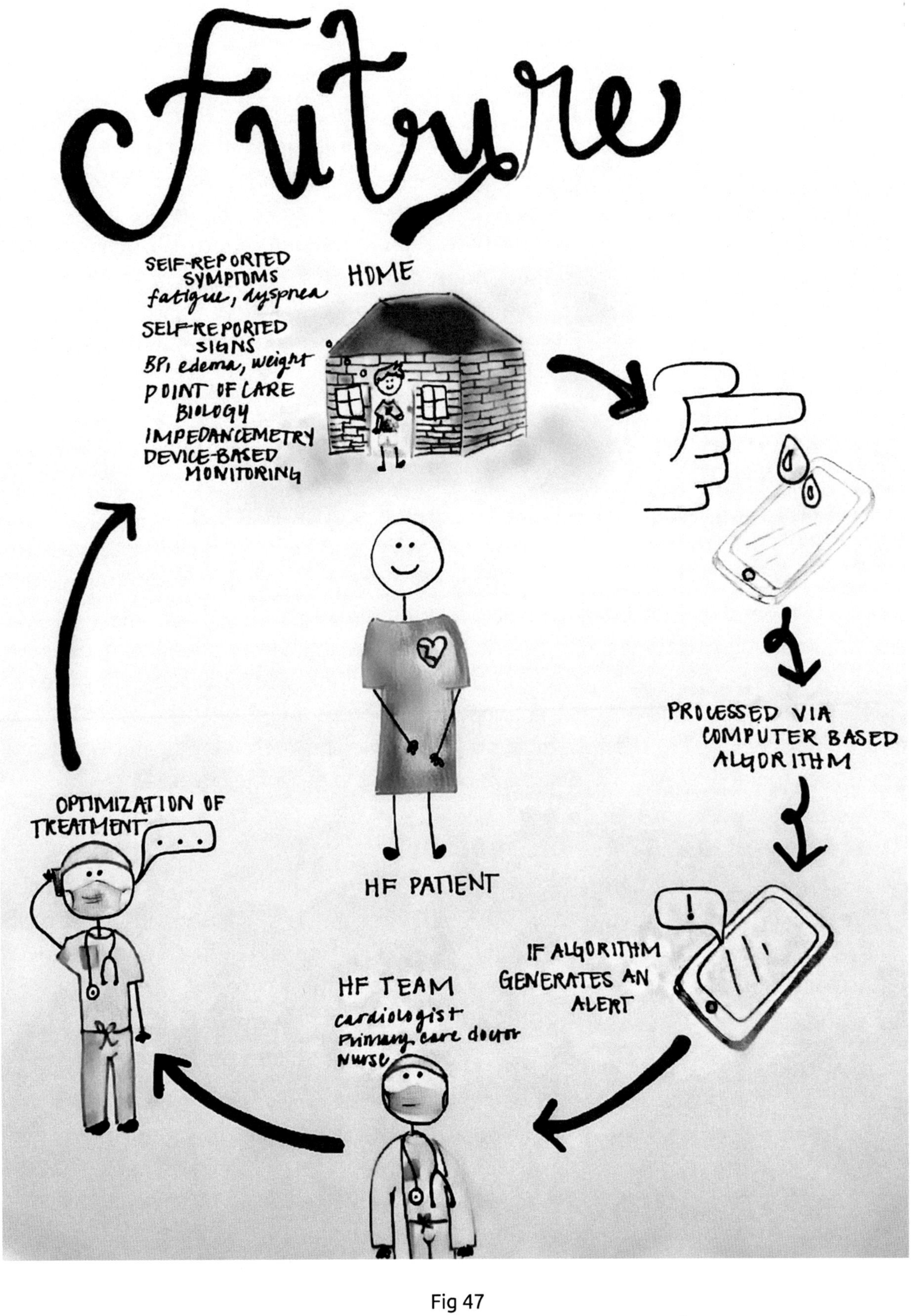
Future
SELF-REPORTED SYMPTOMS
fatigue, dyspnea
HOME
SELF-REPORTED SIGNS
BP, edema, weight
POINT OF CARE BIOLOGY
IMPEDANCEMETRY
DEVICE-BASED MONITORING
PROCESSED VIA COMPUTER BASED ALGORITHM
OPTIMIZATION OF TREATMENT
HF PATIENT
IF ALGORITHM GENERATES AN ALERT
HF TEAM
cardiologist
Primary care doctor
Nurse

Fig 47

Big Data and Structural Reporting

This technology has been becoming increasingly popular over the past 10 years and most of them have been related to the use of electronic medical records and digital reporting systems. While the government road map computerized order entry (CPOE) and clinical decision support, healthcare systems have realized that they can immediately leverage EMR to data-mine their rapidly growing digital archive. Analytic software is now the main priorities for most hospitals, hence, analytical data from structured reporting are being utilized to find workflow bottlenecks, monitor staff workload, track number of procedures, track disease types, track inventory, track outcomes, track costs, track supply chain and track equipment usage. The big data is also mining into the concept of population health care risk factors of patients. They can automatically identify who should be screened or monitored; examples include atrial fibrillation and heart failure.

Holographic Procedural and Navigation in The Cath Lab

Holographic technology is quickly advancing with each pixel. The GE technology using the PEE system projects a hologram of live views of the heart valves and 3D imaging of the left atrial appendage to assess and place devices such as Watchmen or Mitraclip. Robotic catheter navigational systems are here to stay and many of the cardiac cath labs have been using this technology for years. The question of why there is limited adoption includes whether robotic systems are improving outcomes. The robotic systems have allowed controlled manipulations of catheters which takes the operator out of the radiation field and has less exposure to radiation. Also, it allows them to take off their heavy lead aprons and stay at the controlled cockpit area while maneuvering the robotic tools. With time this technology will become more advanced with fewer limitations and more improvement in outcomes overall.

Virtual Image-Based FFR Technology

FFR technology is a fractional flow reserved technology used in the cath lab to assess if an artery needs to be angioplastied or stented. FFR CT imaging is being done in the cath lab as well with 3D imaging is being decreased in the cath lab. Hence, FFR technologies that are FDA approved uses a rotational angiography image acquisition around the patient on the table and the software creates 3D imaging and reconstruction.

In summary, there is a need for evidence that technology is being utilized in cardiac environments that are reliable and accurate. It is important to know if it can be cost-effective and improve patient outcomes. There is also a need for digital solutions in a clinical setting that are designed to address clinical issues that can be integrated into clinical care. The development of technology including digit cells should be at least driven by the users which are the patients and health care providers. Then, they need to be incentivized for use including reimbursement models for digital healthcare and finally the need for data protection regulations including privacy and security to ascertain the attention to detail that would translate to improved outcomes in health care.

CHAPTER 44

New Devices to Treat Heart Failure

WATCH NOW

There are new tools that are being introduced to cardiologists to combat heart failure which include transcatheter left ventricular remodeling, pacemaker devices, pulmonary artery pressure sensors, and percutaneous hemodynamic support devices.

Heartmate 3 has been cleared as a destination therapy which the FDA approved in January 2020. This is a pump that will allow heart failure patients to avoid open-heart surgery. This new approach is designed to provide surgeons a choice in surgical methods. The study was based on a trial called ELEVATE which showed potential complications including bleeding, infections, and arrhythmias.

Another device called a **Precardia SVC Occlusion Balloon** which is a temporary occlusion of the superior vena cava which is done to reset the heart to normal function. The first in man proof of concept device that reduces pressures and volume in the heart effectively. It seems to reduce cardiac filling pressures without reducing cardiac output or systolic blood pressure. While the occlusion is only for 5 minutes, a follow up over a 7-day period showed sustained benefit and FDA is assessing this device therapy at this current time.

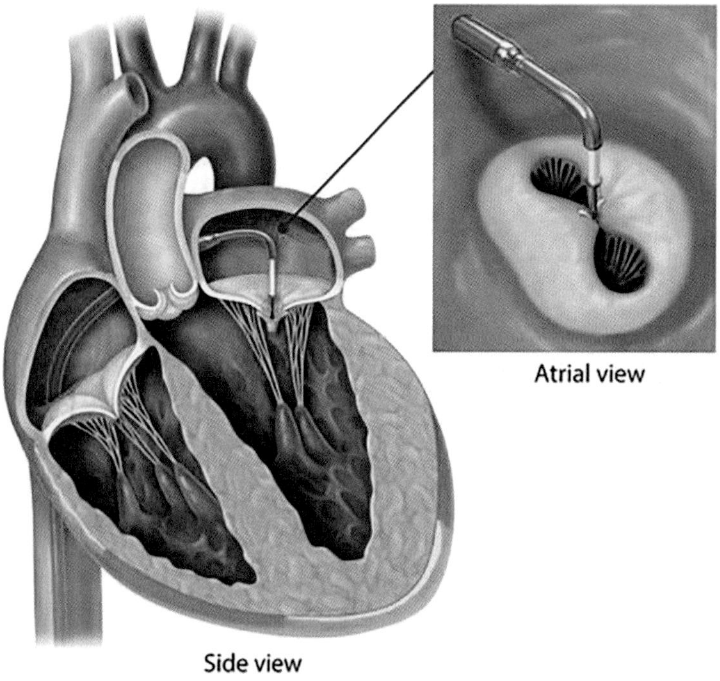

Fig. 48

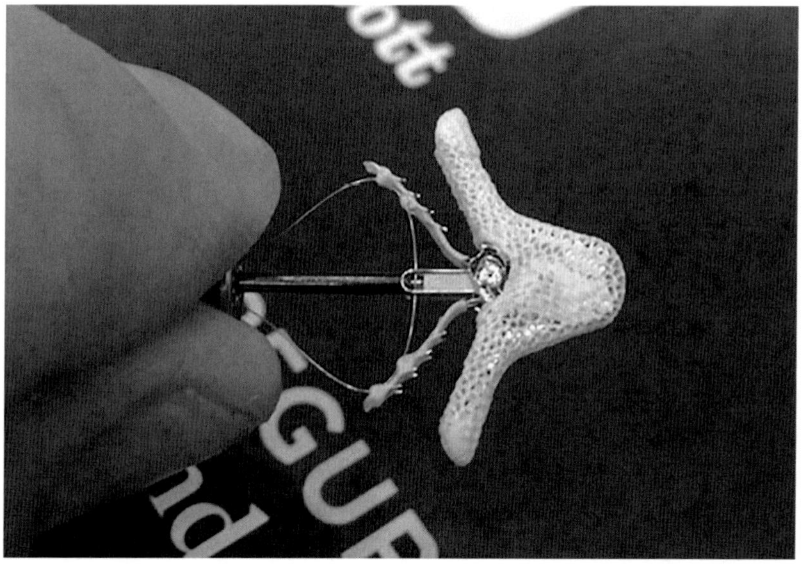

Fig. 49

FDA has approved **Mitraclip** transcatheter mitral valve repair that can be utilized among heart failure patients with mitral valve disorder. A trial called COAPT demonstrated benefit in reducing heart failure hospitalizations and proved to be superior to medical therapy alone.

The **optimizer** is a smart system for contractility modulation which is a pacemaker-like device that delivers pulses rapidly and seems to strengthen heart contractility.

Barostim is another pacemaker-like pulse generator system that was approved by FDA in August 2019 and has leads that deliver electrical signals to the baroreceptors in the carotid artery which send impulses to the brain which in return releases signals to the heart and blood vessels which relaxes the blood vessels and inhibits the production of neurohormones that may cause heart issues. Reducing neurohormones may be indirectly protecting the heart. This is indicated among patients with regular rhythm who are not candidates for resynchronization therapy and have an ejection fraction of less than 35%.

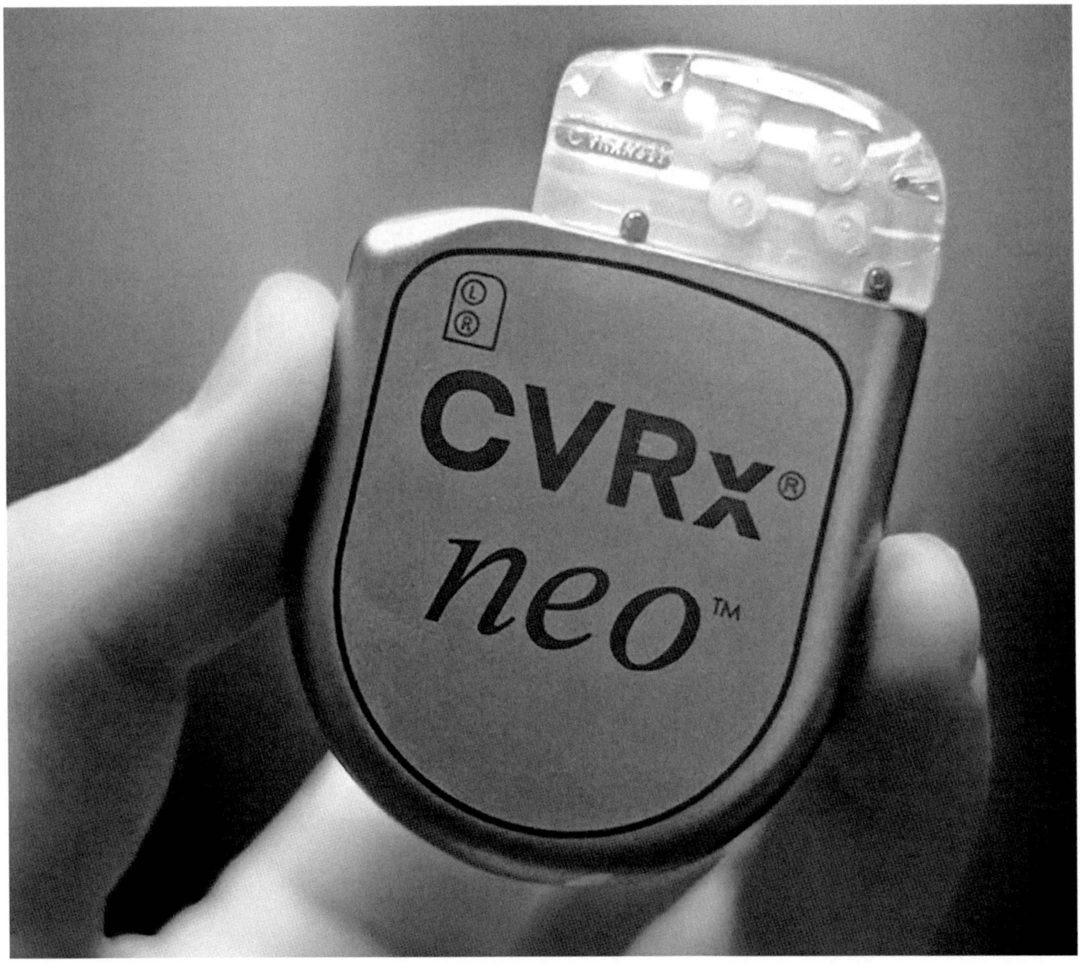

Fig. 50

Interatrial Shunt Device: Interatrial Shunt Device (**CORVIA**) is a transcatheter implant shunt device between the left and right atrium which forms a passage that enables the left atrium to decompress at rest and during physical activity. The main aim is to reduce left atrial pressure which unloads the left atrium and reduces diastolic heart failure. More data is still being found and will be available in the future.

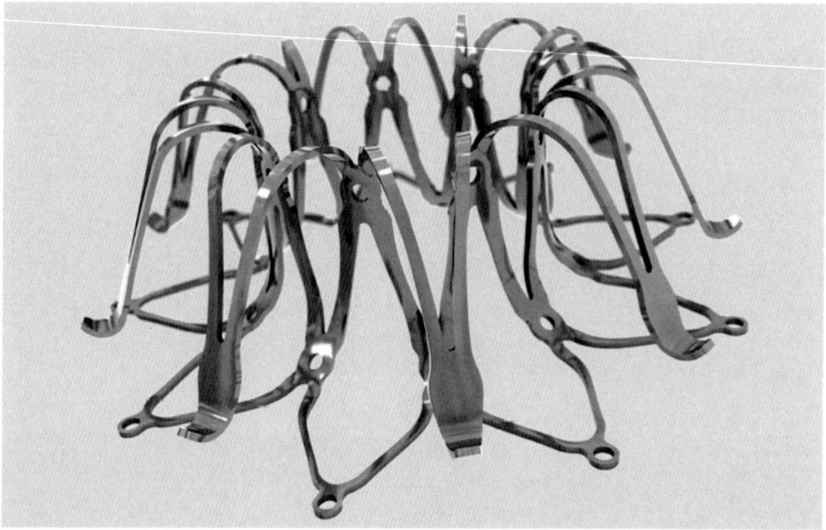

Fig. 51

CORVIA Device

V wave interatrial shunt device is another implantable interatrial shunt device placed in between both atrial chambers in NYHA class II-IV with HFpEF to reduce heart failure and pulmonary artery pressures. This will be entering clinical trials.

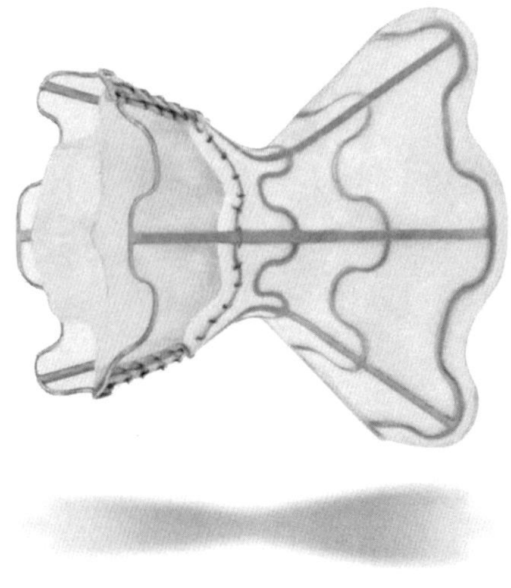

Fig. 52

V Wave Interatrial Device

Another device called **Bioventrix Revivent TC System,** a catheter-based system that can remodel the heart by placing an anchor in the septum and a cord attached to a second anchor on the outside of the ventricle. The cord is pulled to sink the anchor in the infarct area in the heart muscle and helps in remodeling the left ventricle. This seems to have some initial success, but we will wait to have more clinical trials as we continue to research the outcomes.

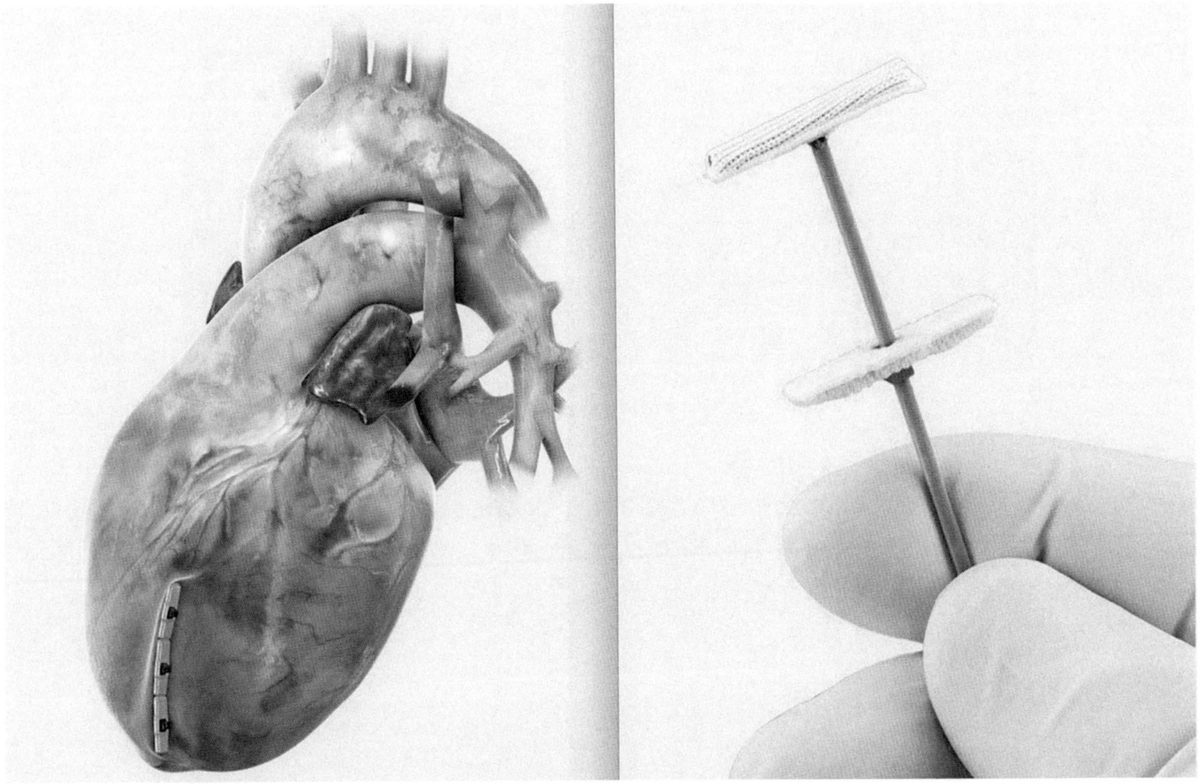

Bioventrix Fig. 53

Accucinch, is a ventricular septal repair system which is another C-shaped wire that is placed in the left ventricle and held in place with anchors and it is then tightened to the left ventricle to improve contractility is a being used in chronic heart failure as a catheter used in patients who have been hospitalized with heart failure.

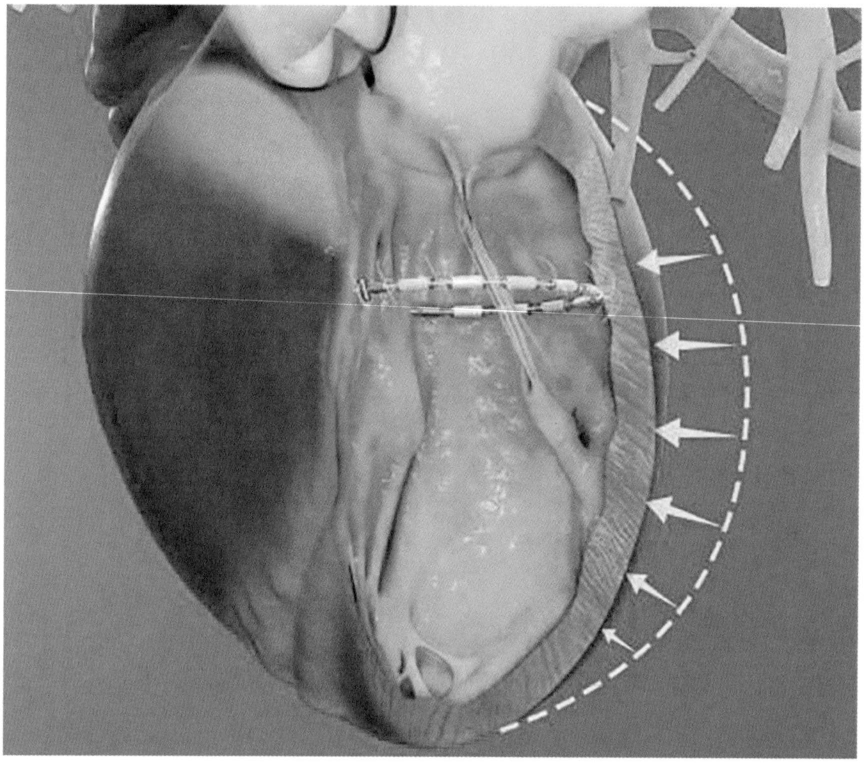

ACCUCINCH Fig. 54

Procyrion Aortix percutaneous hemodynamic support device is a tool to support the heart, rest the heart, and perfuse the kidneys when a patient is decompensated with cardiorenal syndrome. This is in clinical trial.

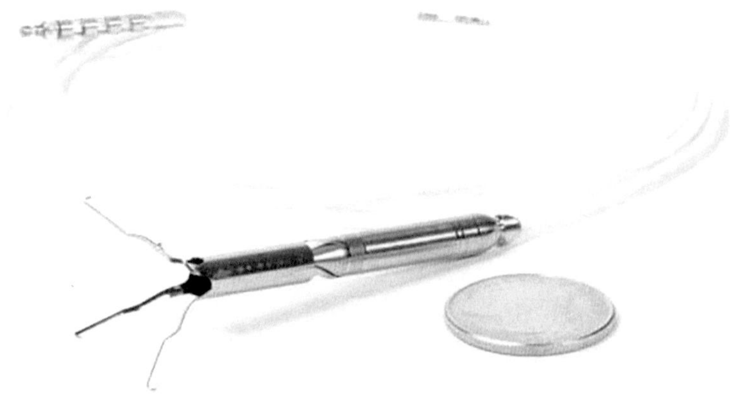

Fig. 55

Reprieve is a personalized volume management system to manage fluid volume in those who are unable to have fluid removed with diuretics. Research is ongoing.

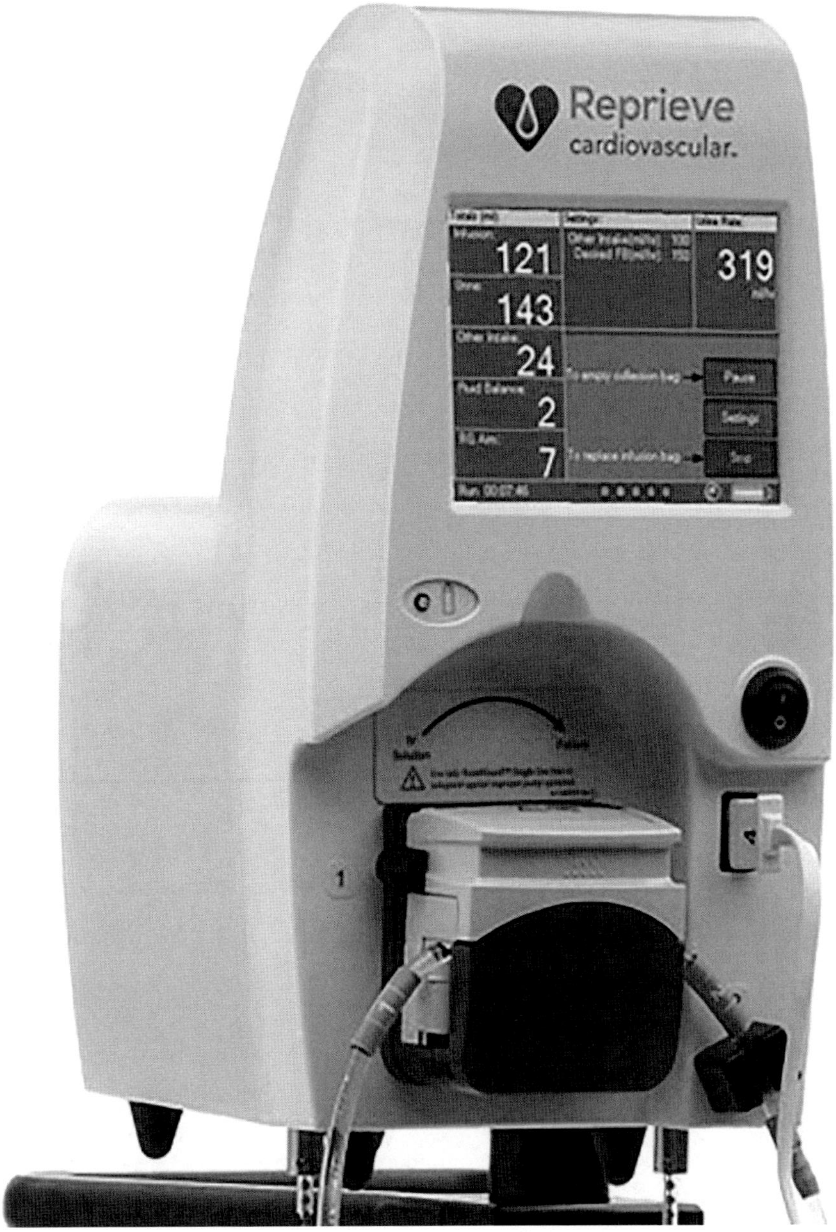

Fig. 56

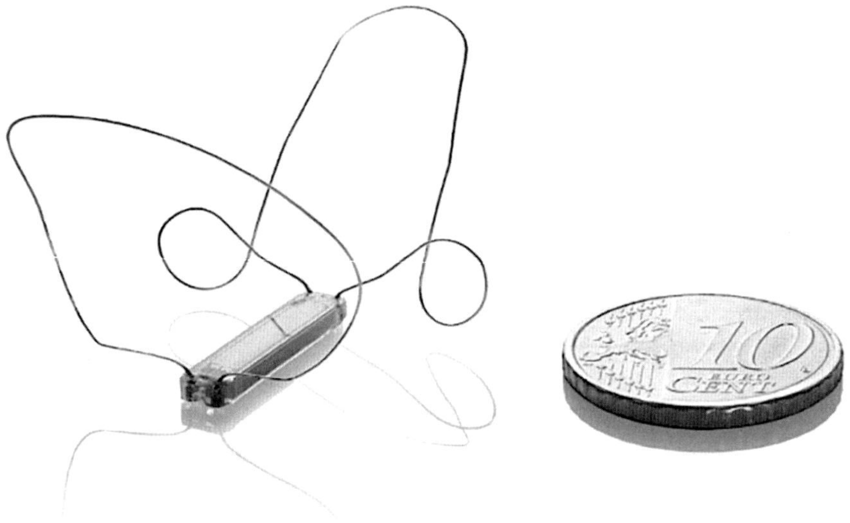

Fig. 57

Cordella pulmonary artery sensor system is a device used for diagnostic measurement and similar to cardiomems by being placed in the pulmonary artery and monitored remotely.

With new devices and drugs used to treat heart failure, the FDA is awaiting clearance on a few. Many patients who are not candidates for a heart transplant will hear this message of hope for improved quality of life and survival as new technologies evolve and get FDA approval.

CHAPTER 45

Stem Cells in Heart Failure

WATCH NOW

Patient Stories

I have had quite a few patients who have been on COQ10, L-carnitine, D-ribose, berberine and some of these had significantly benefited with increased energy. Others have not had a significant benefit and actually made a huge hole in their pocket by spending a lot of money on some of these agents where evidence has been sparse and not backed by scientific vigor.

One caveat about stem cells is that it one of my patients, after having reduced heart muscle function, he was having more symptoms. He was not a candidate for LVAD or heart transplant and decided to seek help in clinical research trials to get stem cell therapy. He did go through a skeletal myoblast stem cell research trial where we take a piece of muscle from the thigh, cultured it, and reintroduce it into the heart muscle with the help of an imaging device that directs to a specific portion. However, this did not make an impact on his ejection fraction or functional capacity as he developed ventricular tachycardia and required amiodarone and a ventricular defibrillator.

No stem cell therapy for the heart has been approved in the United States. Although many other therapies including pharmacologic agents are approved in other places such as Europe, they are not available in the US as FDA has not approved it yet.

There are ongoing clinical trials in the US that would allow these medications or therapies to gain approval. Until such time, one would want to wait, instead of jumping into something unknown.

He then chose to go to Thailand to get a different kind of stem cell used outside of clinical trials. It was not really compassionate use and was essentially touted as a therapy for patients with reduced cardiac muscle function. He thought about this and took a trip down to Bangkok and came back and felt better for about 3 months or so before deteriorating and passed away.

The lesson that we learned from this story is that one needs to be cautious of the marketing of stem cell therapy by many other countries, luring Americans for a big chunk of money. Many of the claims are false and can harm.

This is the reason why the FDA is being more cautious in ascertaining that these agents do not cause any harm. This is the lesson that we learned, and we have not really sent anyone outside of the US to pursue stem cell therapy as we do not know what type of stem cells they are using or if it is genuine.

Stem Cells for Heart Failure

The people who bind themselves to systems, are those who are unable to encompass the whole truth and try to catch it by the tail. A system is like the tail of the truth, but the truth is like a lizard – it leaves its tail in your fingers and runs away knowing full well that it will grow a new one in a twinkling.

—Turgenev to Tolstoy

We have been utilizing stem cell treatments for almost two decades with 200 clinical trials being performed. New technologies that harness the functional capacity of the heart have been explored. The efficacy of stem cell therapy has still not panned for FDA to approve any form of therapy at this time. Safety seems to be an issue. The lessons that they have learned during this period of time include knowledge gained in cell isolation techniques, standardization of conditions, measurement techniques, assessment of multiple endpoints. However, many of these clinical trials have not truly translated into bedside utilization. In this chapter, we will explore the specifics of stem cells and what needs to be explored.

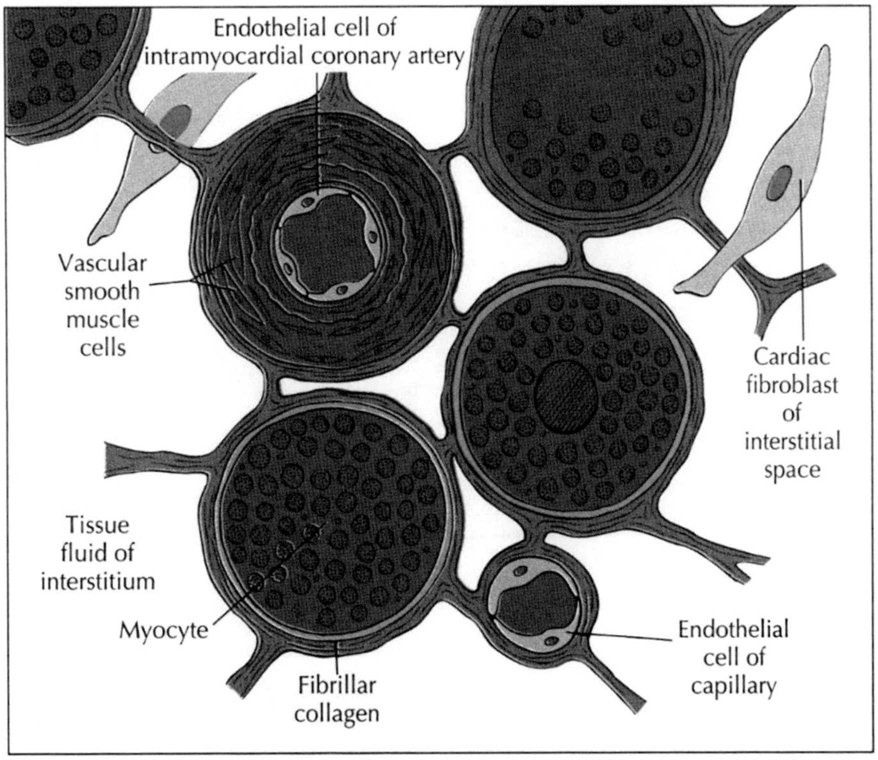

Fig. 58

Extracellular Matrix and Cardiomyocyte Balance

There have been disappointing results in clinical trials in stem cells, but it still peaks the interests of scientists to find newer treatments for patients with ischemic heart disease and congestive heart failure. Heart failure is projected to increase to over 8 million in the next 10 years. Although the mortality attributed to heart failure has fallen over the past few years due to medical optimization, there is still a high prevalence of mortality and the high cost in hospitalizations as well the disability-adjusted life years.

The limited trait of heart disease is because of the misconception that the heart is terminally differentiated and does not have any regional recovery capacity. This is being disputed in stem cell trials where these cells seem to increase the contractile reserve and functional capacity. The stem cells have the ability to self-renew and differentiate into at least one other cell type. The current application of stem cells has been challenging because of the transdifferentiation of any of these stem cells into the cell that may not have the contractile reserve as expected. There are multiple ways of delivering the stem cell, the ones that have been experimented include intravenous delivery, trans-endocardial injection, epicardial injection, and intracoronary infusion.

Cell types that have been studied include skeletal myoblasts, bone marrow, mononuclear cells, adipocyte-derived regenerative cells, purified mesenchymal cells, hematopoietic stem cells, second-generation stem cells, cardio-sphere derived cells, pluripotent stem cells, embryonic stem cells, and pluripotent allogeneic cells. The next-generation form of stem cells includes cardiopoietic stem cells from mesenchymal stem cells and cell combination therapy of some of the specific types as mentioned above.

The endpoints of these clinical trials examined include improvement of ejection fraction, with echocardiograms, nuclear imaging, CT imaging, and cardiac MRI imaging. Other serum biomarkers are being used as BNP, NT pro-BNP, TNF alpha, C reactive protein, and functional capacity. Most of the clinical trials after an acute heart attack used bone marrow mononuclear derived stem cells. Mainly, they have harvested this from the same patient 1-12 days after an intervention has been performed. Since the bone marrow, mononuclear bone cells have the advantage of not requiring it to be cultured, for it to be harvested, isolated, and reinfused into the body very quickly.

Multiple trials have been examined after an acute heart attack and include: TOPCARE AMI, BOOST REPAIR AMI, SWISS AMI, BOOST 2, and PRESERVE AMI. So far, bone marrow mononuclear stem cells have not shown much efficacy. In patients with refractory angina without experiencing a heart attack, CD34, CD33, and CD30 showed initial promise; however, long term data has not supported this to be useful. Different types of stem cells have been studied among patients with ischemic cardiomyopathy.

Some studies include TOPCARE CHD, SCIPIO, POSEIDEN, CADUCEUS, CHART 1, RHYME CARE and Athena, to mention a few. All these studies have evaluated stem cells in this population including adipose-derived regenerative cells. Nonischemic dilated cardiomyopathy has also been studied in clinical trials. So far, while many of the stem cells are deemed to be safe, the efficacy is still up in the air.

Due to early inflammation which leads to stretching and thinning of the heart walls, multiple biochemical effects go on during these processes and are targets for stem cell research. They include **paracrine** signaling and exoenzyme release. The paracrine signaling leads to immune modulation, **extracellular matrix** remodeling, and **apoptosis**. There is new revascularization which means new blood vessels are being formed which may do harm and

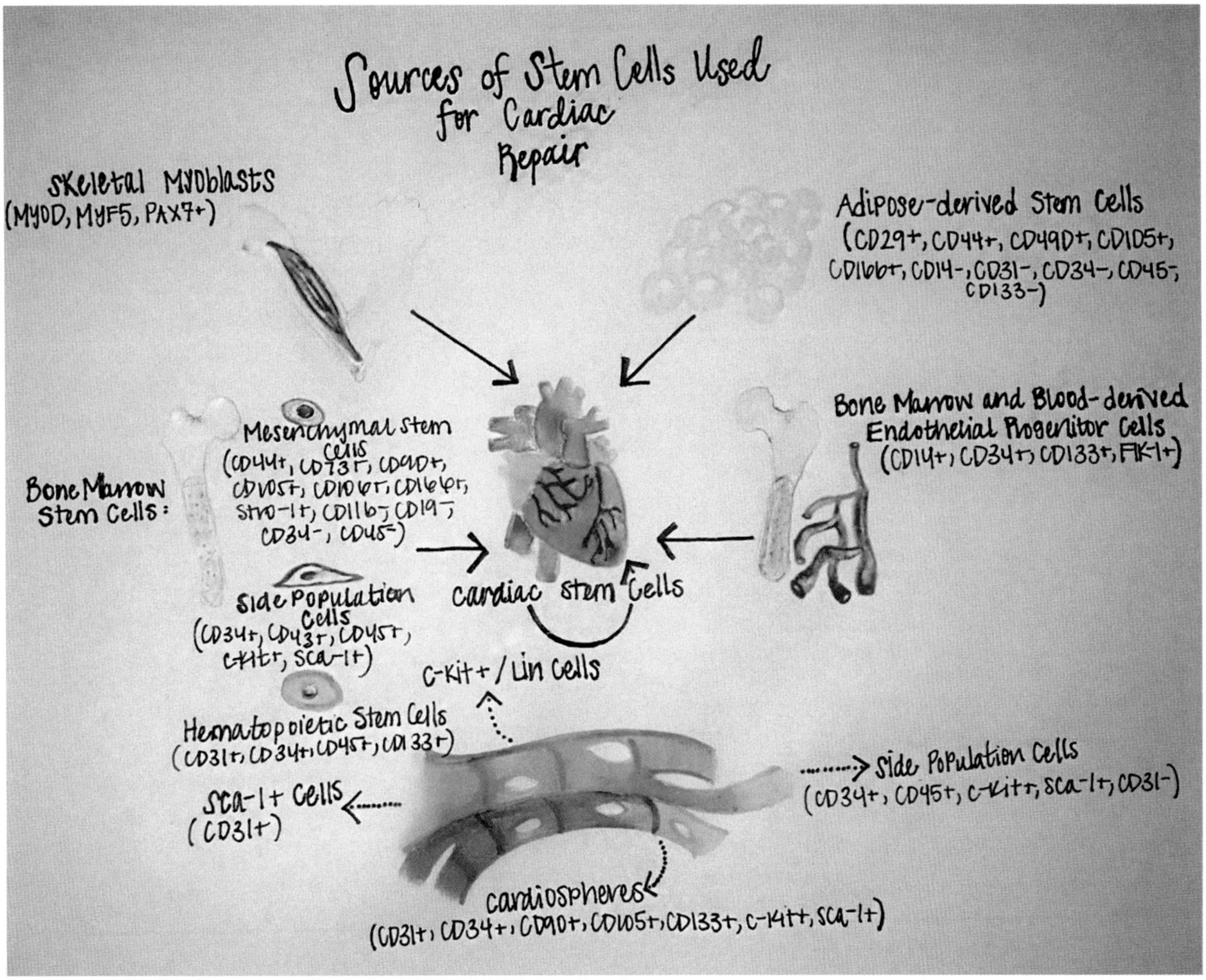

Fig. 59

increase oxidative stress. The exoenzyme release includes impaired calcium handling and stimulation of abnormal stem cells inside the heart.

In addition, these cells may transdifferentiate into other cells inside the heart and may not have the capacity to perform. All of these are targets for newer stem cell therapies. It is still not clear which type of stem cells is most effective and there is still confusion behind the mechanistic behavior of these stem cells differentiating into cardiac cells and having an increased function. We are also not sure about the number and capacity of stem cells that need to be injected into the area in question. We are not sure of the mobilization of these stem cells and unclear if it is from the bone marrow, mesenchyme, or adipose tissue and if too much mobilization can be an issue as well.

We are not sure about how many needs to retain in the heart muscle or how many need to survive. Many of these stem cells are dying shortly after injection and there may be other mechanisms that allow these cells to sustain their survival. We are not sure about the effect of engraftment after a percentage of stem cells have been used and the consequence of cells that are not engrafted. Do they die, transform, release paracrine hormone (unwanted) factors, cause cancer, or organ disease?

The ability to track stem cells has increased; however, it has not quite clear whether we are adequately tracking all of the injected stem cells. It is not clear if there is a decrease in cell death or increasing collagen, (different kinds of stem cells) which may be ineffective. The proliferation of cardiac myocytes into to a functioning cell has been the main goal when injecting stem cells but has not been studied enough.

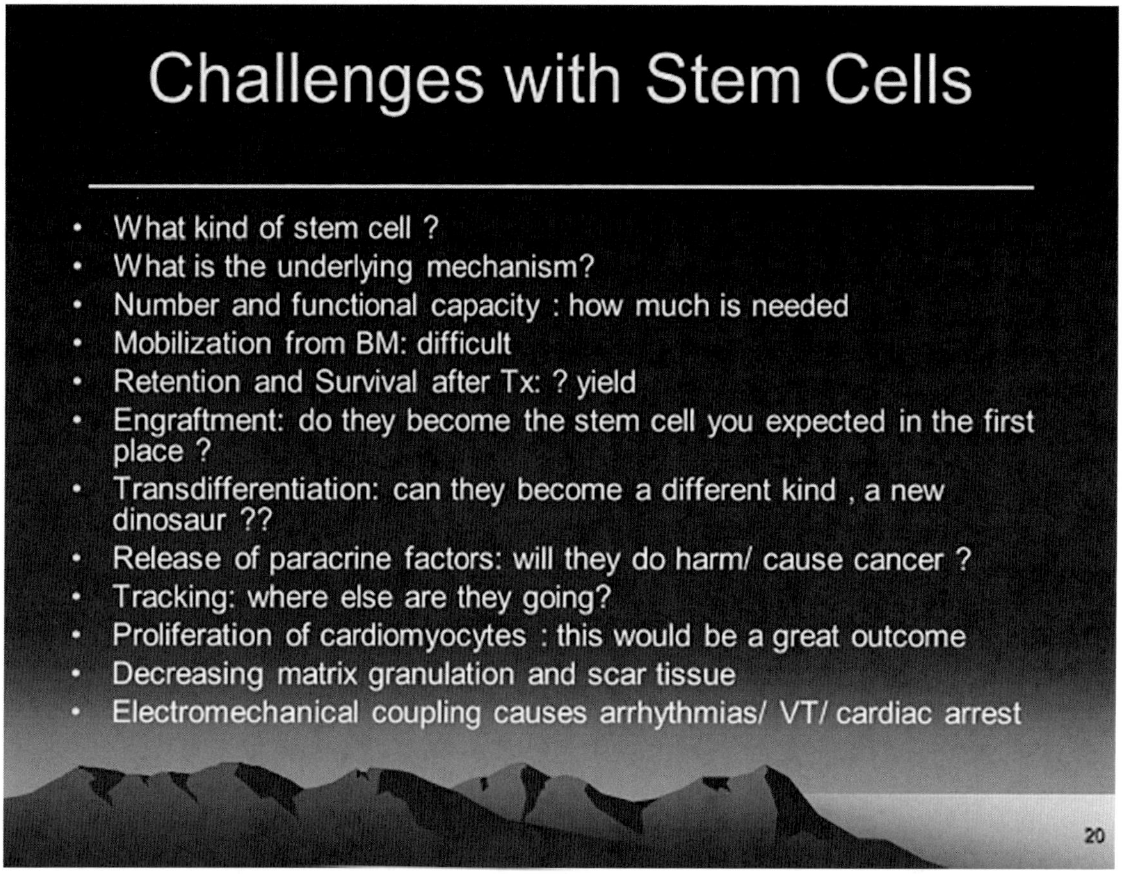

Fig. 60

The extracellular matrix may have a role in transporting and sustaining the viability of some stem cells. Once stem cells are injected, there is an **electromechanical coupling** that occurs which can lead to ventricular tachycardia, arrhythmias, or death. Hence, we need to be sure that the alteration of electrolytes is kept to a minimum. As we raise questions, there will be opportunities that will address each challenge mentioned. At present, the human pluripotent stem cells and endothelial-derived stem cells may have the capacity to stimulate the inner cell mass of blastocysts.

However, this is limited due to ethical concerns such as immunosuppression, tumor stimulation and possible arrhythmias. The human embryonic stem cell-derived progenitors in heart failure revealed no significant increase in arrhythmias. Whether these cells along with an extracellular matrix patch can be useful is being studied in future clinical trials. The translation of pluripotent stem cells has caused clinical investigations and will require future research. Mature cardiac myocytes for repairing stem cells that can couple electromechanically with the cardiac myocytes is being researched as well. The Cell-Wave trial which combines electro extracorporeal shockwave therapy and intracoronary stem cell therapy in patients who have ischemic cardiomyopathy is ongoing. A combination of stem cell and gene therapy may also be useful in future clinical trials.

There is a situation where lack of blood flow and thus less oxygen to the tissue leads to hypoxia. Hypoxic preconditioning of some stem cells in low oxygen environments may improve survival as it becomes conditioned similar to how one becomes conditioned when exercising in high elevations. Utilizing these stem cells which already have resistance to low oxygen environments is being studied in phase 2 clinical trials. Multiple other hypotheses are being addressed in newer clinical trials. MicroRNA along with specific stem cells that increases specific hormones mimicking microparticles to improve heart pump function are in clinical trials. The quantity and frequency of stem cell injections that one might need to raise the question if we should treat stem cell treatment similarly to pharmaceutical methods by using them daily. The repeated injections may itself be an issue with procedure induce complications and is being addressed.

Conclusion:

Over the last two decades, we have come a long way in understanding some of the mechanistic behavior, and hypothesis in stem cell therapy. As technology improves, more modified stem cell types and engineered stem cells with certain combinations of supplements should be the concepts we should use in clinical trials. Hopefully, we can expect results of stem cell therapy in heart disease in phase 2 and 3 clinical trials in the next 5 years.

CHAPTER 46

Gene Therapy in Heart Failure

WATCH NOW

While the new drugs and devices have shown improvement in overall outcomes in heart failure, mortality and morbidity are still extremely high up to 40% in affected individuals in a year and 75% within 5 years of diagnosis. Hence, the concept that gene therapy might improve outcomes is exciting. Can a noninfectious viral vector carry a gene of interest into a cell in the heart and make it perform and function long term? This was demonstrated two decades ago at the University of Michigan which showed that the vector can transfer DNA into an arterial wall. It was found in a medical center in Boston that using a plasmid containing human vascular endothelial growth factor gene applied to angioplasty balloons and delivered to an area of interest may be effective.

There are 2 topics of interest in gene therapy: The first one includes a **vector** that is capable of carrying genetic material and the second includes the genetic material itself. The vector that carries genetic material which has been studied include lentivirus, adenovirus, and adeno associated virus (AAV). At present, these 3 viral vectors have had challenges due to safety, toxicity, immunogenicity, and increasing antibodies that develop against adeno associated virus that may cause serious adverse side effects.

There are alternate methods of gene induction and delivery which have been studied and include plasmid vectors, synthetically modified mRNA. The method of delivering viral vectors also has been a focus on research. Questions are whether one needs to go into the heart through catheters and perform intracoronary injections or intravenously without inserting catheters into the heart or are there other successful ways that genes can be delivered.

The second involves **genetic material**. Gene therapy itself has also been studied extensively. Certain genes show significant promise which targets cardiac excitation-contraction coupling. (See Fig. 59) There are multiple players in this signal transduction model. The genes that are being studied include the ryanodine receptor **(RYR2)** in the sarcoplasmic reticulum or the **SERCA 2a** which is the sarcoplasmic reticulum protein which binds to calcium to initiate contraction.

Figure below depicts some areas of target for gene therapy research

Phospholamban is a modulator of the serca2a, and the beta-adrenergic receptor (BAR) itself may be a target. Cyclic AMP that is generated uses more energy and increases contractile strength. **BAG3** associated genes seem to have multiple downstream effects including effects on myofilaments and mitochondria, maintaining nuclear envelope integrity, and cell to cell communication, which may all be positively regulated. Gene therapy among patients with heart failure is close to making a major impact but is not an obscure topic anymore. Challenges of implementation include a better understanding of the viral vectors such AAV vector which may have immunogenic properties.

Perhaps the development of nonimmunogenic AAVs can be used among patients with AAV antibodies. The second construct that is being packaged includes large genes that may facilitate the generation of newer biomarkers and molecules that improve the contractile reserve of the heart.

Finally, a large study called ALL-OF-US is ongoing which may identify new therapies causing mutations expanding to a large number of agents that can benefit from utilizing gene therapy.

FINAL NOTE

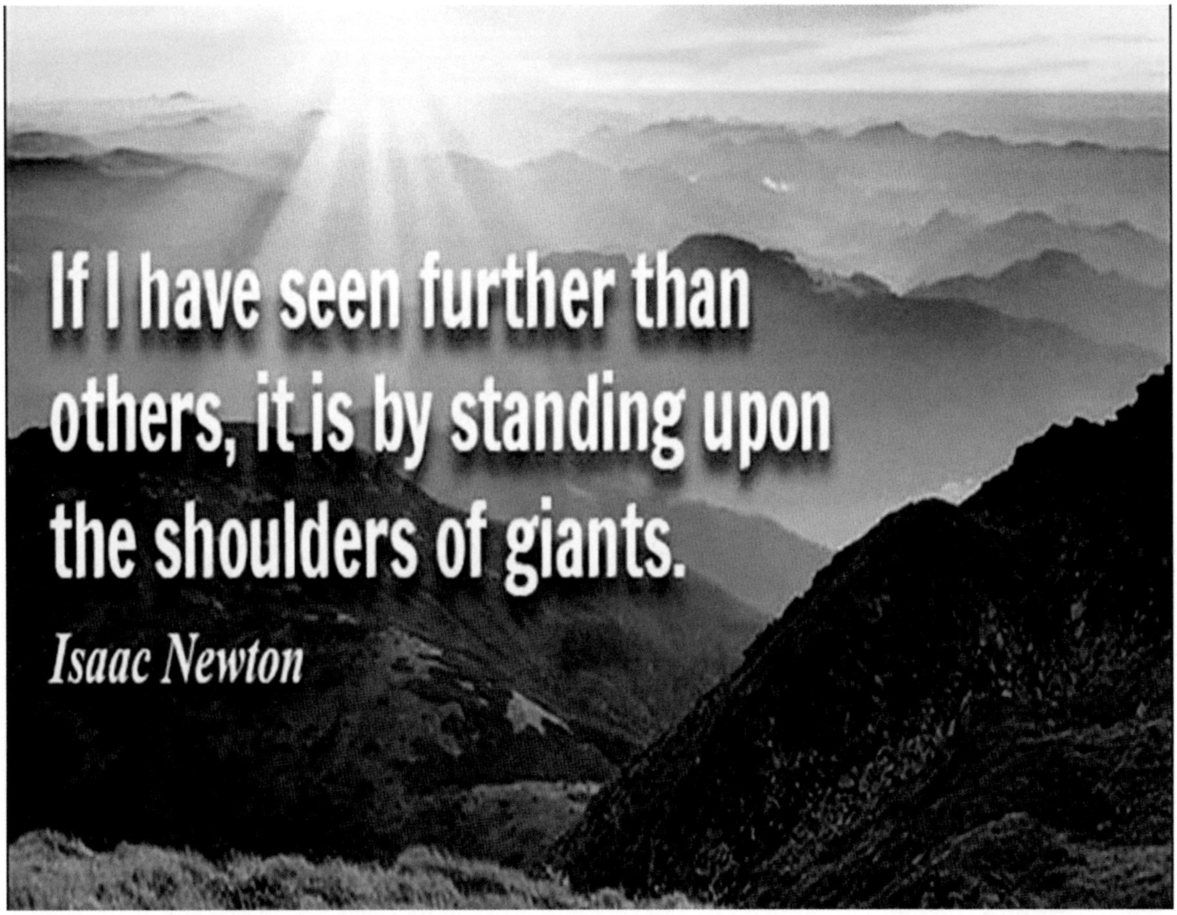

Fig. 61

It has been a fantastic roller coaster ride. With more than 40 years of medical practice in patient care, and spending more than 20 years of that in Heart Failure education, patient care and research, I feel so honored and humbled to have had the opportunity to serve those in need, and indebted to my patients for giving me the chance to help them and in turn become a better person than my previous self. To you, I say "Namaste" as in saluting the Godliness in you!!

I have used all my God given skills to connect with each of you, to heal through touch and embrace, by just not reaching out but by pulling in. You have taught me to find my own happiness in your smiling faces, your laughter, and your improvement towards a better health. Your trials and tribulations match so many peoples' struggles including mine. Yet, you have allowed me to be personally secure but not complacent. Rather you have given me an option to be driven by passion and have strong faith in the positive aspects of believing in recovery and restoration. You have permitted me to freely expose my strengths and weaknesses and yet display humanity in its full spectacle!

Hopefully, this book has provided you with many points to ponder : From the physical aspects of the Heart to the metaphysical; from the colossal societal economic burden at large to the individual struggle in getting prescriptions filled; from having the health care provider control your risk factors for heart failure to your own toils to grapple them; from the neurohormonal perturbations inside your blood stream to your neurocognitive efforts to subside the storm; from abnormal rhythms of the electrical conduction pathways to your determination to get your cadence in sequence; from endothelial dysfunction to your attempts to stabilize the inner lining so as to prevent morbidity associated with it; and from HFpEF, HFrEF, Right Heart Failure and beyond to your inner therapist invoking your psychosocial abilities to rise up to beat the odds of mortality and morbidity associated with the disease.

I would also like to believe you had an interesting glimpse into the newer therapies, advances in technology in heart failure diagnosis and management as well as stem cell therapy and where we stand in gene therapy in Heart failure and their potential. I would like to reiterate the topic of nursing care and the complexities that involves a meticulous management of our patients , making themselves available 24/7, enhancing the affordability of diagnostics and therapeutics, enabling accessibility to care and ascertaining the acceptability from a patient perspective, cognizant of the ethnic nuances and maintaining a cultural humility for best patient outcomes.

I do want to want to emphasize the reasons for narrating patient stories and experiences. First, in this telling, I hope it will facilitate you in remembering and recalling your own deliberations from the past and recent; second, I hope it might embolden your conscious allegiance each day to values that bolster our better natures; and thirdly, that, in illuminating these stories, it might help you in embracing a positive approach towards the potential for prevention and recovery from heart disease and evoke a sense of hope and dream towards rejuvenation.

INSPIRE HF Manifesto is a model we would like to live by. Truly, our patient stories make me and my team members a better person every day. These stories have evolved and jumped out of the blue, only to beg the question: “Are you making a living, or, Are you making a life?” I would like to believe that, indeed, there is a chasm between the two questions and that we are bridging the gap in between. No matter how positive I am, one must tackle the ambiguity of life and death, for life and loss are as defenseless as they are durable. My alacrity to respond at times of crisis places me in great demand; and yet, my ability to survive and thrive should reflect a unique attitude towards loss.

In essence, fundamentally, I must learn as if it is a new lesson with each experience. I should be able to see the world as overflowing with opportunity for all and understand that procrastinating an opportunity in the interest of a more demanding commitment is not a lost prospect for ever; but a new opening for another window to get unlocked in making an impact on one's life with more vigor and enthusiasm. I ask the higher powers to give me more faith and memory which would allow me to feel and experience the presence of loved ones even in their absence. And finally, all I ask of you is to give me the strength to uniquely fill the void in the lives of my patients and families , my near and dear ones, and give me the courage to find productive ways towards a net contribution to society, to those who are in need and to those who are underserved. And most importantly I ask that all my readers get the boon from above to attain a sense of tranquility and to be at peace with oneself!!

WATCH NOW

Glossary

WATCH NOW

Abdomen – The area of the body between the bottom of the ribs and the top of the thighs.

Abdominal Aorta – The portion of the aorta in the abdomen.

Ablation – Elimination or removal.

ACE (angiotensin-converting enzyme) Inhibitor – A medicine that lowers blood pressure by interfering with the breakdown of a protein-like substance involved in blood pressure regulation. It is also used in Heart Failure

Acetylcholine – A type of chemical (called a neurotransmitter) that transmits messages among nerve cells and muscle cells.

Acquired Heart Disease – Heart disease that arises after birth, usually from infection or through the build-up of fatty deposits in the arteries that feed the heart muscle.

AGE – Advanced Glycation End products that result from uncontrolled diabetes causing target organ damage

Aldosterone – A neurohormone released by kidney and adrenal glands causing damage to blood vessels

Alveoli – Air sacs in the lungs where oxygen and carbon dioxide are exchanged.

Amiodarone – A kind of medicine (called an antiarrhythmic) used to treat irregular heart rhythms such as atrial fibrillation and ventricular tachycardia. It works by regulating nerve impulses in your heart. Amiodarone is mainly given to patients who have not responded to other antiarrhythmic medicines.

Aneurysm – A sac-like protrusion from a blood vessel or the heart, resulting from a weakening of the vessel wall or heart muscle.

Angina or Angina Pectoris – Chest pain that occurs when diseased blood vessels restrict blood flow to the heart.

Angiography – An x-ray technique in which dye is injected into the chambers of your heart or the arteries that lead to your heart (the coronary arteries). The test lets doctors measure the blood flow and blood pressure in the heart chambers and see if the coronary arteries are blocked.

Angioplasty – A nonsurgical technique for treating diseased arteries by temporarily inflating a tiny balloon inside an artery.

Angiotensin II Receptor Blocker – A medicine that lowers blood pressure by blocking the action of angiotensin II, a chemical in the body that causes the blood vessels to tighten (constrict). Also used in heart failure

Annulus – The ring around a heart valve where the valve leaflet merges with the heart muscle.

Antiarrhythmics – Medicines used to treat patients who have irregular heart rhythms.

Anticoagulant – Any medicine that keeps blood from clotting, a blood thinner.

Antihypertensive – Any medicine or other therapy that lowers blood pressure.

Antiplatelet Therapy – Medicines that stop blood cells (called platelets) from sticking together and forming a blood clot.

Aorta – The largest artery in the body and the main vessel to supply blood from the heart.

Aortic Valve – The valve that regulates blood flow from the heart into the aorta.

Aphasia – The inability to speak, write, or understand spoken or written language because of brain injury or disease.

Arrhythmia (or dysrhythmia) – An abnormal heartbeat.

Arrhythmogenic Right Ventricular Dysplasia (ARVD) – ARVD is a type of cardiomyopathy with no known cause. It appears to be a genetic condition (passed down through a family's genes). ARVD causes ventricular arrhythmias.

Arteriography – A test that is combined with cardiac catheterization to visualize an artery or the arterial system after injection of a contrast dye.

Arterioles – Small, muscular branches of arteries. When they contract, they raise resistance to blood flow, and blood pressure in the arteries increases.

Artery – A vessel that carries oxygen-rich blood to the body.

Arteritis – Inflammation of the arteries.

Arteriosclerosis – A disease process, commonly called "hardening of the arteries", which includes a variety of conditions that cause artery walls to thicken and lose elasticity.

Artificial Heart – A manmade heart. Also called a total artificial heart (TAH).

ASCVD: Atherosclerotic Cardiovascular Disease

Ascending Aorta – The first portion of the aorta, emerging from the heart's left ventricle.

Aspirin – Acetylsalicylic acid; a medicine used to relieve pain, reduce inflammation, and prevent blood clots.

Atherectomy – A nonsurgical technique for treating diseased arteries with a rotating device that cuts or shaves away material that is blocking or narrowing an artery.

Atherosclerosis – A disease process that leads to the buildup of a waxy substance, called plaque, inside blood vessels.

Atrium (right and left) – The two upper or holding chambers of the heart (together referred to as atria).

Atrial Fibrillation – A type of irregular heartbeat in which upper chamber and lower chambers are disconnected placing one at high risk for heart failure and stroke

Atrial Flutter – A type of arrhythmia in which the upper chambers of the heart (the atria) beat extremely fast, causing the walls of the lower chambers (the ventricles) to beat inefficiently as well.

Atrial Septal Defect – See septal defect.

Atrial Tachycardia – A type of arrhythmia that begins in the heart's upper chambers (the atria) and causes an extremely fast heart rate of 160 to 200 beats a minute. A resting heart rate is normally 60 to 100 beats a minute.

Atrioventricular Block – An interruption or disturbance of the electrical signal between the heart's upper two chambers (the atria) and the lower two chambers (the ventricles).

Atrioventricular (AV) Node – A group of cells in the heart located between the upper two chambers (the atria) and the lower two chambers (the ventricles) that regulates the electrical current that passes through it to the ventricles.

Atrium – Either one of the heart's two upper chambers.

Autologous – Relating to self. For example, autologous stem cells are those taken from the patient's own body.

Autoregulation – When blood flow to an organ stays the same although the pressure in the artery that delivers blood to that organ may have changed.

Bacteria – Germs that can lead to disease.

Bacterial Endocarditis – A bacterial infection of the lining of the heart's chambers (called the endocardium) or of the heart's valves.

Balloon Catheter – A long tube-like device with a small balloon on the end that can be threaded through an artery. Used in angioplasty or valvuloplasty.

Balloon Valvuloplasty – A procedure to repair a heart valve. A balloon-tipped catheter is threaded through an artery and into the heart. The balloon is inflated to open and separate any narrowed or stiffened flaps (called leaflets) of a valve.

Beta-Blocker – An antihypertensive medicine that limits the activity of epinephrine, a hormone that increases blood pressure.

Beta Receptor – a receptor protein that attaches to a beta blocker to initiate action downstream

Biopsy – The process by which a small sample of tissue is taken for examination.

Blalock-Taussig Procedure – A shunt between the subclavian and pulmonary arteries used to increase the supply of oxygen-rich blood in "blue babies" (see below).

Blood Clot – A jelly-like mass of blood tissue formed by clotting factors in the blood. Clots stop the flow of blood from an injury. Clots can also form inside an artery when the artery's walls are damaged by atherosclerotic buildup, possibly causing a heart attack or stroke.

Blood Pressure – The force or pressure exerted by the heart in pumping blood; the pressure of blood in the arteries.

Body Mass Index (BMI) – A number that indicates an increased risk of cardiovascular disease from a person being overweight. BMI is calculated using a formula of weight in kilograms divided by height in meters squared (BMI = W [kg]/H [m^2]). Click here for a BMI calculator: https://www.texasheart.org/heart-health/know-your-numbers/

Bradycardia – Abnormally slow heartbeat.

Bridge to Transplant – Use of mechanical circulatory support to keep heart failure patients alive until a donor's heart becomes available.

Bruit – A sound made in the blood vessels resulting from turbulence, perhaps because of a buildup of plaque or damage to the vessels.

Bundle Branch Block – A condition in which parts of the heart's conduction system are defective and unable to conduct the electrical signal normally, causing an irregular heart rhythm (arrhythmia).

Bypass – Surgery that can improve blood flow to the heart (or other organs and tissues) by providing a new route, or "bypass" around a section of the clogged or diseased artery.

Calcium Channel Blocker (or calcium blocker) – A medicine that lowers blood pressure by regulating calcium-related electrical activity in the heart.

Capillaries – Microscopically small blood vessels between arteries and veins that distribute oxygen-rich blood to the body's tissues.

Cardiac – Pertaining to the heart.

Cardiac Amyloidosis – A disorder caused by deposits of an abnormal protein (amyloid) in the heart tissue, which makes it hard for the heart to work properly. Also called "stiff heart syndrome."

Cardiac Arrest – The stopping of the heartbeat, usually because of interference with the electrical signal (often associated with coronary heart disease).

Cardiac Cachexia – A term for the muscle and weight loss caused by severe heart disease. It is often related to the depressed cardiac output associated with end-stage heart failure, but it can also occur with severe coronary artery disease.

Cardiac Catheterization – A procedure that involves inserting a fine, hollow tube (catheter) into an artery, usually in the groin area, and passing the tube into the heart. Often used along with angiography and other procedures, cardiac catheterization has become a primary tool for visualizing the heart and blood vessels and diagnosing and treating heart disease.

Cardiac Enzymes – Complex substances capable of speeding up certain biochemical processes in the heart muscle. Abnormal levels of these enzymes signal a heart attack.

Cardiac Output – The amount of blood the heart pumps through the circulatory system in one minute.

Cardiologist – A doctor who specializes in the study of the heart and its function in health and disease.

Cardiology – The study of the heart and its function in health and disease.

Cardiomegaly – An enlarged heart. It is usually a sign of an underlying problem, such as high blood pressure, heart valve problems, or cardiomyopathy.

Cardiomyopathy – A disease of the heart muscle that leads to generalized deterioration of the muscle and its pumping ability.

Cardiopulmonary Bypass – The process by which a machine is used to do the work of the heart and lungs so the heart can be stopped during surgery.

Cardiopulmonary Resuscitation (CPR) – An emergency measure that can maintain a person's breathing and heartbeat. The person who performs CPR actually helps the patient's circulatory system by breathing into the patient's mouth to give them oxygen and by giving chest compressions to circulate the patient's blood. Hands-only CPR involves only chest compressions.

Cardiovascular (CV) – Pertaining to the heart and blood vessels that make up the circulatory system.

Cardiovascular Disease (CVD) – A general term referring to conditions affecting the heart (cardio) and blood vessels (vascular system). May also simply be called heart disease. Examples include coronary artery disease, valve disease, arrhythmia, peripheral vascular disease, congenital heart defects, hypertension, and cardiomyopathy. Refer to specific conditions for detailed explanations.

Cardioversion – A technique of applying an electrical shock to the chest to convert an abnormal heartbeat to a normal rhythm.

Carotid Artery – A major artery (right and left) in the neck supplying blood to the brain.

Cerebral Embolism – A blood clot formed in one part of the body and then carried by the bloodstream to the brain, where it blocks an artery.

Cerebral Hemorrhage – Bleeding within the brain resulting from a ruptured blood vessel, aneurysm, or head injury.

Cerebral Thrombosis – Formation of a blood clot in an artery that supplies part of the brain.

Cerebrovascular – Pertaining to the blood vessels of the brain.

Cerebrovascular Accident – Also called cerebral vascular accident, apoplexy, or stroke. Blood supply to some part of the brain is slowed or stopped, resulting in injury to brain tissue.

Cerebrovascular Occlusion – The blocking or closing of a blood vessel in the brain.

Cholesterol – An oily substance that occurs naturally in the body, in animal fats, and dairy products, and that is transported in the blood. Limited amounts are essential for the normal development of cell membranes. Excess amounts can lead to coronary artery disease.

Cineangiography – The technique of using moving pictures to show how a special dye passes through blood vessels, allowing doctors to diagnose diseases of the heart and blood vessels.

Circulatory System – Pertaining to the circulation of blood through the heart and blood vessels.

CKD – Chronic Kidney Disease. There are many stages: Stage 5-6 is End stage and may require dialysis

Claudication – A tiredness or pain in the arms and legs caused by an inadequate supply of oxygen to the muscles, usually due to narrowed arteries or peripheral arterial disease (PAD).

Collateral Circulation – Blood flow through small, nearby vessels in response to blockage of the main blood vessel.

Commissurotomy – A procedure used to widen the opening of a heart valve that has been narrowed by scar tissue.

Computed Tomography (CT or CAT Scan) – An x-ray technique that uses a computer to create cross-sectional images of the body.

Conduction System – Special muscle fibers that conduct electrical impulses throughout the heart muscle.

Congenital – Refers to conditions existing at birth.

Congenital Heart Defects – Malformation of the heart or its major blood vessels present at birth.

Congestive Heart Failure – A condition in which the heart cannot pump all the blood returning to it, leading to a backup of blood in the vessels and an accumulation of fluid in the body's tissues, including the lungs.

Coronary Arteries – Two arteries arising from the aorta that arch down over the top of the heart and divide into branches. They provide blood to the heart muscle.

Coronary Artery Anomaly (CAA) – A congenital defect in one or more of the coronary arteries of the heart.

Coronary Artery Bypass (CAB) – Surgical rerouting of blood around a diseased vessel that supplies blood to the heart. Done by grafting either a piece of vein from the leg or a piece of the artery from under the breastbone.

Coronary Artery Disease (CAD) – A narrowing of the arteries that supply blood to the heart. The condition results from a buildup of plaque and greatly increases the risk of a heart attack.

Coronary Heart Disease – Disease of the heart caused by a buildup of atherosclerotic plaque in the coronary arteries that can lead to angina pectoris or heart attack.

Coronary Occlusion – An obstruction of one of the coronary arteries that hinder blood flow to the heart muscle.

Coronary Thrombosis – Formation of a clot in one of the arteries carrying blood to the heart muscle. Also called coronary occlusion.

Cryoablation – The removal of tissue using an instrument called a cold probe.

Cyanosis – Blueness of the skin caused by a lack of oxygen in the blood.

Cyanotic Heart Disease – A birth defect of the heart that causes oxygen-poor (blue) blood to circulate to the body without first passing through the lungs.

Cytokine: proteins that cause harm to many parts of the body released by abnormal endothelium

Death Rate (Age-Adjusted) – A death rate that has been standardized for age so different populations can be compared or the same population can be compared over time.

Deep Vein Thrombosis – A blood clot in a deep vein in the calf (DVT).

Defibrillator – A device that helps restore a normal heart rhythm by delivering an electric shock.

Diabetes (Diabetes Mellitus) – A disease in which the body doesn't produce or effectively use insulin. Insulin is needed to convert sugar and starch into the energy used in daily life.

Diastole – A phase of relaxation of the heart muscle.

Diastolic Blood Pressure – The lowest blood pressure measured in the arteries. It occurs when the heart muscle is relaxed between beats.

Digitalis – A medicine made from the leaves of the foxglove plant. Digitalis is used to treat congestive heart failure (CHF) and heart rhythm problems (arrhythmias).

Dissecting Aneurysm – A condition in which the layers of an artery separate or are torn, causing blood to flow between the layers. Dissecting aneurysms usually happen in the aorta, the large vessel that carries blood from the heart to other parts of the body and can cause sudden death.

Diuretic – A drug that lowers blood pressure by causing fluid loss. Diuretics promote urine production.

Doppler Ultrasound – A technology that uses sound waves to assess blood flow within the heart and blood vessels and to identify leaking valves.

Dysarthria – A speech disorder resulting from muscular problems caused by damage to the brain or nervous system.

Dyspnea – Shortness of breath.

Echocardiography – A method of studying the heart's structure and function by analyzing sound waves bounced off the heart and recorded by an electronic sensor placed on the chest. A computer processes the information to produce a one, two, or three-dimensional moving picture that shows how the heart and heart valves are functioning.

Edema – Swelling caused by fluid accumulation in body tissues.

Ejection fraction – A measurement of the rate at which blood is pumped out of a filled ventricle. The normal rate is 50% or more.

Electrocardiogram (ECG or EKG) – A test in which several electronic sensors are placed on the body to monitor electrical activity associated with the heartbeat.

Electroencephalogram (EEG) – A test that can detect and record the brain's electrical activity. The test is done by pasting metal disks, called electrodes, to the scalp.

Electrophysiological Study (EPS) – A test that uses cardiac catheterization to study patients who have arrhythmias (abnormal heartbeats). An electrical current stimulates the heart in an effort to provoke an arrhythmia, determine its origin, and test the effectiveness of medicines to treat the arrhythmias.

Embolus – Also called embolism; a blood clot that forms in a blood vessel in one part of the body and travels to another part.

Endarterectomy – Surgical removal of plaque deposits or blood clots in an artery.

Endocardium – The smooth membrane covering the inside of the heart. The innermost lining of the heart.

Endothelium – The smooth inner lining of many body structures, including the heart (endocardium) and blood vessels.

Endocarditis – A bacterial infection of the heart's inner lining (endothelium).

Enlarged Heart – A state in which the heart is larger than normal because of heredity, long-term heavy exercise, or diseases and disorders such as obesity, high blood pressure, and coronary artery disease.

Enzyme – A complex chemical capable of speeding up specific biochemical processes in the body.

Epicardium – The thin membrane covering the outside surface of the heart muscle.

ESRD – End Stage Renal Disease

Estrogen – A female hormone produced by the ovaries that may protect premenopausal women against heart disease. Estrogen production stops after menopause.

Estrogen (or Hormone) Replacement Therapy (ERT or HRT) – Hormones that some women may take to offset the effects of menopause.

Etiology – Cause

Exercise Stress Test – A common test to help doctors assess blood flow through coronary arteries in response to exercise, usually walking, at varying speeds, and for various lengths of time on a treadmill. A stress test may include the use of electrocardiography, echocardiography, and injected radioactive substances. Also called exercise test, stress test, nuclear stress test, or treadmill test.

Familial Hypercholesterolemia – A genetic predisposition to dangerously high cholesterol levels.

Fatty Acids (fats) – Substances that occur in several forms in foods; different fatty acids have different effects on lipid profiles.

Fibrillation – Rapid, uncoordinated contractions of individual heart muscle fibers. The heart chamber involved can't contract all at once and pumps blood ineffectively, if at all.

First-degree heart block – Occurs when an electrical impulse from the heart's upper chambers (the atria) is slowed as it moves through the atria and atrioventricular (AV) node.

Flutter –The rapid, ineffective contractions of any heart chamber. A flutter is considered to be more coordinated than fibrillation.

Fusiform Aneurysm – A tube-shaped aneurysm that causes the artery to bulge outward. Involves the entire circumference (outside wall) of the artery.

Gated Blood Pool Scan – An x-ray analysis of how blood pools in the heart during rest and exercise. The test uses a radioactive substance to tag red blood cells to allow doctors to estimate the heart's overall ability to pump and its ability to compensate for one or more blocked arteries. Also called MUGA (multiple gated acquisition scan) or nuclear ventriculography.

Genetic Testing – Blood tests that study a person's genes to find out if he or she is at risk for certain diseases that are passed down through family members.

GLP1 Agonist – Glucagon Like Peptide 1 agonist; a diabetes medication that is now showing benefit in reducing risk of cardiovascular disease

Guidewire – A small, bendable wire that is threaded through an artery; it helps doctors position a catheter so they can perform angioplasty or stent procedures.

Gynecomastia – enlargement of breast in men

Heart Assist Device – A mechanical device that is surgically implanted to ease the workload of the heart.

Heart Attack – Death of, or damage to, part of the heart muscle caused by a lack of oxygen-rich blood flowing to the heart.

Heart Block – General term for conditions in which the electrical impulse that activates the heart muscle cells is delayed or interrupted somewhere along its path.

Heart Failure – See congestive heart failure.

HFpEF – Heart Failure with Preserved Ejection Fraction

HFrEF – Heart Failure with Reduced Ejection Fraction

Heart-Lung Machine – An apparatus that oxygenates and pumps blood to the body during open-heart surgery; see cardiopulmonary bypass.

Heart Murmur – An abnormal heart sound caused by turbulent blood flow. The sound may indicate that blood is flowing through a damaged or overworked heart valve, that there may be a hole in one of the heart's walls, or that there is a narrowing in one of the heart's vessels. Some heart murmurs are a harmless type called innocent heart murmurs.

Hematocrit – A measure of the percentage of red blood cells in a given amount (or volume) of whole blood.

Hemochromatosis – A disease in which too much iron builds up in your body (iron overload). Too much iron in the heart can cause irregular heartbeats (arrhythmias) and heart failure. Too much iron in the pancreas can lead to diabetes.

Heredity – The genetic transmission of a particular quality or trait from parent to child.

High Blood Pressure – A chronic increase in blood pressure above its normal range.

High Density Lipoprotein (HDL) – A component of cholesterol, HDL helps protect against heart disease by promoting cholesterol breakdown and removal from the blood; hence, its nickname "good cholesterol."

Holter Monitor – A portable device for recording heartbeats over a period of 24 hours or more.

Homocysteine – An amino acid (one of the building blocks that makes up a protein) normally found in small amounts in the blood. Too much homocysteine in the blood may promote the buildup of fatty plaque in the arteries. For some people, high homocysteine levels are genetic. For others, it is because they do not get enough of certain B vitamins in their diet. (Common misspelling: homocysteine)

Hormones – Chemicals released into the bloodstream that control different functions in the body, including metabolism, growth, sexual development, and responses to stress or illness.

Hypertension – High blood pressure.

Hypertrophic Obstructive Cardiomyopathy (HOCM) – An overgrown heart muscle that creates a bulge into the ventricle and impedes blood flow.

Hypertrophy – Enlargement of tissues or organs because of increased workload.

Hyperventilation – Rapid breathing usually caused by anxiety. People feel like they can't get enough air, so they breathe heavily and rapidly, which can lead to numb or tingly arms and legs, or fainting.

Hypoglycemia – Low levels of glucose (sugar) in the blood.

Hypokinesia – Decreased muscle movement. In relation to the heart, hypokinesia refers to decreased heart wall motion during each heartbeat. It is associated with cardiomyopathy, heart failure, or heart attack. Also called hypokinesis.

Hypotension – Abnormally low blood pressure.

Hypoxia – Less than normal content of oxygen in the organs and tissues of the body.

Idiopathic – No known cause.

Immunosuppressants – Any medicine that suppresses the body's immune system. These medicines are used to minimize the chances that the body will reject a newly transplanted organ, such as a heart.

Impedance Plethysmography – A noninvasive diagnostic test used to evaluate blood flow through the leg.

Incompetent valve – Also called insufficiency; a valve that is not working properly, causing it to leak blood back in the wrong direction.

Infarct – The area of heart tissue permanently damaged by an inadequate supply of oxygen.

Infective Endocarditis – An infection of the heart valves and the innermost lining of the heart (the endocardium), caused by bacteria in the bloodstream.

Inferior Vena Cava – The large vein returning blood from the legs and abdomen to the heart.

Inotropes – Positive inotropes: Any medicine that increases the strength of the heart's contraction. Negative inotropes: Any medicine that decreases the strength of the heart's contraction and the blood pressure in the vessels.

Internal Mammary Artery – A durable artery in the chest wall often used as a bypass graft in coronary artery bypass surgery.

Intravascular echocardiography – A combination of echocardiography and cardiac catheterization. A miniature echo device on the tip of a catheter is used to generate images inside the heart and blood vessels.

Introducer Sheath – A catheter-like tube that is placed inside a patient's vessel during an interventional procedure to help the doctor with insertion and proper placement of the actual catheter.

Ischemia – Decreased blood flow to an organ, usually due to constriction or obstruction of an artery.

Ischemic Heart Disease – Also called coronary artery disease and coronary heart disease, this term is applied to heart problems caused by narrowing of the coronary arteries, thereby causing a decreased blood supply to the heart.

Ischemic Stroke – A type of stroke that is caused by a blockage in a blood vessel.

Jugular Veins – The veins that carry blood back from the head to the heart.

Left Ventricular Assist Device (LVAD) – A mechanical device that can be placed outside the body or implanted inside the body. An LVAD does not replace the heart—it "assists" or "helps" it pump oxygen-rich blood from the left ventricle to the rest of the body.

Lesion – An injury or wound. An atherosclerotic lesion is an injury to an artery due to the hardening of the arteries.

Lipid – A fatty substance that is insoluble (cannot be dissolved) in the blood.

Lipoprotein – A lipid surrounded by a protein; the protein makes the lipid-soluble (can be dissolved) in the blood.

Low-Density Lipoprotein (LDL) – The body's primary cholesterol-carrying molecule. High blood levels of LDL increase a person's risk of heart disease by promoting cholesterol attachment and accumulation in blood vessels; hence, the popular nickname "bad cholesterol."

Lumen – The hollow area within a tube, such as a blood vessel.

Magnetic Resonance Imaging (MRI) – A technique that produces images of the heart and other body structures by measuring the response of certain elements (such as hydrogen) in the body to a magnetic field. MRI can produce detailed pictures of the heart and its various structures without the need to inject a dye.

Maze Surgery – A type of heart surgery that is used to treat chronic atrial fibrillation by creating a surgical "maze" of new electrical pathways to let electrical impulses travel easily through the heart. Also called the Maze procedure.

Mitral Stenosis – A narrowing of the mitral valve, which controls blood flow from the heart's upper left chamber to its lower left chamber. May result from an inherited (congenital) problem or from rheumatic fever.

Mitral Valve – The structure that controls blood flow between the heart's left atrium (upper chamber) and left ventricle (lower chamber).

Mitral Valve Prolapse – A condition that occurs when the leaflets of the mitral valve between the left atrium and left ventricle bulge into the atrium and permit the backflow of blood. The condition can be associated with progressive mitral regurgitation.

Mitral Valve Regurgitation – Failure of the mitral valve to close properly, causing blood to flow back into the heart's upper left chamber (the left atrium) instead of moving forward into the lower left chamber (the left ventricle).

mm Hg – An abbreviation for millimeters of mercury. Blood pressure is measured in units of mm Hg—how high the pressure inside the arteries would be able to raise a column of mercury.

Monounsaturated Fats – A type of fat found in many foods but mainly in avocados and canola, olive, and peanut oils. Monounsaturated fat tends to lower LDL cholesterol levels, and some studies suggest that it may do so without also lowering HDL cholesterol levels.

Mortality – The total number of deaths from a given disease in a population during an interval of time, usually a year.

Murmur – Noises superimposed on normal heart sounds. They are caused by congenital defects or damaged heart valves that do not close properly and allow blood to leak back into the chamber from which it has come.

Myocardium – Heart Muscle

Myocardial Infarction – A heart attack. The damage or death of an area of the heart muscle (myocardium) resulting from a blocked blood supply to the area. The affected tissue dies, injuring the heart. Symptoms include prolonged, intensive chest pain and a decrease in blood pressure that often causes shock.

Myocardial Ischemia – Occurs when a part of the heart muscle does not receive enough oxygen.

Myocarditis – A rare condition in which the heart muscle becomes inflamed as a result of infection, toxic drug poisoning, or diseases like rheumatic fever, diphtheria, or tuberculosis.

Myocardium – The muscular wall of the heart. It contracts to pump blood out of the heart and then relaxes as the heart refills with returning blood.

Myxomatous Degeneration – A connective tissue disorder that causes the heart valve tissue to weaken and lose elasticity.

Natriuretic Peptide – BNP or NT ProBNP: A protein released by ventricles due to stretch from heart failure: A biomarker that is elevated > 300 in CHF

Nitroglycerin – A medicine that helps relax and dilate arteries; often used to treat cardiac chest pain (angina).

Necrosis – Refers to the death of tissue within a certain area.

Nitric Oxide – A good biomarker released by the endothelium causing vasodilatation

Noninvasive Procedures – Any diagnostic or treatment procedure in which no instrument enters the body.

NSTEMI – Non-ST-segment-elevation myocardial infarction. The milder form of the 2 types of heart attack, an NSTEMI does not produce an ST-segment elevation on an electrocardiogram. See also STEMI.

NYHA – New York Heart Association Class: A prognostic marker in CHF

Obesity – The condition of being significantly overweight. It usually applies when a person is 30% or more over ideal body weight. Obesity puts a strain on the heart and can increase the risk of developing high blood pressure and diabetes.

Occluded Artery – An artery in which the blood flow has been impaired by a blockage.

Open Heart Surgery – An operation in which the chest and heart are opened surgically while the bloodstream is diverted through a heart-lung (cardiopulmonary bypass) machine.

Pacemaker – A surgically implanted electronic device that helps regulate the heartbeat.

Palpitation – An uncomfortable feeling within the chest caused by an irregular heartbeat.

Pancreas – The organ behind the stomach that helps control blood sugar levels.

Pancreatitis – Swelling (inflammation) of the pancreas.

Paralysis – Loss of the ability to move muscles and feel in part of the body or the whole body. Paralysis may be temporary or permanent.

Parasympathetic – One of the 2 major components of Autonomic nervous system that works in conjunction with cardiac pathology

Paroxysmal Supraventricular Tachycardia (PSVT) – An occasional rapid heart rate (150-250 beats per minute) that is caused by events triggered in areas above the heart's lower chambers (the ventricles). See also supraventricular tachycardia (SVT).

Patent Ductus Arteriosus – A congenital defect in which the opening between the aorta and the pulmonary artery does not close after birth.

Patent Foramen Ovale – An opening between the left and right atria (the upper chambers) of the heart. Everyone has a PFO before birth, but in 1 out of every 3 or 4 people, the opening does not close naturally, as it should, after birth.

Percutaneous Coronary Intervention (PCI)– Any of the noninvasive procedures usually performed in the cardiac catheterization laboratory. Angioplasty is an example of a percutaneous coronary intervention. Also called a transcatheter intervention.

Percutaneous Transluminal Coronary Angioplasty (PTCA) – See angioplasty.

Pericarditis – Inflammation of the outer membrane surrounding the heart. When pericarditis occurs, the amount of fluid between the two layers of the pericardium increases. This increased fluid presses on the heart and restricts its pumping action.

Pericardiocentesis – A diagnostic procedure that uses a needle to withdraw fluid from the sac or membrane surrounding the heart (pericardium).

Pericardium – The outer fibrous sac that surrounds the heart.

Plaque – A deposit of fatty (and other) substances in the inner lining of the artery wall characteristic of atherosclerosis.

PICC Line – Peripherally Inserted Central Catheter: Access to infuse medications into the vein

Platelets – One of the three types of cells found in blood; they aid in the clotting of blood.

Polyunsaturated Fat – The major fat in most vegetable oils, including corn, safflower, sunflower, and soybean oils. These oils are liquid at room temperature. Polyunsaturated fat actually tends to lower LDL cholesterol levels but may reduce HDL cholesterol levels as well.

Positron Emission Tomography (PET) – A test that uses information about the energy of certain elements in your body to show whether parts of the heart muscle are alive and working. A PET scan can also show if your heart is getting enough blood to keep the muscle healthy.

Postural Orthostatic Tachycardia Syndrome (POTS) – A disorder that causes an increased heart rate when a person stands upright.

Premature Ventricular Contraction (PVC) – An early or extra heartbeat that happens when the heart's lower chambers (the ventricles) contract too soon, out of sequence with the normal heartbeat.

Prevalence – The total number of cases of a given disease that exists in a population at a specific time.

Pulmonary – Refers to the lungs and respiratory system.

Pulmonary Embolism – A condition in which a blood clot that has formed elsewhere in the body travels to the lungs.

Pulmonary Valve – The heart valve between the right ventricle and the pulmonary artery that controls blood flow from the heart into the lungs.

Pulmonary Vein – The blood vessel that carries newly oxygenated blood from the lungs back to the left atrium of the heart.

RAAS – Renin Angiotensin Aldosterone System

Radial Artery Access – Using the radial artery in the wrist as the entry point for the catheter in an angioplasty or stent procedure. Also called trans radial access, the trans radial approach, or trans radial angioplasty.

Radionuclide Imaging – A test in which a harmless radioactive substance is injected into the bloodstream to show information about blood flow through the arteries. Damaged or dead heart muscle can often be identified, as can serious narrowing in an artery.

Radionuclide Studies – Any of the diagnostic tests in which a small amount of radioactive material is injected into the bloodstream. The material makes it possible for a special camera to take pictures of the heart.

Radionuclide Ventriculography – A diagnostic test used to determine the size and shape of the heart's pumping chambers (the ventricles).

Regurgitation – Backward flow of blood through a defective heart valve.

Renal – Pertains to the kidneys.

Restenosis– The re-closing or re-narrowing of an artery after an interventional procedure such as angioplasty or stent placement.

Revascularization – A procedure to restore blood flow to the tissues. Coronary artery bypass surgery is an example of a revascularization procedure.

Rheumatic Fever – A disease, usually occurring in childhood, that may follow a streptococcal infection. Symptoms may include fever, sore or swollen joints, skin rash, involuntary muscle twitching, and development of nodules under the skin. If the infection involves the heart, scars may form on heart valves, and the heart's outer lining may be damaged.

Rheumatic Heart Disease – A disease of the heart (mainly affecting the heart valves) caused by rheumatic fever.

Right Ventricular Assist Device (RVAD) – A mechanical device that can be placed outside the body or implanted inside the body. An RVAD does not replace the heart—it "assists" or "helps" it pump oxygen-poor blood from the right ventricle to the lungs.

Risk Factor – An element or condition involving a certain hazard or danger. When referring to heart and blood vessels, a risk factor is associated with an increased chance of developing cardiovascular disease, including stroke.

Rubella – Commonly known as German measles.

Saccular Aneurysm – A round aneurysm that bulges out from an artery; involves only part of the circumference (outside wall) of the artery.

Sarcoidosis – An inflammatory disease that starts as tiny, grain-like lumps called granulomas, which most often appear in your lungs or lymph nodes. The granulomas can clump together and form larger lumps that attack other organs. Sarcoidosis often affects your skin, eyes, or liver, but it can lead to heart problems, such as irregular heartbeats (arrhythmias) or restrictive cardiomyopathy.

Saturated Fat – Type of fat found in foods of animal origin and a few vegetable origins; they are usually solid at room temperature. Abundant in meat and dairy products, saturated fat tends to increase LDL cholesterol levels, and it may raise the risk of certain types of cancer.

Second-Degree Heart Block – Impulses traveling through the heart's upper chambers (the atria) are delayed in the area between the upper and lower chambers (the AV node) and fail to make the ventricles beat at the right moment.

Septal Defect – A hole in the wall of the heart separating the atria or in the wall of the heart separating the ventricles.

Septum – The muscular wall dividing a chamber on the left side of the heart from the chamber on the right.

SGLT2 Inhibitor – Sodium Glucose cotransporter Protein 2: A protein and molecule triggered by the same receptor in the kidneys; an inhibitor of the receptor is used for treating diabetes. Recently, now approved for CV risk reduction and heart failure.

Sheath – A catheter-like tube that is placed inside a patient's vessel during an interventional procedure to help the doctor with insertion and proper placement of the actual catheter. Also called an introducer sheath.

Shock – A condition in which body function is impaired because the volume of fluid circulating through the body is insufficient to maintain normal metabolism. This may be caused by blood loss or by a disturbance in the function of the circulatory system.

Shunt – A connector that allows blood to flow between two locations.

Sick Sinus Syndrome – The failure of the sinus node to regulate the heart's rhythm.

Silent Ischemia – Episodes of cardiac ischemia that are not accompanied by chest pain.

Sinus (SA) Node – The "natural" pacemaker of the heart. A node is a group of specialized cells in the top of the right atrium which produces the electrical impulses that travel down to eventually reach the ventricular muscle, causing the heart to contract.

Sodium – A mineral essential to life found in nearly all plant and animal tissue. Table salt (sodium chloride) is nearly half sodium.

Sphygmomanometer – An instrument used to measure blood pressure.

Stem Cells – Special cells in the body that can transform into other cells. Stem cells can transform into heart cells, nerve cells, or other cells of the body, possibly helping to improve the function of failing organs, including the heart.

STEMI – ST-segment-elevation myocardial infarction. The more severe form of the 2 types of a heart attack. See also NSTEMI. A STEMI produces a characteristic elevation in the ST segment on an electrocardiogram.

Stent – A device made of expandable, metal mesh that is placed (by using a balloon catheter) at the site of a narrowing artery. The stent is then expanded and left in place to keep the artery open.

Stenosis – The narrowing or constriction of an opening, such as a blood vessel or heart valve.

Stethoscope – An instrument for listening to sounds within the body.

Stokes-Adams Disease – Also called third-degree heart block; a condition that happens when the impulses that pace your heartbeat do not reach the lower chambers of your heart (the ventricles). To make up for this, the ventricles use their own "backup" pacemaker with its slower rate. This rhythm can cause severe dizziness or fainting and can lead to heart failure or death.

Streptococcal Infection ("strep" infection) – An infection, usually in the throat, resulting from the presence of streptococcus bacteria.

Streptokinase – A clot-dissolving medicine used to treat heart attack patients.

Sternum – The breastbone.

Stress – Bodily or mental tension resulting from physical, chemical, or emotional factors. Stress can refer to physical exertion as well as mental anxiety.

Stroke – A sudden disruption of blood flow to the brain, either by a clot or a leak in a blood vessel.

Subarachnoid Hemorrhage – Bleeding from a blood vessel on the surface of the brain into the space between the brain and the skull.

Subclavian Arteries – Two major arteries (right and left) that receive blood from the aortic arch and supply it to the arms.

Sudden Death – Death that occurs unexpectedly and instantaneously or shortly after the onset of symptoms. The most common underlying reason for patients dying suddenly is cardiovascular disease, in particular coronary heart disease.

Superior Vena Cava – The large vein that returns blood from the head and arms to the heart.

Supraventricular Tachycardia (SVT) – A regular rapid heart rate (150-250 beats per minute) that is caused by events triggered in areas above the heart's lower chambers (the ventricles); see also paroxysmal supraventricular tachycardia (PSVT).

Sympathetic – One of the 2 components of Autonomic Nervous system that works in synergy to the heart

Syncope – A temporary, insufficient blood supply to the brain which causes a loss of consciousness. Usually caused by a serious arrhythmia.

Systole – A phase of cardiac contraction

Systolic Blood Pressure – The highest blood pressure measured in the arteries. It occurs when the heart contracts with each heartbeat.

Tachycardia – Accelerated beating of the heart. Paroxysmal tachycardia is a particular form of rapid heart action, occurring in seizures that may last from a few seconds to several days.

Tachypnea – Rapid breathing.

Tamponade – Also called cardiac tamponade. A condition in which the heart is compressed or constricted because of a large amount of fluid or blood in the space between the heart muscle and the sac that surrounds the heart (the pericardium).

Thallium-201 Stress Test – An x-ray study that follows the path of radioactive potassium carried by the blood into the heart muscle. Damaged or dead muscle can be defined, as can the extent of narrowing in an artery.

Third-degree Heart Block – A serious condition also called Stokes-Adams disease; impulses from the heart's upper chambers (the atria) are completely blocked from reaching the heart's lower chambers (the ventricles). To make up for this, the ventricles use their own "backup" pacemaker with its slower rate.

Thrombolysis – The breaking up of a blood clot.

Thrombosis – A blood clot that forms inside the blood vessel or cavity of the heart.

Thrombolytic Therapy – Intravenous or intra-arterial medicines that are used to dissolve blood clots in an artery.

Thromboxane – An enzyme active in clotting/bleeding aspects

Thrombus – A blood clot.

Thyroid – A gland located in the front of the neck, just below the voice box.

Tissue Plasminogen Activator (tPA) – A clot-dissolving medicine that is used to treat heart attack and stroke patients.

TNF Alpha – A protein activated in Heart Failure

Trans Fat – Created when hydrogen is forced through an ordinary vegetable oil (hydrogenation), converting some polyunsaturated to monounsaturated, and some monounsaturated to saturated. Trans fat, like saturated fat, tends to raise LDL cholesterol levels, and, unlike saturated fat, trans fat also lowers HDL cholesterol levels.

Transcatheter Aortic Valve Implantation (TAVI) – A minimally invasive procedure to repair a damaged or diseased aortic valve. A catheter is inserted into an artery in the groin and threaded to the heart. A balloon at the end of the catheter, with a replacement valve folded around it, delivers the new valve to take the place of the old. Also called TAVR (Transcatheter aortic valve replacement).

Transcatheter Intervention – Any of the noninvasive procedures usually performed in the cardiac catheterization laboratory. Angioplasty is an example of a transcatheter intervention. Also called a percutaneous coronary intervention (PCI).

Transesophageal Echocardiography – A diagnostic test that analyzes sound waves bounced off the heart. The sound waves are sent through a tube-like device inserted in the mouth and passed down the esophagus (food pipe), which ends near the heart. This technique is useful in studying patients whose heart and vessels, for various reasons, are difficult to assess with standard echocardiography.

Transient Ischemic Attack (TIA) – A stroke-like event that lasts only for a short time and is caused by a temporarily blocked blood vessel.

Transplantation – Replacing a failing organ with a healthy one from a donor.

Tricuspid Valve – The structure that controls blood flow from the heart's upper right chamber (the right atrium) into the lower right chamber (the right ventricle).

Triglyceride – The most common fatty substance found in the blood; normally stored as an energy source in fat tissue. High triglyceride levels may thicken the blood and make a person more susceptible to clot formation. High triglyceride levels tend to accompany high cholesterol levels and other risk factors for heart disease, such as obesity.

Ultrasound – High-frequency sound vibrations, which cannot be heard by the human ear, used in medical diagnosis.

Valve Replacement – An operation to replace a heart valve that is either blocking normal blood flow or causing blood to leak backward into the heart (regurgitation).

Valvuloplasty – Reshaping of a heart valve with surgical or catheter techniques.

Varicose Vein – Any vein that is abnormally dilated (widened).

Vascular – Pertains to the blood vessels.

Vasodilators – Any medicine that dilates (widens) the arteries.

Vasopressors – Any medicine that elevates blood pressure.

Vein – Any one of a series of blood vessels of the vascular system that carries blood from various parts of the body back to the heart, returning oxygen-poor blood to the heart.

Ventricle (right and left) – One of the two lower chambers of the heart.

Ventricular Assist Device (VAD) – A mechanical pump that helps the ventricles pump blood, easing the workload of the heart in patients with heart failure.

Ventricular Fibrillation – A condition in which the ventricles contract in a rapid, unsynchronized fashion. When fibrillation occurs, the ventricles cannot pump blood throughout the body.

Ventricular Tachycardia – An arrhythmia (abnormal heartbeat) in the ventricle characterized by an extremely fast heartbeat.

Vertigo – A feeling of dizziness or spinning.

WHO – World Health Organization

Wolff-Parkinson-White Syndrome – A condition in which an extra electrical pathway connects the atria (two upper chambers) and the ventricles (two lower chambers). It may cause a rapid heartbeat.

X-ray – Form of radiation used to create a picture of internal body structures on film.

Resources

Associations and Organizations

- AAHFN 2018: https://www.togetherinhf.com/
- American College of Cardiology: https://www.cardiosmart.org/
- American Heart Association: https://www.heart.org/
- American Diabetes Association: https://www.diabetes.org/
- American Kidney Fund: https://www.kidneyfund.org/
- Life Options: https://lifeoptions.org/
- National Diabetes education program: https://www.cdc.gov/diabetes/ndep/index.html
- National Institute of Diabetes and Digestive and Kidney Disease: https://www.niddk.nih.gov/
- National Kidney Foundation: https://www.kidney.org/
- Heart Failure Society of America: https://hfsa.org/
- Twinepidemic.com: https://twinepidemic.com/
- National Lipid Association: https://www.lipid.org/
- Cardiorenal Society of America: https://www.cardiorenalsociety.org/
- Center for Disease Control: https://www.cdc.gov/heartdisease/about.htm
- World Health Organization: https://www.who.int/news-room/fact-sheets/detail/cardiovascular-diseases-(cvds)
- Mayo Clinic https://www.mayoclinic.org/diseases-conditions/heart-failure/symptoms-causes/syc-20373142:

References and Suggested Readings

- Jackson G, Gibbs CR, Davies MK, Lip GY. ABC of heart failure. Pathophysiology. *BMJ.* 2000;320(7228):167-170. doi:10.1136/bmj.320.7228.167
- https://www.medicalnewstoday.com/articles/150109
- https://www.webmd.com/diabetes/heart-blood-disease
- https://www.ahajournals.org/doi/10.1161/CIRCRESAHA.118.311371Helena C. Kenny, E. Dale Abel. Heart Failure in Type 2 Diabetes Mellitus. Impact of Glucose-Lowering Agents, Heart Failure Therapies, and Novel Therapeutic Strategies, 2019https://doi.org/10.1161/CIRCRESAHA.118.311371Circulation Research. 2019; 124:121–141
- American College of Radiology Information Site: www.radiologyinfo.org/en/info.cfm?PG=ct_calscoring
- *Blake GJ, Ridker PM (October 2002). "Inflammatory bio-markers and cardiovascular risk prediction". Journal of Internal Medicine. 252 (4): 283–94. doi:10.1046/j.1365-2796.2002.01019.x. PMID 12366601.*
- *^ Mizuno Y, Jacob RF, Mason RP (2011). "Inflammation and the development of atherosclerosis". Journal of Atherosclerosis and Thrombosis. 18 (5): 351–8. doi:10.5551/jat.7591. PMID 21427505.*
- Vijayaraghavan K, Deedwania PC. The renin angiotensin system as a therapeutic target to prevent diabetes and its complications. Cardiol Clin. 2005;23(2):165-183. doi: 10.1016/j.ccl.2004.11.003Takatoshi Kasai, T. Douglas Bradley, Obstructive Sleep Apnea and Heart Failure, J Am Coll Cardiol. 2011 Jan, 57 (2) 119-127.
- Janani Rangaswami, Vivek Bhalla, Claudio Ronco, Peter A. McCullough, et al. On behalf of the American Heart Association Council on the Kidney in Cardiovascular Disease and Council on Clinical Cardiology, 2019 https://doi.org/10.1161/CIR.0000000000000664 Circulation. 2019;139: e840–e878
- House AA, Wanner C, Sarnak MJ, et al. Heart failure in chronic kidney disease: conclusions from a Kidney Disease: Improving Global Outcomes (KDIGO) Controversies Conference. Kidney Int. 2019;95(6):1304-1317. doi: 10.1016/j.kint.2019.02.022
- Vijayaraghavan K, McCullough PA, Singh B, et al. Cardiometabolic-Renal Disease in South Asians: Consensus Recommendations from the Cardio Renal Society of America. Cardiorenal Med. 2019;9(4):240-251. doi:10.1159/000499341
- Peter A. McCullough, James A. Tumlin , Harold Szerlip , Krishnaswami Vijayaraghavan, Sathya Jyothinagaram , John F. Rausch Jr , Bhupinder Singh , Jun Zhang and Mikhail Kosiborod. Cardiorenal Syndromes: Advances in Determining Diagnosis, Prognosis, and Therapy. 2015, 3:5 DOI: 10.4172/2329-9517.1000221

- 2017 ACC/AHA/HFSA Focused Update of the 2013 ACCF/AHA Guideline for the Management of Heart Failure, A Report of the American College of Cardiology/American Heart Association Task Force on Clinical Practice Guidelines and the Heart Failure Society of America, Clyde W. Yancy, Mariell Jessup, Biykem Bozkurt, Javed Butler, Donald E. Casey Jr., Monica M. Colvin, Mark H. Drazner, Gerasimos S. Filippatos, Gregg C. Fonarow, Michael M. Givertz, Steven M. Hollenberg, JoAnn Lindenfeld, Frederick A. Masoudi, Patrick E. McBride, Pamela N. Peterson, Lynne Warner Stevenson and Cheryl Westlake. Journal of the American College of Cardiology, Volume 70, Issue 6, August 2017DOI: 10.1016/j.jacc.2017.04.025
- https://www.mayoclinic.org/diseases-conditions/atrial-fibrillation/symptoms-causes/syc-20350624
- Philippe Pibarot, Jean G. Dumesnil. Prosthetic Heart Valves, Selection of the Optimal Prosthesis and Long-Term Management, 2009https://doi.org/10.1161/CIRCULATION AHA.108.778886Circulation. 2009; 119:1034–1048
- Cicero AFG, Colletti A, von Haehling S, et al. Nutraceutical support in heart failure: a position paper of the International Lipid Expert Panel (ILEP) [published online ahead of print, 2020 Mar 16]. *Nutr Res Rev.* 2020;1-25. doi:10.1017/S0954422420000049
- Yancy CW, Fonarow GC. Coronavirus Disease 2019 (COVID-19) and the Heart—Is Heart Failure the Next Chapter? *JAMA Cardiol.* Published online July 27, 2020. doi:10.1001/jamacardio.2020.3575
- Koutsoukis A, Ntalianis A, Repasos E, Kastritis E, Dimopoulos MA, Paraskevaidis I. Cardio-oncology: A Focus on Cardiotoxicity. Eur Cardiol. 2018;13(1):64-69. doi:10.15420/ecr.2017:17:2
- Baman JR, Ahmad FS. Heart Failure. *JAMA.* Published online August 04, 2020. doi:10.1001/jama.2020.13310
- https://nurseslabs.com/heart-failure-nursing-care-plans/
- Richardson LG. Psychosocial issues in patients with congestive heart failure. Prog Cardiovasc Nurs. 2003;18(1):19-27. doi:10.1111/j.0889-7204.2003. 00835.x

OTHER RESOURCES

1. **DESIDERATA**: I would like to share a beautiful poem framed and given to me by one of my patients. We have learned this in high school. It is just a reminder to all of us to be grateful for being alive and why the message of "joie de vivre" should be engrained in our DNA.

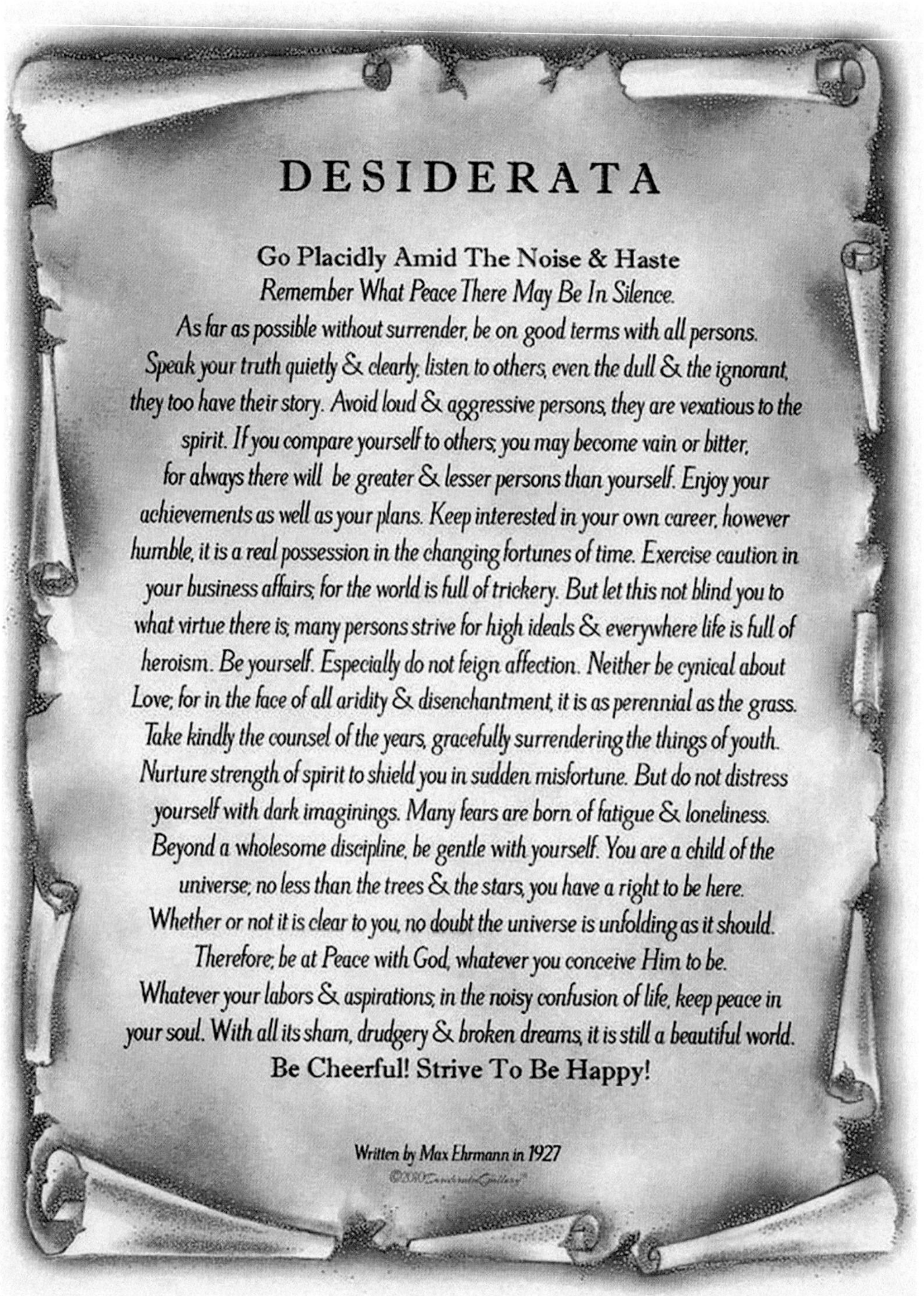

DESIDERATA

Go Placidly Amid The Noise & Haste

Remember What Peace There May Be In Silence.

As far as possible without surrender, be on good terms with all persons. Speak your truth quietly & clearly; listen to others, even the dull & the ignorant, they too have their story. Avoid loud & aggressive persons, they are vexatious to the spirit. If you compare yourself to others, you may become vain or bitter, for always there will be greater & lesser persons than yourself. Enjoy your achievements as well as your plans. Keep interested in your own career, however humble, it is a real possession in the changing fortunes of time. Exercise caution in your business affairs; for the world is full of trickery. But let this not blind you to what virtue there is; many persons strive for high ideals & everywhere life is full of heroism. Be yourself. Especially do not feign affection. Neither be cynical about Love; for in the face of all aridity & disenchantment, it is as perennial as the grass. Take kindly the counsel of the years, gracefully surrendering the things of youth. Nurture strength of spirit to shield you in sudden misfortune. But do not distress yourself with dark imaginings. Many fears are born of fatigue & loneliness. Beyond a wholesome discipline, be gentle with yourself. You are a child of the universe; no less than the trees & the stars, you have a right to be here. Whether or not it is clear to you, no doubt the universe is unfolding as it should. Therefore, be at Peace with God, whatever you conceive Him to be. Whatever your labors & aspirations, in the noisy confusion of life, keep peace in your soul. With all its sham, drudgery & broken dreams, it is still a beautiful world.

Be Cheerful! Strive To Be Happy!

Written by Max Ehrmann in 1927

Fig. 62

2. **The Library:** This section is to provide resources that will magnify knowledge boundaries and unlock new channels, the domains of which are primarily dependent on the reader's willingness to invest time and vigor in a lifelong and enriching exploration. This may empower one's mind and deploy the energy generated towards healing. Many are medically related to inspirational.

   I have divided these into 3 sections:

   - Movies with messages that enthrall.
   - Books of fiction in the medical genre that may exhilarate you.
   - Books on nonfiction that may cosmically turbocharge your psyche.

A. MOVIES

1. The English Patient - 1996
2. Kumare - 2011
3. Lost in Translation - 2003
4. Perks of Being a Wallflower - 2012
5. Lagaan - 2001
6. 12 Monkeys - 1995
7. The Usual Suspects - 1995
8. Awake - 2007
9. Doctor Zhivago - 1965
10. The Hospital - 1971
11. Awakenings - 1990
12. Coma - 1978
13. Dead Ringer - 1988
14. Shutter Island - 2010
15. Outbreak - 1995
16. One Flew Over the Cuckoo's Nest - 1975
17. Sicko - 2007
18. Red Beard - 1965
19. Gandhi - 1982
20. Mother Teresa - 2003
21. Braveheart - 1995
22. Remember the Titans - 2000
23. Hotel Rwanda - 2004

24. Florence Nightingale - 1985
25. Front of Class - 2008
26. A Beautiful Mind - 2001
27. Mandela - 2013
28. Pay it Forward- 2000
29. Pursuit of Happyness - 2006
30. Mr. Holland's Opus - 1995
31. Anne Frank - 2001
32. Million Dollar Arm - 2014
33. Not as a Stranger - 1955
34. Into the Wild - 2007
35. Gully Boy - 2019
36. It's a Wonderful Life - 1946
37. October Sky - 1999
38. Life of Pi - 2012
39. Good Will Hunting - 1997
40. Dead Poets Society - 1989
41. 3 Idiots - 2009
42. Shawshank Redemption - 1994
43. Life is Beautiful - 1998
44. Billy Elliot - 2000
45. Erin Brockovich - 2000
46. Slumdog Millionaire - 2008
47. To Kill a Mockingbird - 1962
48. Cast Away - 2000
49. Lawrence of Arabia - 1962
50. Rain Man - 1988
51. Forest Gump - 1994
52. The Pianist - 2002
53. My Left Foot - 1989

54. Charlie - 1968
55. 127 Hours - 2010
56. Khamoshi: The Musical - 1996
57. Taare Zameen Par - 2007
58. Munna Bhai MBBS - 2003
59. Iqbal - 2005
60. Bhopal: A Prayer for Rain - 2014

B. Fiction books

1. Cutting for Stone by Abraham Verghese - 2010
2. Virus Hunters, Bobby Akart - 2020
3. Magic Hour, Kristin Hannah - 2006
4. A Case of Need, Michael Crichton - 1969
5. Arrowsmith, Sinclair Lewis - 1925
6. An Irish Country Doctor, Patrick Taylor - 2007
7. Not as a Stranger, Morton Thompson - 1955
8. The Atlantis Gene, A.G. Riddle - 2013
9. Becoming Mrs. Lewis, Pat Callahan - 2018
10. The Alchemist, Paulo Coelho - 1988
11. Gilead, Marilynne Robinson - 2004
12. Toxin, Robin Cook - 1998
13. The Andromeda Strain, Michael Crichton - 1969
14. The Physician, Noah Gordon - 1986
15. Doctors, Erich Segal - 1988
16. Miracle Cure, Michael Palmer - 1988
17. Life Support, Tess Gerritsen - 1997
18. Flowers for Algernon, Daniel Keyes - 1966
19. The Final Diagnosis, Arthur Hailey - 1959
20. The Dream Daughter, Diane Chamberlain - 2018
21. The Citadel, A.J Cronin - 1937

22. Heart Failure, Richard Mabry - 2013
23. Cider House Rules, John Irving - 1985
24. The Hot Zone, Richard Preston - 1994
25. The English Patient, Michael Ondaatje - 1992

Non-Fiction

1. When breath becomes air, Paul Kalanithi - 2016
2. The Last Lecture, Randy Pausch - 2012
3. Complications, Atul Gawande - 2002
4. The Intern Blues, Robert Marion - 2001
5. Anatomy of Hope, Jerome Groopman - 2005
6. The Immortal Life of Henrietta Lacks, Rebecca Skloot - 2011
7. White Coat, Ellen Rothman - 2000
8. Emperor of all Maladies: A Biography of Cancer, Siddhartha Mukherjee - 2011
9. Becoming a Doctor, Melvin Konner - 1988
10. One Doctor: Close Calls, Cold Cases and Mysteries of Medicine, Brendan Reilly - 2014
11. Hospital, Julie Salamon - 2008
12. Measure of Our Days, Jerome Groopman - 1998
13. God's Hotel, Victoria Sweet - 2013
14. Being Mortal, Atul Gawande - 2014
15. Mountain Beyond Mountains: The Quest of Dr. Paul Farmer, Tracy Kidder - 2003
16. The Body Keeps the Score: Mind and Body in the Healing of Trauma - 2014
17. Awakenings, Oliver Sacks - 1973
18. Love, Medicine, Miracles, Erich Segal - 1986
19. The Doctor's Kidney Diets, Mandip Kang - 2015
20. 1 in 9 Tribe, Analyn and Raymond Scott - 2019
21. Awaken the Giant Within, Anthony Robbins - 1992
22. Sky is the Limit, Wayne Dyer - 1980
23. The Third Pillar, Raghuram Rajan - 2019
24. Long Walk Out of the Woods, Adam Hill - 2019
25. Rebuilding the Front Porch of America, Patrick Overton – 2017

C. Another poem that inspired me was given to me by a patient who was struggling with alcoholic cardiomyopathy. He had recovered totally and normalized his heart function due to his self-discipline and evoking the power from within.

Just for Today

Just for today, I will try to live through this day only,
and not tackle all my problems at once.
I can do something for twelve hours that would appall me
if I felt I had to keep it up for a lifetime.
Just for today, I will be happy.
This assumes to be true what Abraham Lincoln said that,
"Most folks are as happy as they make up their minds to be."
Just for today, I will adjust myself to what is,
and not try to adjust everything to my own desires.
I will take my "luck" as it comes and fit myself to it.
Just for today, I will try to strengthen my mind. I will study.
I will learn something useful.
I will not be a mental loafer.
I will read something that requires effort, thought, and concentration.
Just for today, I will exercise my soul in three ways:
I will do somebody a good turn, and not get found out.
if anyone knows of it, it will not count.
I will do at least two things I don't want to do – just for exercise.
I will not show anyone that my feelings are hurt.
they may be hurt, but today I will not show it.
Just for today, I will be agreeable.
I will look as well as I can, dress becomingly,
keep my voice low, be courteous, criticize not one bit.
I won't find fault with anything, nor try to improve or regulate anybody but myself.
Just for today, I will have a program.
I may not follow it exactly, but I will have it.
I will save myself from two pests: hurry and indecision.
Just for today I will have a quiet half-hour all by myself and relax.

During this half-hour, sometime, I will try to get a better perspective of my life.
Just for today, I will be unafraid.
Especially I will not be afraid to notice what is beautiful
and to believe that as I give to the world, so the world will give to me.

About the Author

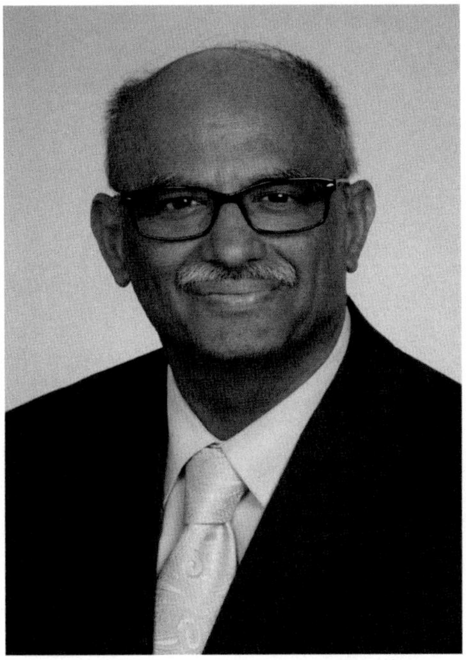

Kris Vijay (Krishnaswami Vijayaraghavan, MD, MS, FACC, FACP, FNLA, FHFSA) is the Medical Director of the Institute of Congestive Heart Failure at Abrazo Arizona Heart Hospital and Abrazo Health Network in Arizona. He is a Non-invasive Cardiologist, a trained endocrinologist, clinical lipidologist, an ardent researcher and a Heart Failure specialist. A native of India, Vijay earned his medical degree from Kasturba Medical College, University of Mysore. He completed postgraduate training in medicine in Bombay, India; Oxford, United Kingdom; and Rochester, New York, and has completed fellowships in endocrinology and diabetes at the University of Southampton, United Kingdom, and in cardiology at Banner University Medical Center Phoenix. He also holds a Master's degree in clinical research design and statistical analysis from the University of Michigan's School of Public Health.

Dr. Vijay serves as a Clinical Professor of Medicine at University of Arizona, Phoenix and as an adjunct Professor of Medicine at Midwestern University Arizona College of Osteopathic Medicine (AZCOM)

He has been in clinical practice for more than 40 years since Medical School and in Arizona for more than 30 years. Dr. Vijay is a past Governor of the American College of Cardiology, Arizona Chapter, Past President of the National Lipid Association, South West Chapter, immediate past Executive Council Chair of National Lipid Association, a founding member and past President of the Cardio Renal Society of America and current President of the TWINEPIDEMIC, Inc., a nonprofit organization addressing Diabetes and Heart disease among Ethnic Communities all over the world.

He is a Fellow of the American College of Cardiology, the American College of Physicians, National Lipid association and Heart Failure Society of America. Dr. Vijay was named a fellow of the prestigious Heart Failure Society of America based on his professional success, outstanding credentials, achievements and contributions to heart failure clinical practice, research, publications, and educational expertise.

He is a member of the clinical cardiology council as well as council for Atherosclerosis, Thrombosis and Vascular Biology at American Heart Association, a member of Prevention and Cardio-metabolic committee at American College of Cardiology and an Executive Board member of the National Lipid Association. He is currently an Associate Editor for the Journal of Clinical Lipidology.

Dr. Vijay has participated in more than 180 clinical trials and his research is focused on such disorders as congestive heart failure, hypercholesterolemia, hypertension, coronary artery disease, plaque regression, Atrial Fibrillation, peripheral vascular disease, and diabetes/ metabolic syndrome. He has published numerous articles in peer reviewed journals.

Dr. Vijay is a founding member of the Arizona Managed Care Quality Enhancement Program (AMCQEP), 1992, and received the Governor's award from Health Services Advisory Group (HSAG), October 2002, an innovation award through the Center for Health Innovation and Clinical Trial (CHI&CT) at Arizona State University from the President of Arizona State University in 2010 and the Jerome Markowitz award for a distinguished career from South Asian Society of Atherosclerosis and Thrombosis in 2013. He was one of the three nominees of Healthcare Heroes award for Phoenix Business Journal towards Lifetime achievement in 2017.He received a Lifetime achievement award from American College of Cardiology, Arizona Chapter in 2018.

He was recognized as one of the AZ TOP DOCS in 2020.

He has presented at numerous national and International meetings on diabetes and heart disease. His professional activities also include serving on Editorial Boards of medical journals, reviewing, and contributing towards landmark guidelines and policy statements as well as serving on many important advisory boards dealing with Quality initiatives of national organizations.

Dr. Vijay takes a holistic view of heart failure, using a variety of treatment options along with motivating, inspiring and coaching to encourage patients to modify their lifestyles. His mission has been in prevention of risk factors of heart disease and diabetes at primordial, primary, secondary, and tertiary care levels. Prevention of Heart Failure has been his main goal. In addition to spending countless hours caring for patients, he has dedicated himself to improving medical education, research, and the overall quality of care. His special brand of care is making a positive and measurable difference in keeping patients healthy, and importantly, out of the hospital.

He is a Medical Sherpa, volunteering his services to serve the underserved in attempts to mitigate diabetes, heart disease and kidney disease around the world through his nonprofit organization, Twinepidemic, Inc. He is also a Needs-Ambassador for a large multinational nonprofit organization, Project C.U.R.E, providing services for the Dalai Lama Heart Foundation, in Ladakh, India, in the Himalayas. He lives with his wife in Phoenix Arizona. They have 2 sons, also living and working in Phoenix, AZ. His parents-in-law have been living with them for the last 28 years.

More Endorsements

It gives me great pleasure to recommend the new book titled, "Invoking Your Inner Therapist in Heart Failure." As indicated on the cover page, it describes evolving strategies from 'Prevention to End Stage.' The author has used untold patient experiences, to illustrate his knowledge – base on this complex topic. The monograph has six sections and covers all aspects of heart failure including the salient features of heart, such as electrical properties, role in promoting circulation, and as the most powerful, efficient, biological pump. Other sections include epidemiology, pathophysiology, various categories of heart failure; risk factors and comorbid conditions; diagnostics in heart failure; management of heart failure, and miscellaneous topics in heart failure.

To create awareness and develop educational and prevention strategies, I started a professional society called South Asian Society on Atherosclerosis and Thrombosis (www.sasat.org) at the University of Minnesota in 1993. Since then, we have organized 15 international conferences and published ten books on topics of interest, which include four monographs on Coronary Artery Disease. The author of this book, Dr. Kris Vijay has participated in our efforts to educate the public, clinicians, and researchers on this topic of great public health importance. I was asked to review two recent books on Emerging Technologies for Heart Disease (Elsevier Publishers) by Udi Nussinovitch, Faulty of Applicative Cardiovascular Research Center, Meir Medical Center, Cardiology Department, Tel Aviv University. Despite my personal experience in editing and publishing several books on this topic, as well as reviewing books published by other experts on this topic, I must confess that the monograph by Dr Kris Vijay on "Heart Failure" is unique.

The uniqueness can be seen right from the introduction, which is a fascinating personal story of his early life in Mumbai, struggles of day to day life in the metropolis, emotional upheavals, dedication, and determination to become a doctor, a cardiologist to serve the patients with a variety of heart ailments. What impressed me most is the way he describes each chapter, with highlighted information to capture the attention of the readers. The very style of writing a medical book in such a simple language, with a unique approach of storytelling, makes this monograph extremely useful.

Furthermore, including patient stories, explaining the underlying causes, and presenting management strategies makes this book a unique reference book for students, researchers, clinicians and to some extent even to the patients who want to know more about their heart ailments.

I have never had the experience of reviewing a medical monograph, which includes emotions, passion, compassion, empathies to illustrate a case in point. Just reading this monograph will make you feel that every doctor you see for your consultation, should have the qualities that Kris expresses in this work of art.

Gundu H.R. Rao
Emeritus Professor
Laboratory Medicine and Pathology
Director, Thrombosis Research
Lillehei Heart Institute, University of Minnesota

A Testimonial for the Pearl of Wisdom!

Having practiced Neurology for almost over 45 years of my life and evaluating countless patients suffering from a myriad of neurological illnesses, I am acutely aware of strong connection between heart and neurological disorders. In fact, a healthy heart is a must for healthy neurological functions and general well-being. When a Cardiologist talks about heart failure to an ill-informed patient, the latter might not comprehend the jargon fully and thus may be left at a dead end.

And that is where the importance of a physician of the cadre of Dr. Kris Vijay, my Cardiologist par excellence, comes to mind. Having worked with him as a colleague for some years and being under his expert care for over quarter of a century, I had the opportunities to listen to his countless seminars and lectures delivered to health care workers including physicians, nurses as well as public at-large. The topics ranged from cardiac illnesses, chronic heart failure and the management of lipid disorders as well as Hypertension. I always felt from the core of my heart that if there were a physician in the real sense of the word, it is him. His rapport, empathy, and tireless patience in listening to his patients is not much in existence in modern day hurried world.

And then all of a sudden, the scenario changed for the better when I received a manuscript of his first book related to his field of expertise titled "Invoking your Inner Therapist in Heart Failure – Evolving Strategies from Prevention to End Stage, and Untold Patient Experiences and lessons learnt". Written with a deep flavor and fervor, it truly hit the apex of my heart where it should. Here he dwells upon newer research, including what happens around the world in relation to these disorders, his field of expertise, answering clearly and precisely all the questions the experts and patients might have!

Besides being a Neurologist myself, I also wear a hat of a Writer and have personally penned five books with sixth one in the pipeline. My field pertains to the diaspora issues and my write-up mostly emanates from "Eastern Reflections in Western Mirror", in which the emphasis is primarily upon 'Adapting to the Adopted Culture' rather than merely trying to fit in the society as "Square Peg in a Round Hole'. After all, we all are "One Coin with Two Sides". In my opinion, this book has an extraordinary socio-medical appeal for universal reading, far and beyond the borders, for after all, it is written by a caring saint-like physician.

If I could suggest one thing to my readers and public-at-large, it will be not just to peruse this book, but rather to own a copy for your personal library. Not doing so, one could miss a treasure of knowledge based on scientific facts made easy, as well as the social milieu.

Dr. Jaswant Singh Sachdev, M.D., F.A.A.N.
Diplomat in American Board of Psychiatry and Neurology
Retired Neurologist
Writer of 5 books on Diaspora Issues,
A Senior Sikh Advisor to Local Gurdwara Sahib Management
Selected as One of the Fifty Prominent Sikhs of USA
Member Advisory Board, Arizona Inter Faith Movement
Chair, Experience Interfaith Annual Event
A Community Volunteer
Sikh Awareness Worker
jaswantsachdev@gmail.com

In the pages of this book you will find invaluable information.

It is Dr. Kris Vijay's deep desire that this book get placed in University bookstores and classrooms around the world.

If you would like to connect with Dr. Kris, please go to: www.elevatebi.com/KrisVijay. This will give a reliable way to get in touch with him.

Also, reviews are the lifeblood of all great books. We ask that you leave a review in the bookseller section of Amazon and other book resellers.

Made in the USA
Monee, IL
13 October 2020

44902207R00224